Infectious Diseases of the Liver

FALK SYMPOSIUM 54

Infectious Diseases of the Liver

EDITED BY

L. Bianchi
University of Basel
Switzerland

W. Gerok
University Medical Clinic
Freiburg im Breisgau
Federal Republic of Germany

K.-P. Maier
Medical Clinic Esslingen
Federal Republic of Germany

F. Deinhardt
Max V. Pettenkofer Institute
Munich
Federal Republic of Germany

Proceedings of the 54th Falk Symposium held at Basel, Switzerland, October 12–14, 1989

KLUWER ACADEMIC PUBLISHERS
DORDRECHT / BOSTON / LONDON

Distributors

for the United States and Canada: Kluwer Academic Publishers, PO Box 358, Accord Station, Hingham, MA 02018-0358, USA
for all other countries: Kluwer Academic Publishers Group, Distribution Center, PO Box 322, 3300 AH Dordrecht, The Netherlands

British Library CIP Data is available
ISBN 0-7923-8902-6

Library of Congress Cataloging in Publication Data

Falk Symposium (54th: 1989: Basel, Switzerland)
Infectious diseases of the liver: proceedings of the 54th Falk Symposium held at Basel, Switzerland, October 12–14, 1989 / edited by L. Bianchi, W. Gerok, K.-P. Maier, F. Deinhardt.
p. cm.
Includes bibliographical references.
ISBN 0-7923-8902-6 (U.S.)
1. Liver—Infections—Congresses. I. Bianchi, Leonardo. II. Gerok, W. (Wolfgang), 1926– . III. Maier, Klaus-Peter. IV. Title.
[DNLM: 1 Hepatitis, Viral, Human—congresses. 2. Infection—congresses. 3. Liver Diseases—congresses. WI 700 F191i 1989]
RC846.F35 1989
616.3'62—dc20
DLC 90-4383
for Library of Congress CIP

Published in the United Kingdom by Kluwer Academic Publishers, PO Box 55, Lancaster, UK.

Kluwer Academic Publishers BV incorporates the publishing programmes of D. Reidel, Martinus Nijhoff, Dr W. Junk and MTP Press.

Printed in Great Britain by Butler and Tanner Ltd., Frome and London

Contents

Preface

This volume comprises the lectures presented at the 8th Congress of Liver diseases held in Basel, Switzerland, on October 12–14, 1989 under the heading "infectious diseases of the liver".

The liver may be involved in different ways when infectious agents invade the organism: first, it can be the target organ of an infectious agent. It is the unique target organ if a specific reaction between the infectious agent and the liver takes place. More frequently, however, several other organs of the host will be invaded by the infectious agent in addition to the liver, so there is only a reaction of the liver concomitant to the reactions of other organs. Second, the liver is also involved in extrahepatic infections. Any major extrahepatic infection induces the so-called acute phase response. This means that, at the site of local injury, signal substances ("mediators", "inflammation hormones") are released and transported in the blood to their target organs. In the liver they induce the synthesis and secretion of the acute phase proteins, which interact with the extrahepatic infectious process and its systemic consequences. The significance of the liver in these non-specific defence mechanisms is elucidated by the observation that liver diseases with reduced organ function influence the occurrence and the course of extrahepatic infectious diseases.

The symposium brought together representatives of different specialties in order to give them the possibility of exchanging information and experiences. This volume contains the text of lectures in greater detail than is possible in oral presentation. Its speedy publication therefore gives "state-of-the-art lectures" about the various topics. Assured facts as well as still open questions are included, thus stimulating further scientific work and improving the understanding of clinical phenomena.

We are deeply indebted to Dr Herbert Falk and the Falk Foundation whose generous sponsorship formed the basis for this symposium.

We also thank all those behind the scenes for the assistance in organization. We wish to express our appreciation to all the speakers and moderators. Last but not least we thank Phil Johnstone from Kluwer Academic Publishers for his cooperation in preparing this volume for publication within a short time after the symposium.

The Editors

List of Principal Contributors

J. P. ACKERS
London School of Hygiene and Tropical Medicine
Department of Medical Parasitology
Keppel Street
London WC1E 7HT
UK

H. J. ALTER
NIH, Department of Health and Human Services
Department of Transfusion Medicine
Clinical Center, Building 10, Room 5D56
Bethesda, MD 20892
USA

P. D. BERK
Division of Liver Diseases
Box 1079
Mount Sinai School of Medicine
One Gustave L Levy Place
New York, NY 10029
USA

L. BIANCHI
Department of Pathology
University of Basel
Schonbeinstrasse 40
CH-4003 Basel
Switzerland

H. E. BLUM
Massachusetts General Hospital
MGH Cancer Center
Molecular Hepatology Laboratory
MGH East, 149 13th Street
Charlestown, MA 02129
USA

D. W. BRADLEY
Hepatitis Branch
Centers for Disease Control
1600 Clifton Road, NE
Atlanta, GE 30333
USA

A. D. M. BRYCESON
Hospital for Tropical Diseases
4 St Pancras Way
London NW1 0PE
UK

G. C. COOK
London School of Hygiene and Tropical Medicine
Keppel Street
London WC1E 7HT
UK

K. DECKER
Biochemisches Institut
Albert-Ludwigs-Universität
Hermann-Herder-Strasse 7
D-7800 Freiburg-im-Breisgau
FRG

F. DEINHARDT
Max von Pettenkofer Institute
Pettenkoferstrasse 9a
D-8000 Munich 2
FRG

V. J. DESMET
Universitair Ziekenhuis Sint Raphael
Pathologische Ontleedkunde B
Minderbroedersstraat 12
B-3000 Leuven
Belgium

W. H. GERLICH
Georg-August-Universität Göttingen
Hygiene-Institut der Universität
Kreuzbergring 57
D-3400 Göttingen
FRG

W. GEROK
Medizinische Universitäts Klinik
Hugstetter Strasse 55
D-7800 Freiburg-im-Breisgau
FRG

F.-D. GOEBEL
Medizinische Poliklinik der Universität München
Pettenkoferstrasse 9a
D-8000 Munich 2
FRG

A. J. GREENSTEIN
Mount Sinai Medical Center
One Gustave L Levy Place
New York, NY 10029
USA

A. HOLSTEGE
Medizinische Universitätsklinik
Hugstetterstrasse 55
D-7800 Freiburg-im-Breisgau
FRG

J. H. HOOFNAGLE
NIH, Department of Health and Human Sciences
National Institute of Diabetes, Digestive and Kidney Diseases
Building 31, Room 9A-23
Bethesda, MD 20892
USA

M. HU
The Hygiene and Anti-epidemic Center of Shanghai
280 Road Chang Shu
Shanghai
People's Republic of China

S. IWARSON
Department of Infectious Diseases
University of Goteborg
Ostra Hospital
S-415 85 Goteborg
Sweden

R. C. JOHNSON
Department of Microbiology
Medical School
1460 Mayo Memorial Building
University of Minnesota
Minneapolis, MN 55455-0312
USA

R. N. M. MacSWEEN
University of Glasgow
Department of Pathology
Western Infirmary
Glasgow G11 6NT
UK

K.-P. MAIER
Department of Medicine
Division of Gastroenterology
City Hospital Esslingen
Hirschlandstrasse 97
D-7300 Esslingen
FRG

R. MÜLLER
Abteilung für Gastroenterologie und Hepatologie
Zentrum für Innere Medizin und Dermatologie der Medizinische Hochschule Hannover
Hannover
FRG

J. REICHEN
Department of Clinical Pharmacology
University of Berne
Murtenstrasse 35
CH-3010 Berne
Switzerland

M. RIZZETTO
Ospedale Molinette
Institute of Internal Medicine
Corso Bramante 88
I-10126 Torino
Italy

S. SHERLOCK
The Royal Free Hospital
Pond Street
Hampstead
London NW3 2QG
UK

D. SHOUVAL
Liver Unit
Hadassah University Hospital
PO Box 12000
Jerusalem, IL 91120
Israel

J. SUMMERS
University of New Mexico School of Medicine
Department of Cell Biology
UNM Cancer Center
900 Camino de Salud, NE
Albuquerque, NM 87131
USA

H. C. THOMAS
St Mary's Hospital Medical School
Department of Medicine
Praed Street, Paddington
London W2 1NY
UK

K. S. WARREN
Director for Science
Maxwell Communication Corporation
866 Third Avenue
New York, NY 10022
USA

1
Memorial Lecture: Tribute to Dr Hans Popper

DAME SHEILA SHERLOCK

Today we meet together to honour Dr Hans Popper, who was born in Vienna in 1903 and died in New York in 1988. He was a man of colossal intellect, profound knowledge and great humanity. He founded our discipline – hepatology. He was my personal friend over so many years. He had a classical education in Vienna, he was the bright boy in the gymnasium and the brilliant medical student. He soon realized the importance of making original observations rather than paying too much attention to lectures and was investigating glycoproteins in the late 1920s. He became very well qualified in medicine, spending 5 years in pathology, where again he made basic observations, particularly on the serosal cells of the liver, now known to be Kupffer cells. Things were proceeding very smoothly indeed. In 1933 Hans was invited by Eppinger, newly appointed Professor in Vienna, to join his department. Everything went well until 1938, when with the possibility of the arrival of the Nazis and the Anschlüss, Hans left for the United States. Earlier he had an offer from Chicago which he refused, but this time he accepted. The Americans bargained with him and gave him a poorer salary than he had been offered the first time; nevertheless, he arrived in the United States and went to the Cook County Hospital in Chicago, which was one of the largest hospitals in the United States, and it served an enormous number of patients with liver disease.

Popper had originally been interested in the kidney, and had, for example, discovered creatinine clearance. Faced with all the patients with liver disease at the Cook County Hospital he turned his attention to the liver and eventually, in 1943, founded the Hektoen Institute for Medical Research. This soon became, particularly just after the war, a Mecca for all who were interested in the liver. In 1943 he became a naturalized American, and showed his gratitude to his adopted country by immediately joining the army and serving for 4 years. He did very interesting research in Korea on the histopathology of viral hepatitis. Somewhere around 1948–9 Hans had become Chairman of the Medical Research Committee of the Surgeon General of the United States. Among his fellow-members were George

Gabuzda (of ascites fame), Robert Kark (of Guy's Hospital London and Chicago), Fred Hofbauer (of Minneapolis), Charles Davidson (of the Thorndike Laboratory, Boston), Paul György (a great nutritionist) and C. G. Child (Professor of Surgery, who later graded liver failure.) (Figure 1).

I first met Hans in 1947, when I was a Research Fellow at Yale, and visited him at the Hektöen Institute. He was very hospitable and immediately took me home to meet Lina. We had a typical jolly Viennese evening, and our family friendship commenced at that time.

Hans Popper founded many societies. In 1948, some of his friends gathered together in the library of the Hektöen Institute to found the American Association for the Study of the Liver. The friends included Dick Capps, Bob Kark, Leon Schiff, Fred Steigmann and Cecil Watson. I was an onlooker at that meeting. Originally the meetings of the AASLD were informal, friendly and great fun. They took place in the Hektöen library, and that meant only about 40–50 people were present. The Association then moved on to the Knickerbocker Hotel in Chicago. Now, two weeks ahead, the meeting will again be held in Chicago, attended by about 1200 people. We shall be remembering Hans.

The next society that he founded was the International Society for the Study of the Liver. This was dreamed up in 1957, when we attended a splendid meeting in Perugia (Italy). The major social event was a visit to Assisi. Adolf Martini (of Marburg), Hans and I, discussed an International Liver Society which we wanted to be elitist. So we began with only four members from each country. Of course this subsequently changed. The first meeting took place in Washington in 1958. The last had about 700 participants in Toronto and the next, in 1990, will be in Brisbane. The emphasis now is on a worldwide society, with particular emphasis on bringing

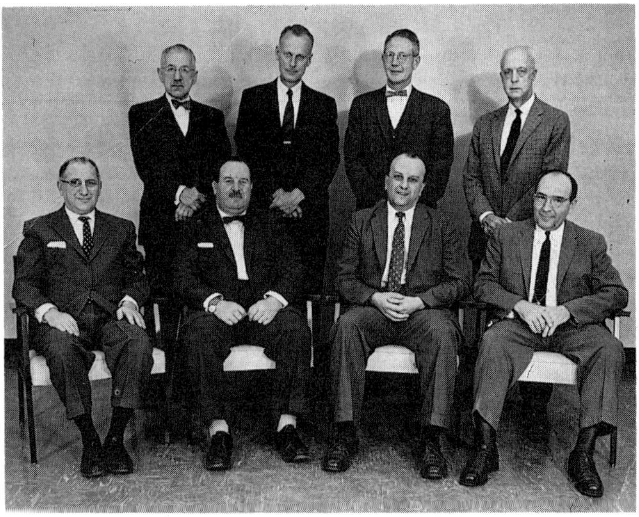

Figure 1 About 1947. The Medical Research Committee of the Surgeon General of the United States. Front row (right to left): Fred Hofbauer, George Gabuzda, Robert M. Kark, Hans Popper

in speakers and attendants from developing countries.

Hans was a great classifier. The first classification meeting I attended with him was in 1956 in Cuba. We classified the basic morphological features of cirrhosis (Figure 2). We had a good social time too (Figure 3). Hans was very jolly and excellent company. Laughter always accompanied him. In Havana we enjoyed the Tropicana Night Club. Hans was a typical Viennese; he liked music – dancing the Viennese waltz with him was something never to be forgotten. He was a founding member of the Playboy Club in Chicago. In 1957 Hans was called to the most prestigious post of Chief Pathologist to the Mount Sinai Hospital in New York. Hans believed it should be a Medical School, and so it was. In 1963 the first students were admitted to the Mount Sinai College of Medicine of the City University of New York. He went on to become Dean and President of the Mount Sinai School of Medicine. In his 70s he was made Gustave Levy Distinguished Professor, a post he held until his death.

At Mount Sinai Dr Popper headed a large pathology department where he trained hundreds of young pathologists. They include Michael Gerber, who is from Germany and is now in New Orleans, Swan Thung, Many Rubin and F. Paronetto, who continues excellent immunological investigations in Sinai. We should also remember our own Piccio Bianchi, who has been so busy with all the Basel meetings, and particularly this one. He spent two years with Hans in New York, as did Peter Scheuer, our Chief of Pathology at the Royal Free Hospital. His real crown prince was Fenton Schaffner, whom he brought with him from Chicago. Their relationship was almost like father and son.

Hans wrote 800 papers and 23 books. I draw attention particularly to

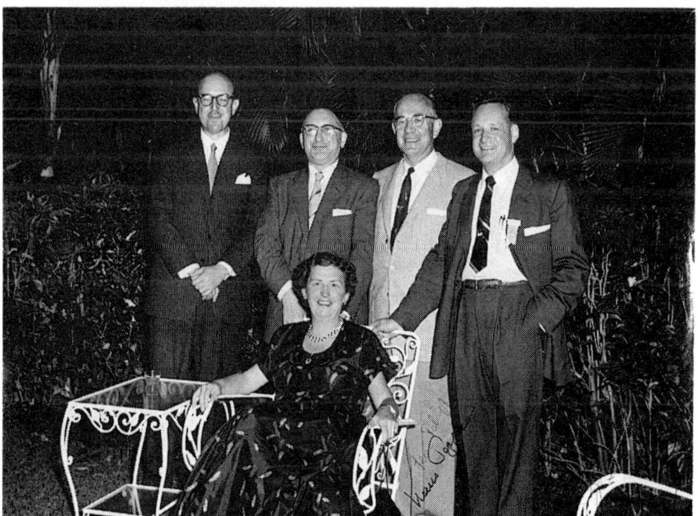

Figure 2 Havana, 1956. Classifying cirrhosis. Bernard Sepulveda, Hans Popper, Leon Schiff, Mitchell Spellberg and Sheila Sherlock

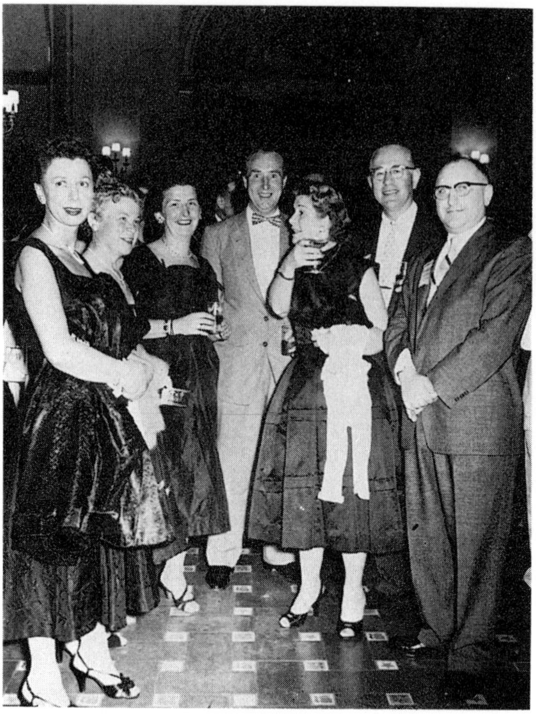

Figure 3 Havana, 1956. At the Tropicana. Right to left, Hans Popper, Leon Schiff, Augusta Schiff, Geraint James, Sheila Sherlock, Mrs Jaffe, Lina Popper

Progress in Liver Disease, edited by Popper and Schaffner. The first volume in 1961 has been followed by eight editions. The ninth one is in press, edited by Fenton Schaffner, but retaining the name of Popper as co-editor. He had many honours: 15 honorary degrees, of which Vienna was perhaps the one he treasured most. He was also delighted when he was made a member of the National Academy of Sciences in the United States and the Deutsche Akademie der Naturforscher Leopoldina, a distinguished Academic German Group.

In 1965 he met Herbert Falk. Dr Falk told me that Hans was coming from Vienna, having been given his honorary degree, and was going on to Freiburg via Basel. Falk was his chauffeur from Basel to Freiburg. From that meeting was built up a wonderful symbiosis of the scientist and the businessman who wanted to benefit medical science. Dr and Mrs Falk become like godchildren to Popper. They really looked after him, and particularly so in his later years (Figure 4). The success of this present Basel meeting emphasizes the contribution that the Falk/Popper combination has made, and is making, to hepatology. It combines the new and the old world, and is the only liver meeting where distinguished American investigators really meet the best of Europe. Hans was forward-looking, he had such exquisite scientific taste in the choice of subjects and speakers, not only for

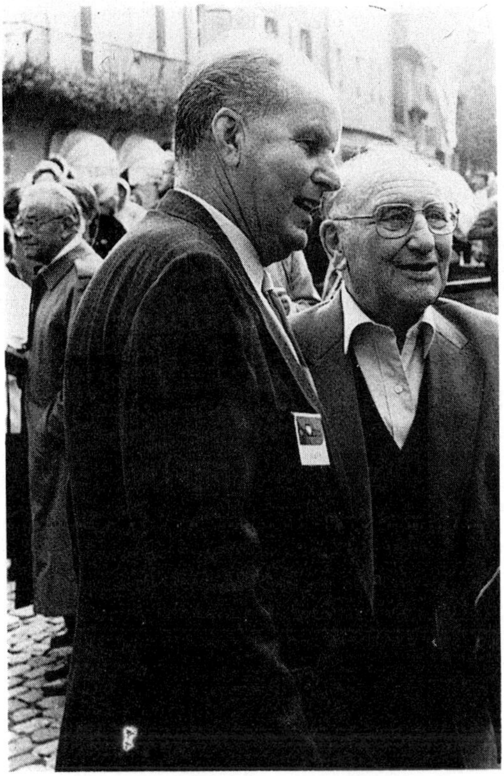

Figure 4 Hans Popper and Herbert Falk planning another Basel Liver Week

this large meeting, but for his little meetings. These were held on such subjects as cell–cell interactions. He set very high scientific standards for hepatology in Europe, and indeed in the world.

Hans's presence could transform a dull meeting into a happening; Hans arrived – that was it. You can see him there, just ready now to leap to his feet to interpret the unclear and to ask the one question the speaker did not want to be asked (Figure 5). He worked incredibly hard, perhaps 12–15 hours a day. When he was travelling he would start off at 6.30 a.m., with Canadian Air Forces exercises, and then go off to a meeting, usually with young pathologists around the microscope. All the difficult slides of the year were brought to him for interpretation. By the time he got back to the hotel at 6 o'clock, he had given two lectures and three seminars and then, after dinner, he would give another lecture and perhaps an after-dinner speech.

Now what about his family? In 1942 he married Lina, also originally from Austria. She does not look any different today than in 1948, when I first met her as a charming hostess in Chicago (Figure 6). The honeymoon took place in Atlantic City where Dr Popper had a poster demonstration at the American Medical Association meeting. Even on her honeymoon Lina was

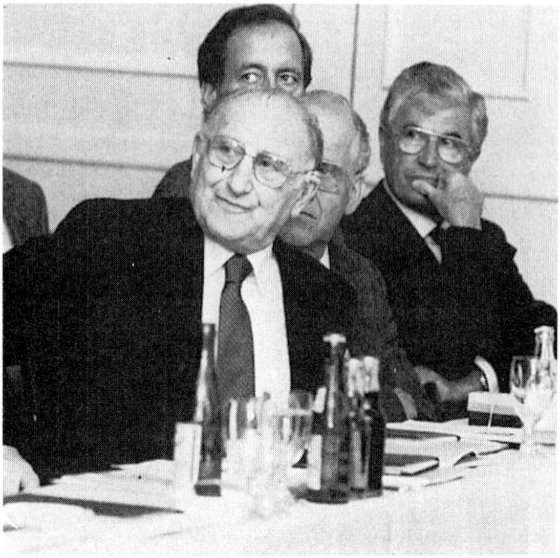

Figure 5 Basel Liver Week 1986. Hans ready to join in discussion

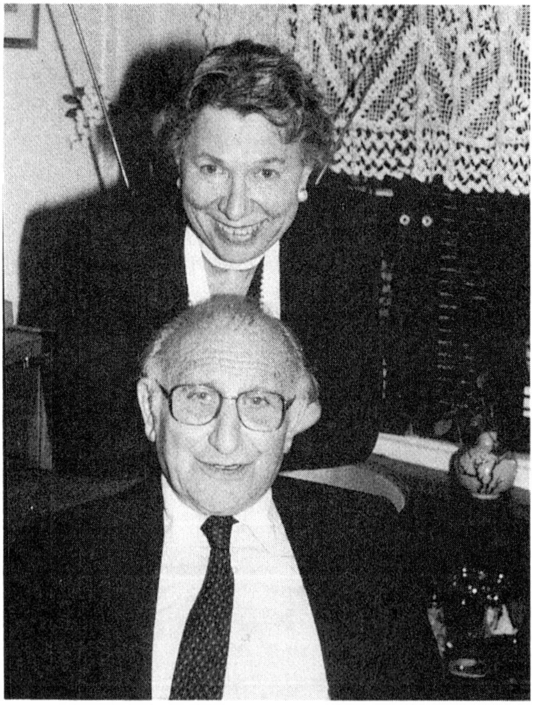

Figure 6 Birthday party 1984, with Lina Popper

busy helping to put up the poster. She knew exactly what her life would be with such a husband. She was his greatest staunch and understanding supporter, with a very high intellect. Hans was extremely lucky with his wife. They have two children, Dr Frank, who is a scientist, and Dr Charley, who is a psychiatrist. There are two grandchildren, and I can see Hans in both of them. So the dynasty goes on. I last saw Hans in 1987, at a meeting in Ancona in Italy. He was talking about viruses and cancer. He had worked terribly hard to embrace molecular biology and had achieved it. At the end of the meeting he said 'I have written a paper on "Viral carcinogenesis in the liver" would you consider it for the *Journal of Hepatology*?' Of course I did, and this was probably the last paper that he had published.

Here then was a man who started with a disciplined academic education in Vienna, a brilliant man of many talents. He coined the term 'cholestasis', he did wonderful work on drug-related liver disease and on viral hepatitis, and latterly he did much work on carcinogenesis.

In a recent obituary Alan Hoffman commented:

> No brief summary can do justice to the accomplishments of this man whose mission in life was to discover, to question, to explain, to teach, to counsel, to inspire, and to bring order and imagination to pathological mysteries. He was a presence at every meeting, listening, enquiring, reminiscing and finally dancing at the farewell ball. His enthusiasm was as contagious as his wisdom was awesome.

In 1979, at the time of his 80th birthday celebrations in Vienna, Hans Popper wrote 'Thanks are due to Goethe who formulated the Faustian bargain with the devil which has become my credo.' In 1984, writing on 'Vienna and the liver' he slightly modified the scene:

> I am grateful to the fates for letting me return once more to Vienna where I was first embued with a restless Faustian drive. Having mellowed through the years, as did Vienna, I may once more quote Goethe, the angels in his Faust:
>
> 'Could I ever say to the moment in time,
> stay still, you are so beautiful,
> then you can put me in chains,
> and I would gladly perish'

Indeed we were all delighted that Hans did not stay still: he worked until the end. Let us think of Hans, and let us think of what he thought and what he made us think: the liver, not so much a living, as a way of life.

2
Award Lecture: The hepatitis B virus and the host response

H. C. THOMAS

Recovery from HBV infection is dependent on the integrated activity of the patient's interferon and immune system. Chronic HBV infections arise because of defects in these defences.

ACUTE HEPATITIS B INFECTION

HBV is not cytopathic, and the liver damage is caused by immune lysis of infected hepatocytes, an essential part of the recovery process. Analysis of the inflammatory infiltrate demonstrates the presence of NK and cytotoxic T cells[1]. Viral antigens are seen on the surface of the hepatocyte[2] and these, in association with the class I MHC proteins, make the cell a target for cytotoxic T-cell lysis[3]. Studies in patients with chronic HBV infection suggest that the nucleocapsid antigens (HBc and HBe – a cleavage product of HBc) are an important target[4,5]. Hepatocytes usually express very little MHC class I glycoprotein[6], but, in the early stage of acute HBV infection, following the production of interferon-α, MHC expression on hepatocytes increases and coincidentally transaminases rise (Figure 1). Recent observations (personal) indicate that the X gene product may activate cellular genes, including those for MHC class I proteins.

Interferon also activates a series of enzymes, including the 2-5A oligoadenylate synthetase/endonuclease system, which leads to inhibition of viral protein synthesis (Figure 2). This would be expected to produce an antiviral state in uninfected regenerating liver cells, preventing reinfection during the lysis of infected hepatocytes.

The virus neutralizing antibodies are directed to epitopes on the envelope of the virus. This is composed of three polypeptides each with the same carboxyl terminus (Figure 3). These are designated the large, middle and major envelope proteins. The aminoterminal 120 amino acid region of the large protein, which is not present in the middle and major proteins, is designated pre-S1. This hydrophilic area is myristilated, and recent data

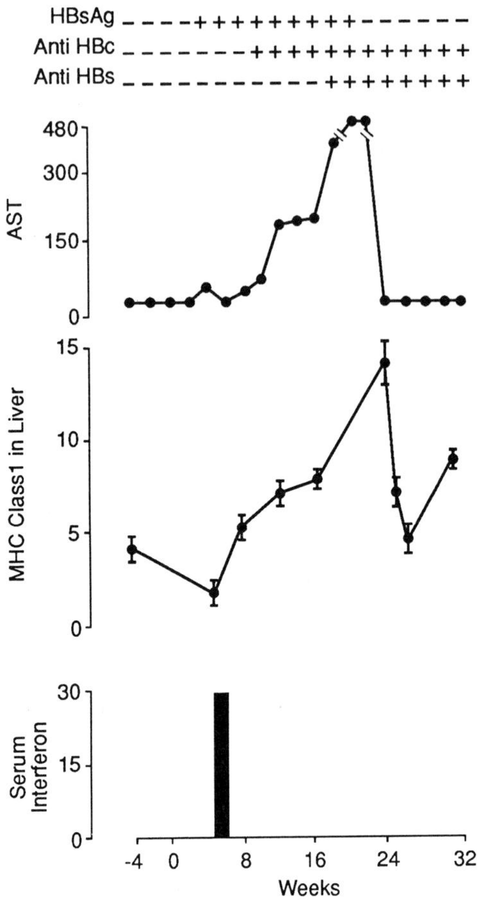

Figure 1 Acute HBV infection in the chimpanzee. Markers of virus infection appear early, coinciding with a detectable pulse of circulating IFN-α.This is followed by enhanced display of MHC class I antigen on hepatocytes. Liver damage as indicated by rising AST coincides with the first appearance of host humoral immunity to HBV (anti-HBc). AST: aspartate aminotransferase (SGOT).

indicate that the region 21–47 amino acids is capable of binding to the membrane of the hepatocyte[7] and is, therefore, probably involved in virus uptake. The pre-S2 region of 55 amino acids, present in the large and middle proteins, binds polymerized human serum albumin (pHSA)[8]. Because this protein also binds selectively to the hepatocytes of species that are susceptible to HBV infection and not to non-susceptible species[9], it has been proposed that pHSA acts as a bridge between the pre-S2 region of the viral envelope and the hepatocyte, facilitating uptake and infection of the cell. More recent observations showing that pHSA is not present in serum, and that native albumin in physiological concentrations blocks the binding of pHSA to HBs antigen[10] make this hypothetical uptake system unlikely to occur *in vivo* in man.

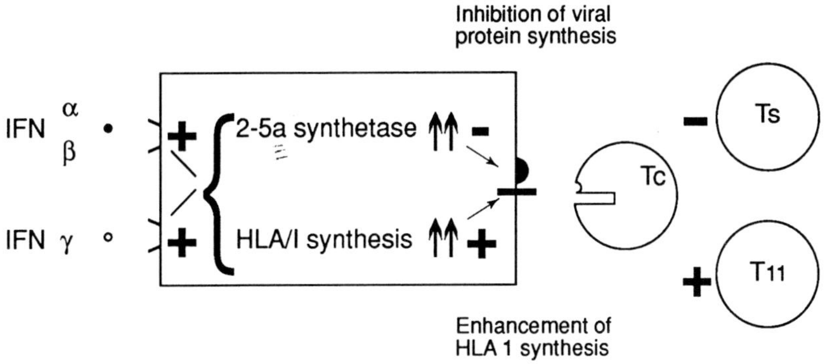

Figure 2 Effect of IFNs on the virus-infected cell. IFN-α and IFN-β acting through a common receptor and IFN-γ acting through a separate receptor activate (+) 2-5A oligoadenylate synthetase. This catalyses production of oligoadenylates which activate an endogenous ribonuclease leading to cleavage of viral RNA. IFN also causes enhanced (+) expression of MHC (HLA) class I proteins on the hepatocyte surface, facilitating recognition of virus-infected cells by the cellular immune mechanisms of the host. HBe and HBc antigens are the target of this component of the host immune response. Tc, Ts, Th: cytotoxic, suppressor and helper T cells. (+) and (−) denote enhancement and suppression, respectively.

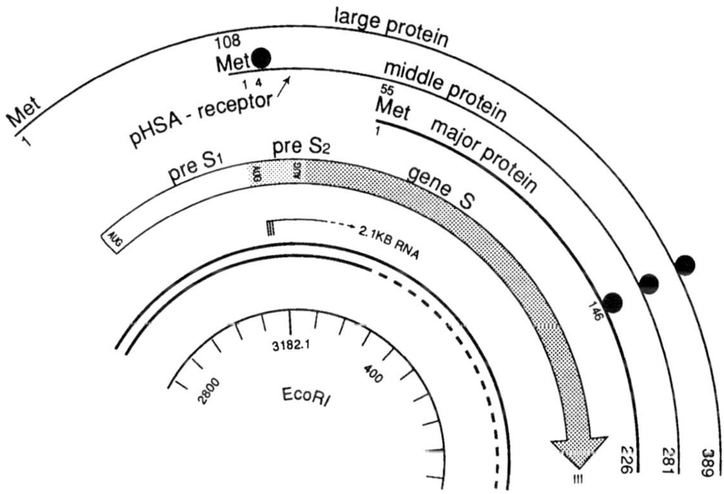

Figure 3 The large, middle and major proteins of the envelope of HBV have the same carboxyl terminal sequence.

The antibodies found in convalescent serum bind predominantly to the epitopes of the HBs gene-encoded region[11], the carboxyl-terminal region of which is present in all the envelope proteins. Two hydrophilic regions of this polypeptide, amino acids 124–147 (Figure 4), form loops because of intramolecular disulphide bridges, and these are the binding region for the majority (>80%) of the antigen-binding capacity of the convalescent sera. Using monoclonal antibodies binding to these regions, it has been possible

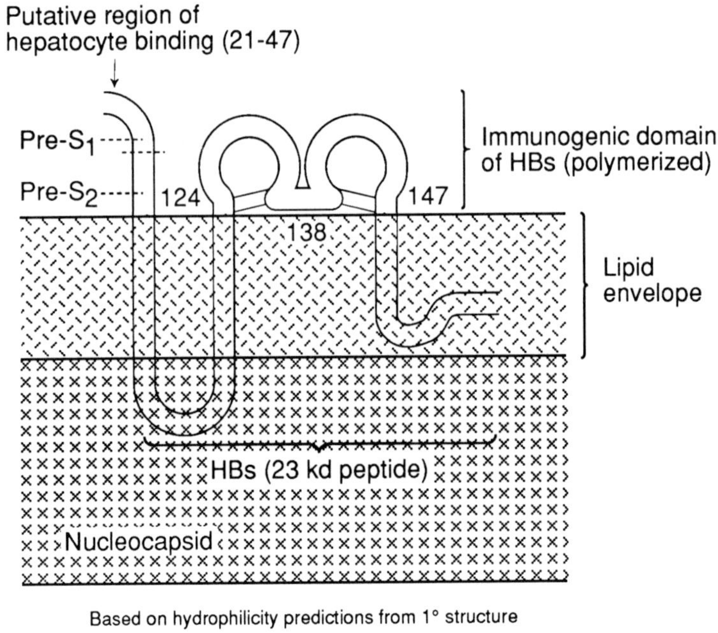

Figure 4 The hydrophilic regions of the pre-S and S gene products are potential immunogenic regions. The pre-S1 amino-terminal sequence binds to the hepatocyte membrane. Antibodies to pre-S1 and the region 124–137 of HBs peptide inhibit infection.

to show that administration of antibody to the region 124–136 to chimpanzees prevents infection[12]. Antibodies to this region, as well as to other epitopes on the S gene-encoded polypeptide, are present in the serum of patients convalescent from HBV infection and in normal subjects immunized with plasma-derived and recombinant DNA-produced HBs vaccine[13].

Although patients recovered from HBV or vaccinated with HBs antigen are protected from further infection, there has been considerable debate on whether the middle pre-S2-bearing and large pre-S1-bearing polypeptides should be added to existing vaccines. During natural infection antibodies to pre-S1 and pre-S2 regions appear before antibodies to the HBs region[14,15] and if pre-S1 is the region of the envelope of the virus that binds to the hepatocyte during infection[7], antibodies to this region might be virus neutralizing and, therefore, inclusion of the pre-S region in a vaccine might be desirable. Furthermore, 15% of normal individuals do not respond to HBs polypeptide and inclusion of pre-S2, by recruiting additional T_h cells, facilitates the development of antibody to the HBs epitopes[16]. More recent data indicate that the inclusion of HBc with HBs antigen further enhances the humoral response to HBs epitopes[17] (Figure 5).

CHRONIC HEPATITIS B INFECTION

It is likely that there are many different reasons why patients develop the chronic carrier state. This exists in several forms.

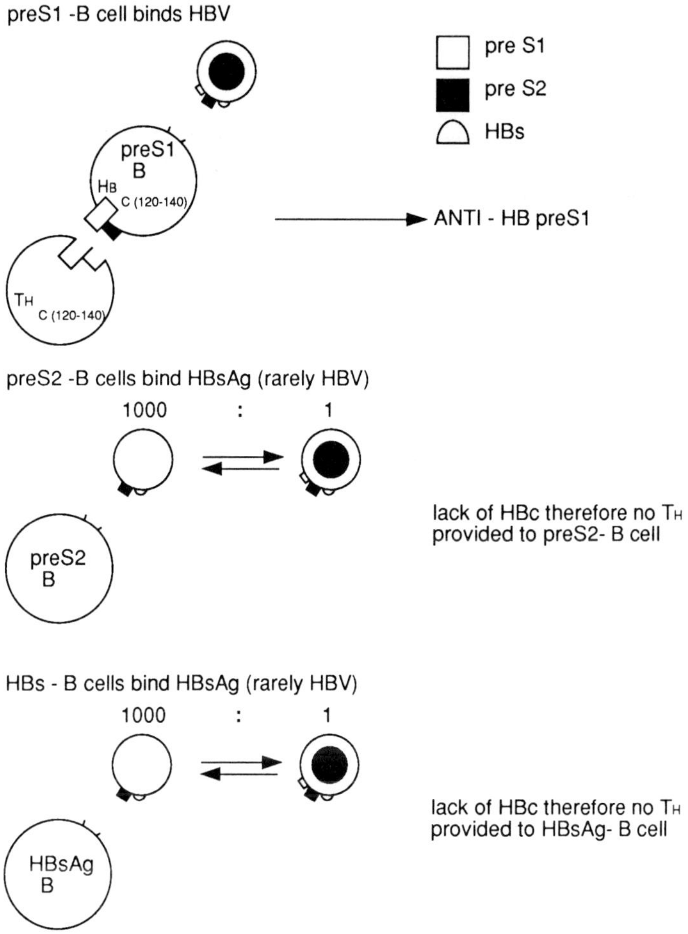

Figure 5 Pre-S1 peptides are only present on HBV particles and not on the non-infectious particles. Pre-S1-reactive B cells will bind and take up HBV particles but not 22 nm HBsAg particles. HBc within B cells will be processed and attract help from HBc reactive T-helper cells[17]. Pre-S2 and S-reactive B cells will take up 22 nm particles as well as HBV, and will therefore be less likely to be able to attract HBc reactive helper T cells.

Chronic HBe antigenaemic patients

This is the first phase of chronic infection and may arise after exposure at any stage of life.

Chronic HBV infection following exposure in neonatal life

Ninety-five per cent of babies born to HBV 'e' antigen positive mothers become infected, and over 95% of these develop a chronic carrier state (Figure 6)[18]. These infants probably receive a large inoculum of virus from maternal blood before or during birth, and by close contact with secretions

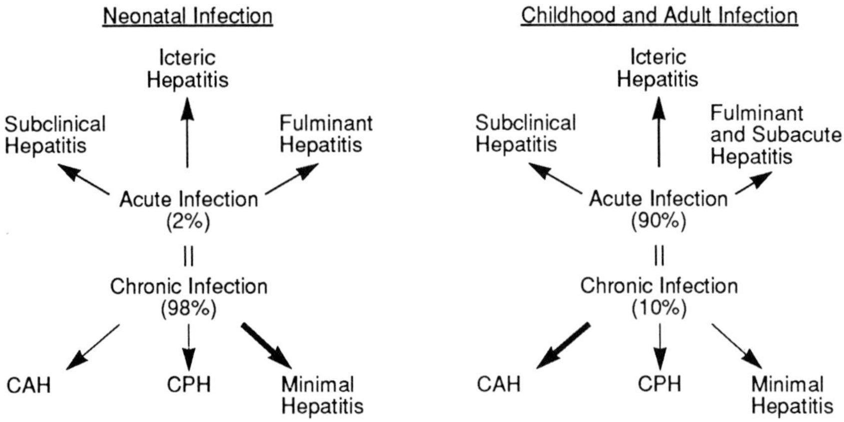

Figure 6 Natural history of HBV infection after neonatal or adult exposure. CPH = chronic persistent hepatitis and CAH = chronic active hepatitis.

soon after birth. The reason for these infants failing to clear the virus is unknown, but likely to relate to the immaturity of the neonatal immune system[19]. HBe antigen, a low molecular weight (15 kd) soluble protein, derived from the pre-core/HBc polypeptide by cleavage of both the amino- and carboxy-terminal ends, passes across the placenta and may suppress the development of the cellular immune response to the nucleocapsid proteins which are the target during immune clearance of infected hepatocytes (Figure 7).

Fulminant hepatitis following exposure in neonatal life

Rarely, children born to HBs antigen anti-HBe positive mothers, develop fulminant hepatitis. The mechanism is once again unknown. One hypothesis is that maternal anti-HBe and anti-HBc pass across the placenta and initially modulate the lysis of infected hepatocytes by the cell-mediated immune response of the child[5]. The virus would spread throughout the liver and as the maternal antibodies disappear at 3–6 months, cytotoxic T cells sensitized to HBe and HBc would then rapidly destroy the infected cells, resulting in hepatic failure.

Chronic HBV infection following exposure after the neonatal period

In marked contrast to the situation at birth, only 50% of subjects infected after this period develop chronic infection (Figure 6). There are probably several different causes for the development of chronic infection at this stage of life. One defect, which has recently been documented, is the production

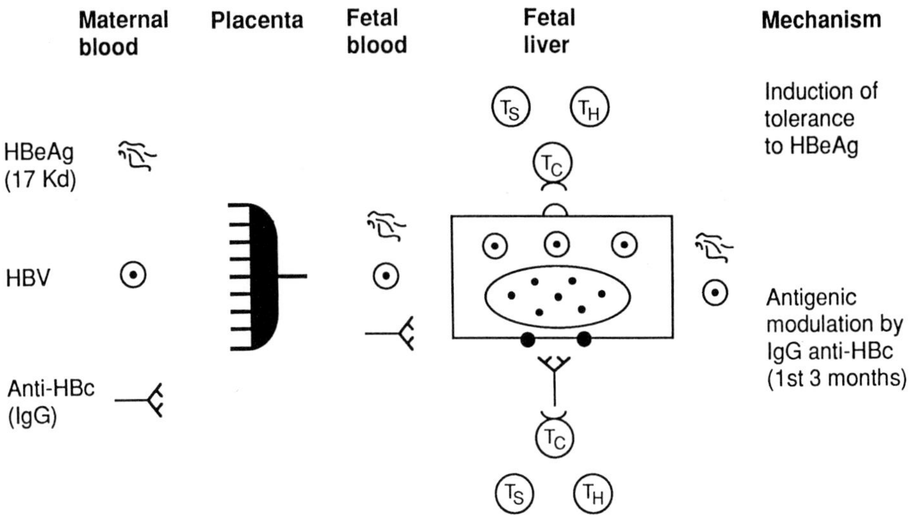

Figure 7 Neonatal HBV infection: postulated mechanism of viral persistence. It is proposed that HBe antigen crosses the placenta from the maternal blood and, in neonates, induces tolerance to HBe antigen which is one of the targets of the cellular immune response. Maternal IgG anti-HBc also crosses the placenta into the neonatal circulation. Persistence of HBV-infected cells in the fetal liver is facilitated as maternal IgG blocks recognition of virus-infected cells by cytotoxic T cells[4,5]. Early exposure to soluble virus protein (HBe) may induce a state of antigenic tolerance to the virus with specific suppressor cells inhibiting the host defence mechanism.

of subnormal quantities of interferon-α by peripheral blood mononuclear cells[20–24]. These individuals also have evidence of abnormal activation of their hepatocytes by interferon: levels of hepatic 2-5A synthetase (an enzyme induced by IFN) are only minimally elevated[22] and MHC class I proteins, which are induced by interferon, are present in very low density on infected hepatocytes[25] whereas levels of 2-5A synthetase and MHC class I display are markedly increased in peripheral blood lymphocytes of chronic HBV carriers[26]. These data suggest interferon activation of peripheral blood lymphocytes but not of infected hepatocytes, and raise the possibility that HBV within the hepatocyte has selectively 'switched off' the responsiveness of the hepatocyte to interferons. *In vitro* transfection of HBV genomes into cells in tissue culture, makes them specifically non-responsive to interferon: they remain susceptible to lysis by Sindbis virus and MHC induction by IFN does not occur[27]. Thus during HBV replication it is hypothesized that T cells cannot lyse infected cells because the virus suppresses the expression of MHC class I proteins (Figure 8).

HBe antigen/antibody seroconversion

It is hypothesized that, as the level of HBV replication within the hepatocytes falls, the suppression of MHC protein display is reduced and infected cells are lysed by cytotoxic T cells probably sensitized to nucleocapsid epitopes:

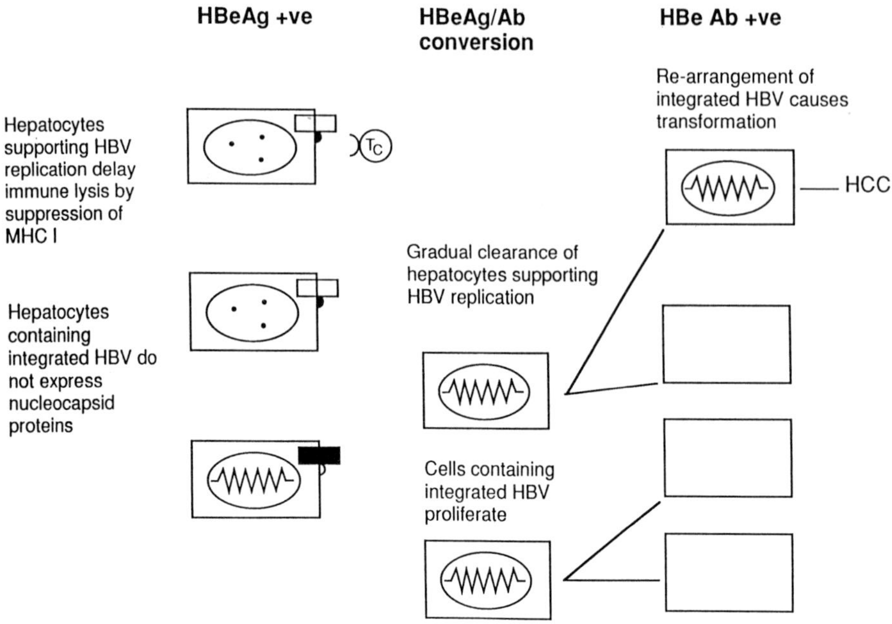

Figure 8 During the HBeAg-positive phase (left-hand column) hepatocytes containing HBV show suppression of MHC class I antigen display and avoid T cell lysis. During the HBe antibody phase (right-hand column) hepatocytes containing integrated HBV sequences avoid T cell lysis because they do not express nucleocapsid proteins. HCC = hepatocellular carcinoma; • = HBV particles; ◗ membrane HBc antigen; ■ membrane MHC I protein; suppressed MHC I protein.

the result is lobular hepatitis. Hepatocytes that contain integrated HBV sequences do not express HBV nucleocapsid proteins because the preferred site of integration within the viral genome is within the regulatory region of the gene encoding for this protein[28]. These cells will therefore avoid immune lysis (Figure 8). The destruction of hepatocytes supporting productive HBV infection results in a reduction in hepatocyte mass. The remaining hepatocytes, including those containing integrated HBV sequences, are stimulated to proliferate to restore liver mass.

Anti-HBe positive patients with no evidence of HBV replication

The sera of these patients do not contain virus particles detectable by dot/blot hybridization. However, in some cases low levels of viraemia can be detected by the polymerase chain reaction. The hepatitis B surface antigen in these patients is encoded by integrated HBV DNA sequences. Ultimately, it is argued that during cell division the integrated sequences rearrange[29] and cause malignant transformation of the hepatocyte. Clinically evident hepatocellular carcinoma then appears within months, and the patients rapidly die.

Chronic anti-HBe positive patients with persistent HBV replication (pre-core HBV mutant)

An HBV mutant with a point mutation generating a novel stop codon at the end of the pre-core sequence has been described[29a] (Figure 9). These

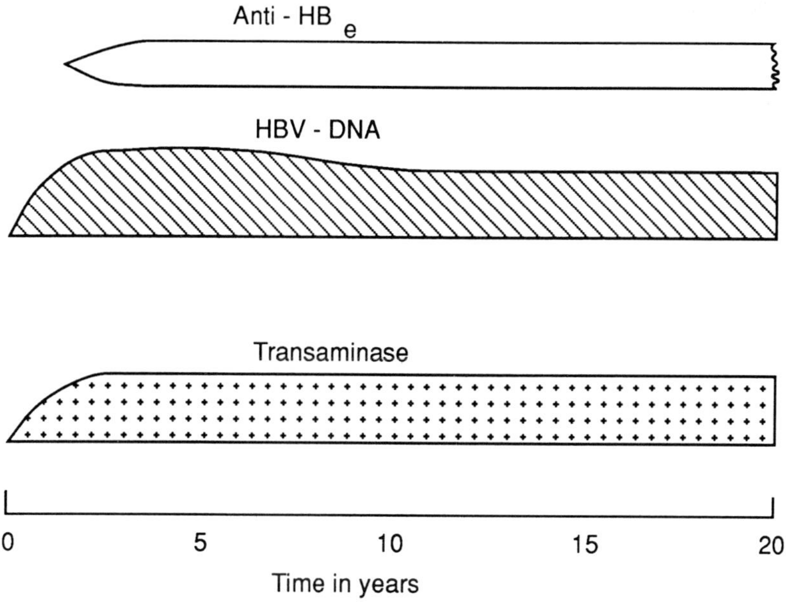

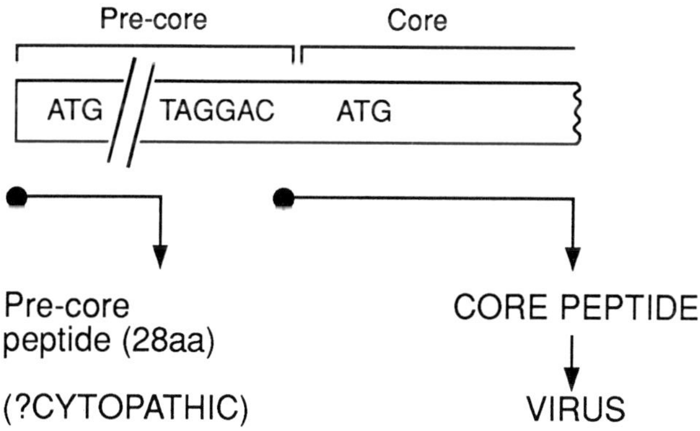

Figure 9 Translation of the pre-core/core transcript may start at either of two AUG sites. When translation starts at the first AUG the pre-core/core peptide is produced. This has a signal peptide at its aminoterminal end and is secreted from the cell to give rise, after cleavage of fragments from the amino and carboxyl ends, to HBe antigen in serum. In the pre-core mutant virus, two mutations in the pre-core region generate a stop codon which prevents translation of the pre-core/core peptide from which HBe antigen is derived, and the second mutation allows efficient translation of the core peptide which is needed for virion production.

patients have significant viraemia but cannot secrete HBe antigen which is derived from the pre-core/core translation product. This nucleocapsid protein is not produced in the presence of the stop codon but translation does occur from the second AUG at the beginning of HBc. This 21 kd HBc is all that is required from virion nucleocapsid and virus particle production.

These patients develop rapidly progressive liver disease and are common in the Mediterranean Basin.

MANAGEMENT OF CHRONIC HBV

There is no established place in treatment of chronic HBV infection for regimens involving solely anti-inflammatory or immunosuppressive drugs[30–32]. A variety of synthetic and natural antiviral compounds have been developed and are being evaluated in clinical trials.

Indications for therapy (not definitively identified)

1. Infectivity – HBe antigen and HBV DNA positivity.
2. Evidence of progressive liver disease – histological evidence of chronic active hepatitis.

Contraindications for therapy

Evidence of decompensated cirrhosis.

Goals of therapy

1. Inhibition of HBV replication (by direct effect or by stimulation of the host antiviral response).
2. Long-term control of inflammatory necrosis of hepatocytes.
3. Prevention of malignant transformation of hepatocytes.

Responses to antiviral therapy may be of three types (Figure 10)

1. Transient response: inhibition of HBV replication – loss of HBV DNA and HBV DNA polymerase – during therapy *but* return of these markers on cessation of therapy.
2. Incomplete response: sustained inhibition of HBV replication – loss of HBV DNA and HBV DNA polymerase – continuing after cessation of therapy, conversion from HBeAg to anti-HBe *but* continued HBs antigenaemia due to translation of integrated HBV DNA.
3. Complete response: sustained inhibition of HBV replication – loss of HBV DNA and HBV DNA polymerase – continuing after cessation of therapy, with permanent seroconversion from HBeAg and HBsAg to anti-HBe and anti-HBs.

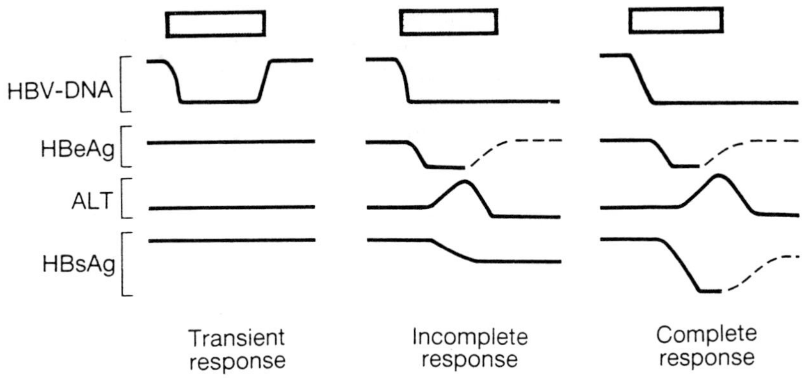

Figure 10 Pattern of response to antiviral treatment.

Active drugs

1. Adenine arabinoside: is a potent inhibitor of HBV replication but its clinical usefulness is limited by poor aqueous solubility. In one small randomized controlled study a 10-day course produced sustained HBe antigen/antibody seroconversion in 40% of cases[33].
2. Adenine arabinoside monophosphate: is an equally effective inhibitor of HBV replication which can be given by i.m. bolus injection[30–32]. A course of 10 mg/kg per day for 3 days followed by 5 mg/kg per day for a further 23 days has been evaluated in three controlled studies[34–36]. Variability of response may be related to heterogeneity of the patient population being studied. In one study, none of 24 homosexual HBV carriers responded, whereas 10/22 heterosexual (predominantly Southern European) carriers did[37] (Figure 11).

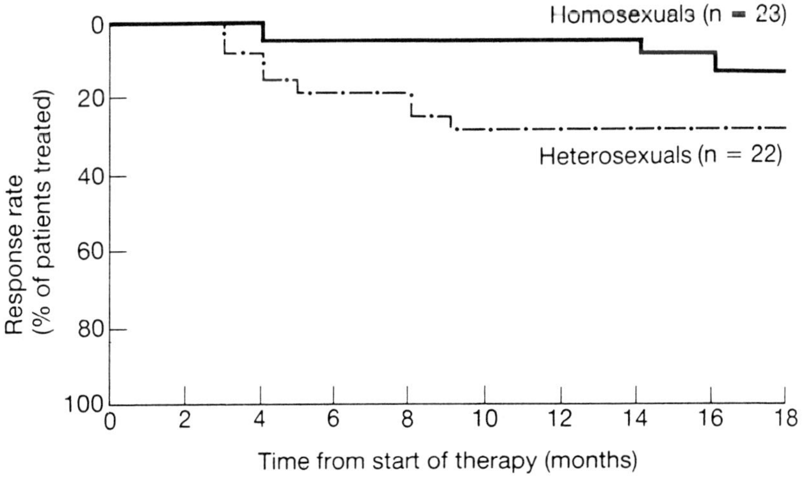

Figure 11 Response to ARA AMP in homosexual and heterosexual men.

3. Acycloguanosine (acyclovir): is active in low concentrations in herpes simplex-infected cells because of phosphorylation to active metabolites by a virus-encoded thymidine kinase. This enzyme is not present in HBV-infected cells so that this mode of action does not operate. Higher concentrations (near the maximum tolerated dose) do partially inhibit HBV replication[38], but this has been shown to be clinically not useful.
4. Type I interferon (α and β): both natural and recombinant DNA produced preparations have been examined.
   (a) Leucocyte IFN-α: has been shown to inhibit HBV replication when given daily in moderate doses (5–10 megaunits/m^2 per day over 3–6 months[39]). A randomized controlled study showed that low doses for 4–6 weeks produced no long-term responses[40].
   (b) Recombinant IFN-α: given daily in high dose inhibits HBV replication but is toxic[41]. Moderate doses (10 megaunits/m^2 daily or thrice weekly) are better tolerated and can be given for 3–6 months[42]. Preliminary analysis of one randomized controlled study shows 45% of patients clearing HBe antigen[42,43].
   (c) Lymphoblastoid IFN-α: given thrice weekly for 3–6 months in moderate doses has been shown, in two randomized controlled studies, to produce HBe antigen clearance in 26–88% of cases, significantly more often than occurred spontaneously in the control groups[44–46]. The response rates were very variable because of heterogeneity of the patients, particularly severity of the liver disease at the start of therapy. The mean response rate is similar to that seen with adenine arabinoside monophosphate (ARA-MP) in heterosexual patients[47] but in homosexual patients ARA-MP does not work, whereas IFN-α does. Additional analysis of some of these studies shows that Chinese carriers (presumably infected from birth) show no response, whereas European carriers exhibit a 55% seroconversion rate[37] (Figure 12). Further studies reveal that 6 months of therapy is no better than three (Figure 13)[48].
   (d) Interferons-β of natural and recombinant types have been used, and shown to have similar activity to IFN-α. No controlled studies are reported.

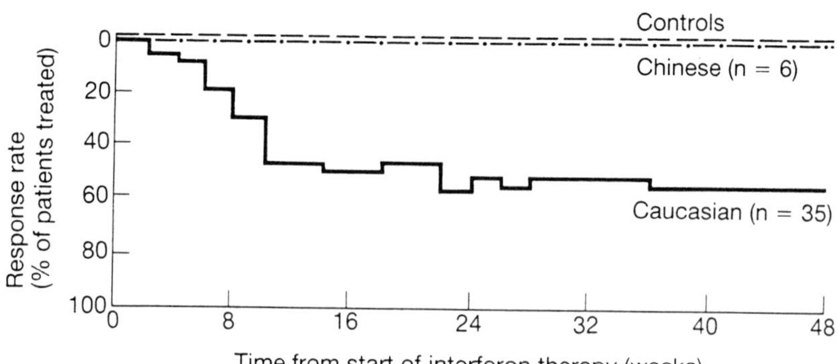

Figure 12 Response to IFN-α in Chinese and Caucasian carriers[56].

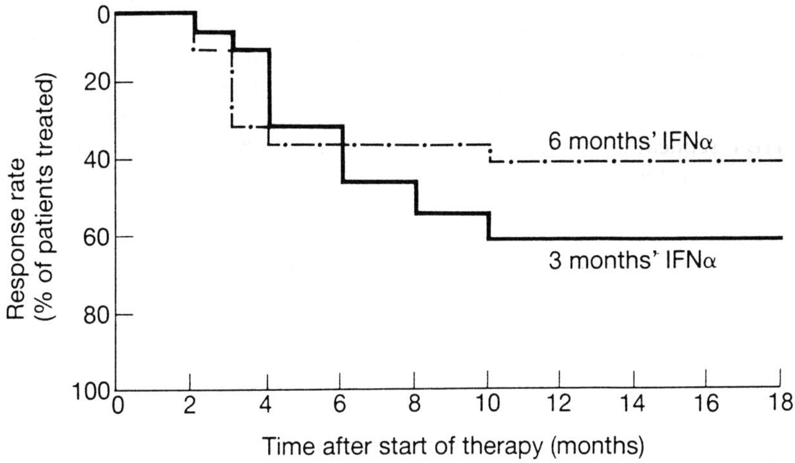

Figure 13 Response to IFN-α: comparison of 3 and 6 months therapy[56].

5. Type II interferon (γ): both natural and recombinant are available. These are predominantly immunostimulant with less direct antiviral activity. Inhibition of HBV replication does occur after several months therapy. Optimal dosaging is not established.
6. Interleukin-2: is a lymphokine which amplifies immune function. It has been tried safely in individual patients but its place has not been established.
7. Combination therapy
   (a) Short-course prednisolone plus antiviral therapy (ARA-MP or IFN-α): withdrawal of immunosuppressant therapy, after several months or years, may result in HBeAg seroconversion[30–32]. However, after short courses of prednisolone, withdrawal does not precipitate seroconversion[49]. When followed by ARA-MP or IFN-α 60–70% seroconversion rates have been reported in small controlled studies[50,51] and in one of these[51] the results were particularly encouraging in that the patients had probably been infected from birth, a group of patients that are resistent to treatment with interferon alone. Care must be taken when withdrawing steroids, particularly in patients with severe liver disease: severe exacerbations have been recorded.
   (b) Acyclovir and IFN-α: preliminary studies did not include appropriate controls and therefore summative or synergistic effects could not be conclusively identified[52].

GENERAL COMMENT

Antiviral therapy has been used principally to treat HBe antigen-positive patients.

The mechanism of action of interferon in inducing seroconversion hepatitis is unknown. Several changes have been noted both in the immune system and in the infected hepatocyte (Figure 14). An increase in MHC class I protein display[53] and alteration in viral protein expression[37] in the hepatocyte occur within 24 h of the start of therapy. An increase in the helper/cytotoxic suppressor cell ratio occurs at 6–8 weeks when the seroconversion hepatitis starts, and is not seen in those that do not respond.

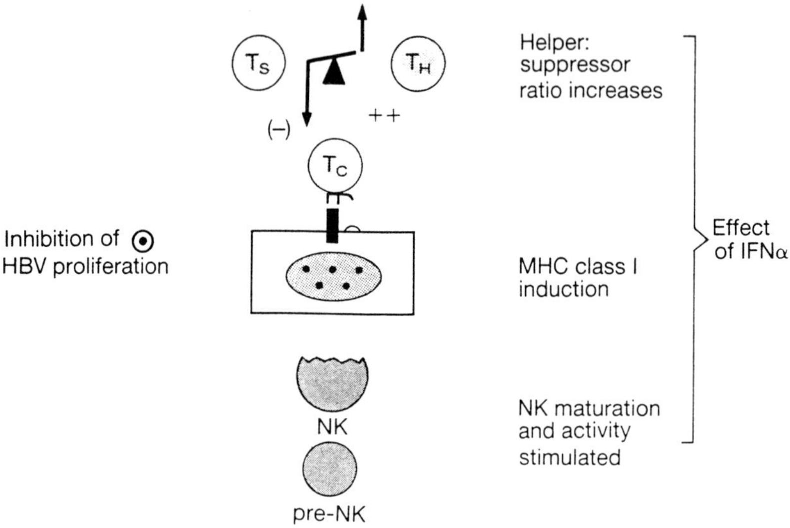

Figure 14 Changes occurring during interferon therapy.

Changes in humoral immunity also occur. Patients who respond to therapy either have IgM anti-HBc present before treatment or develop it during the course of therapy[54]. Changes in cell-mediated immunity may also occur, but have not yet been documented.

Inhibition of viral replication, associated with HBe antigen/antibody seroconversion, is usually long-lasting and accompanied, after a transient exacerbation, by amelioration of the inflammatory liver disease[43]. Reactivation may occur particularly in homosexual patients with or without HIV infection[55].

Patients treated early in the course of the disease will lose HBs antigen from their serum if cessation of HBV replication is achieved (Figure 15a). If integration of HBV sequences into the host cell genome has occurred before starting treatment, HBs antigenaemia will continue after cessation of detectable HBV replication (Figure 15b). However, inflammatory liver disease will ameliorate in these patients if long-term inhibition of HBV replication is achieved.

Histology

Several investigations have shown improvement in alanine aminotransferase levels following clearance of HBeAg and HBV DNA from the serum. A

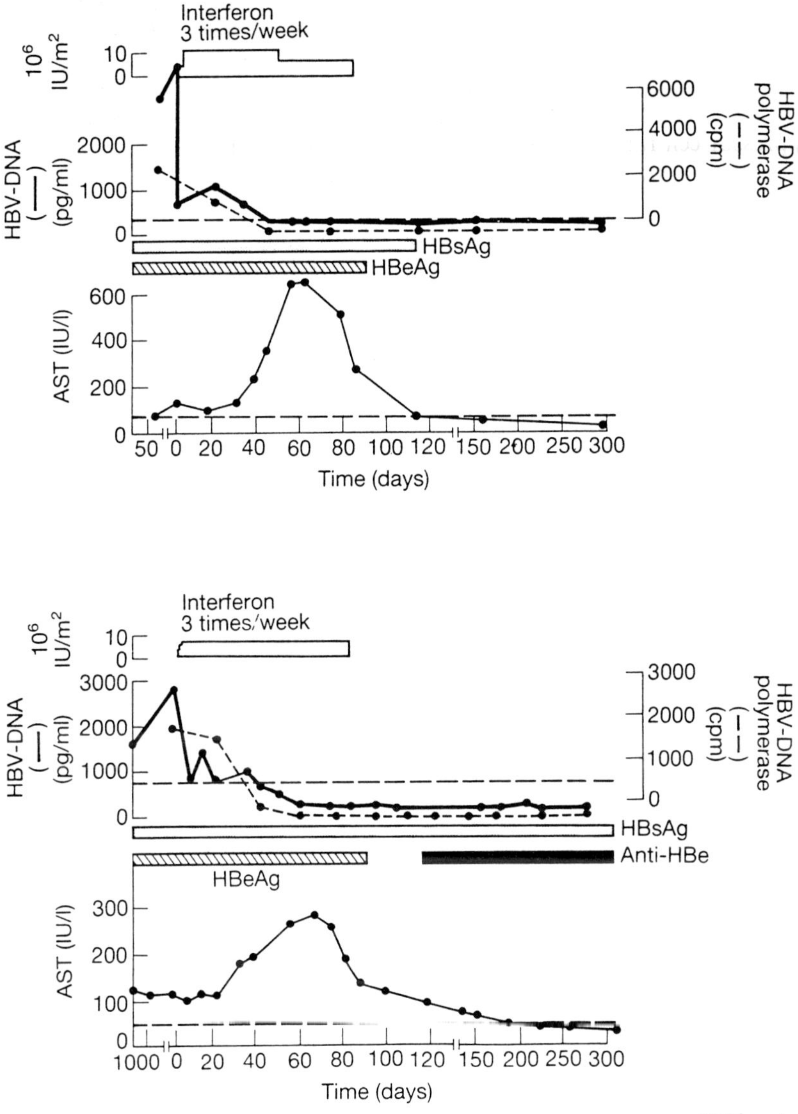

Figure 15 **(a)** Complete response: inhibition of HBV replication and clearance of HBs antigen. **(b)** Incomplete response: inhibition of HBV replication associated with a transient exacerbation and then normalization of the liver function tests. Note the patient remains HBsAg-positive, presumably because of the presence of integrated HBV sequences. Benefits to the patient include infectivity and cessation of inflammatory liver disease.

review of 50 treated and 25 untreated control patients has conclusively shown a reduction in inflammatory necrosis of liver cells and a diminished rate of development of cirrhosis in patients responding to therapy with loss of markers of HBV replication[43].

Whether interferon will also be of value in the treatment of chronic infection with the pre-core mutant remains to be determined. Preliminary data suggest that this is not the case, and that the liver disease in these patients is caused by a cytopathic effect of the virus.

THE NEED TO SELECT PATIENTS FOR TREATMENT

Infectivity and progressive liver disease are the major reasons for attempting therapy with either adenine arabinoside monophosphate or IFN-α. Currently interferons are the most satisfactory therapy, but less than 50% of patients respond and the side-effects of interferon are substantial. For this reason both clinical and serological features, which predict a greater chance of response, have been sought. The clinical features include marked inflammatory activity, high transaminases and more recently the presence of IgM anti-HBc[54] and low serum HBV DNA[42].

SUMMARY

The clearance of HBV-infected cells from the liver is probably dependent on an interplay between the interferon system and the cellular limb of the host immune response. Although the importance of the nucleocapsid proteins as targets for sensitized cytotoxic T cells is established in chronic HBV infection, further studies are needed during the early phase of acute HBV infection. The relative importance of pre-S sequences as inducers and targets of the virus-neutralizing humoral immune response is becoming established, but their precise place will await the development of *in vitro* models of hepadna virus infection and precise definition of the mechanism of viral uptake.

Our understanding of the mechanisms underlying the development of chronic HBV infection is still incomplete. When this occurs in adult life, deficient production of IFN-α and suppression of the ability of the host to respond to interferon, are probably important factors. In the neonate, specific suppression of the cell-mediated immune response, perhaps because of exposure to soluble HBe antigen or to modulating quantities of maternally derived anti-nucleocapsid antibodies at a time when the immune system is 'immature', may be involved.

The presence of a mutation in the pre-core region of some virus isolates has recently been described. Hepatocytes infected with this virus cannot produce HBe antigen and the course of the liver disease is fairly rapid. Whether this mutant causes liver damage in the same way as the wild virus, or is directly cytopathic, needs further study.

In adult acquired chronic HBC infection IFN-α produces HBe antigen clearance in 40–60% of cases and is followed by resolution of the hepatic inflammation. Results in neonatally acquired infection are less impressive and prednisolone priming, followed by interferon, may be needed. Better understanding of the mechanisms resulting in failure to clear this virus should result in improved therapy.

References

1. Eggink, H. F., Houthoff, H. J., Huitema, S., Gips, C. H. and Poppema, S. (1982). Cellular and humoral immune reactions in chronic active liver disease. Lymphocyte subsets in liver biopsies of patients with untreated idiopathic auto-immune hepatitis, chronic active hepatitis B and primary biliary cirrhosis. *Clin. Exp. Immunol.*, **50**, 17–24
2. Gudat, F., Bianchi, L., Sonnabend, W., Thiel, G., Aenishaenslin, W. and Stadler, C. A. (1975). Pattern of core and surface expression in liver tissue reflects state of immune response in hepatitis. *Br. J. Lab. Invest.*, **32**, 1–9
3. Doherty, P. C. and Zinkernagel, R. M. (1975). A biological role for the major histocompatibility antigen. *Lancet*, **1**, 1405–9
4. Eddleston, A. W. L. F., Mondelli, M., Mieli-Vergani, G. and Williams, R. (1982). Lymphocyte cytotoxicity to autologous hepatocytes in chronic hepatitis B virus infection. *Hepatology*, **2**, 122S–127S
5. Pignatelli, M., Waters, J., Lever, A. M. L., Iwarson, S., Gerety, R. and Thomas, H. C. (1987). Cytotoxic T-cell responses to the nucleocapsid proteins of HBV in chronic hepatitis. *J. Hepatol.*, **4**, 15–21
6. Thomas, H. C., Shipton, U. and Montano, L. (1982). The HLA system: its relevance to the pathogenesis of liver disease. In Schaffner, F. and Popper, H. (eds.), *Progress in Liver Disease*, vol. 16. (New York: Grune & Stratton), pp. 517–27
7. Neurath, A. R., Kent, S. B. H., Strick, N. and Parker, K. (1986). Identification and chemical synthesis of a host receptor binding site on hepatitis B virus. *Cell*, **46**, 429–36
8. Machida, A., Kishimoto, S., Ohnuma, H., Miyamoto, H., Baba, K., Oda, K., Nakamura, T., Funatsu, G., Miyakawa, Y. and Mayumi, M. (1983). A hepatitis B surface antigen polypeptide (p31) with the receptor for polymerised human as well as chimpanzee albumin. *Gastroenterology*, **85**, 268–74
9. Trevisan, A., Gudat, F., Guggenheim, R., Krey, G., Durmuller, U., Luond, G., Duggelin, M., Landmann, J., Thomas, H. C., Pignatelli, M. and Lever, A. M. L. (1986). Homology between HBV-DNA and a sequence regulating the interferon induced antiviral system: possible mechanism of persistent infection. *J. Med. Virol.*, **19**, 63–9
10. Ishisara, K., Waters, J., Pignatelli, M. and Thomas, H. C. (1987). Characterisation of the polymerised and monomeric human serum albumin binding sites on hepatitis B surface antigen. *J. Med. Virol.*, **21**, 89–95
11. Brown, S. E., Howard, C. R., Zuckerman, A. J. and Steward, M. W. (1984). Affinity of antibody responses in man to hepatitis B vaccine determined with synthetic peptides. *Lancet*, **2**, 184–7
12. Iwarson, S., Tabor, E., Thomas, H. C., Goodall, A., Waters, J., Snoy, P., Shih, J. W. and Gerety, R. J. (1985). Neutralisation of hepatitis B virus infectivity by a murine monoclonal antibody: an experimental study in the chimpanzee. *J. Med. Virol.*, **16**, 89–96
13. Thomas, H. C., Farci, P., Shein, R., Karayiannis, P., Smedile, A., Caruso, L. and Gerin, L. (1987). Inhibition of hepatitis delta virus (HDV) replication by lymphoblastoid human interferon. In Rizzetto, M., Gerin, J. and Purcell, R. (eds), *The Hepatitis Delta Virus.* (New York: Alan R. Liss), pp. 277–90
14. Neurath, A. R., Kent, S. B. H., Strick, N., Taylor, P. and Stevens, C. E. (1985). Hepatitis B virus contains pre-S gene encoded domains. *Nature*, **315**, 154–6
15. Petit, M. A., Maillard, P., Capel, F. and Pillot, J. (1986). Immunochemical structure of the hepatitis B surface antigen vaccine. II. Analysis of antibody responses in human sera against the envelope proteins. *Mol. Immunol.*, **23**, 511–23
16. Milich, D. R., McNamara, M. K., McLachlen, A., Thornton, G. and Chisari, F. V. (1985). Distinct H-2 linked regulation of T-cell responses to the pre-S and S regions of the same hepatitis B surface antigen polypeptide allows circumvention of non-responsiveness to the S regions. *Proc. Natl. Acad. Sci., USA*, **82**, 8168–72
17. Milich, D. R., McLachlan, A., Thornton, G. B. and Hughes, J. L. (1987). Antibody production to the nucleocapsid and envelope of the hepatitis B virus primed by a single synthetic T-cell site. *Nature*, **329**, 547–9
18. Beasley, R. P., Hwang, L.-Y., Lin, C.-C. *et al.* (1981). Hepatitis B immune globulin (HBIG) efficacy in the interruption of perinatal transmission of hepatitis B carrier state. *Lancet*, **2**, 388–93

19. Nash, A. A. (1985). Tolerance and suppression in virus diseases. *Br. Med. Bull.*, **41**, 41–5
20. Tolentino, P., Dianzani, F. and Zucea, M. (1985). Decreased interferon responses by lymphocytes from children with chronic hepatitis. *J. Infect. Dis.*, **132**, 459–61
21. Kato, Y., Nakagawa, H. and Kobayashi, K. (1982). Interferon production by peripheral lymphocytes in HBsAg positive liver disease. *Hepatology*, **2**, 789–90
22. Ikeda, T., Pignatelli, M., Lever, A. M. L. and Thomas, H. C. (1986a). Relationship of HLA protein display to activation of 2-5A synthetase in HBe antigen or anti-HBe positive chronic HBV infection. *Gut*, **27**, 1498–1501
23. Ikeda, T., Lever, A. M. L. and Thomas, H. C. (1986b). Evidence for a deficiency of IFN production in patients with chronic HBV infection acquired in adult life. *Hepatology*, **6**, 962–5
24. Abb, J., Zachoval, R. and Eisenberg, J. (1985). Production of interferon alpha and interferon gamma by peripheral blood leucocytes from patients with chronic hepatitis B virus infection. *J. Med. Virol.*, **16**, 171–6
25. Montano, L., Miescher, G. C., Goodhall, A. H., Weidmann, K. H., Janossy, G. and Thomas, H. C. (1982). Hepatitis B virus and HLA display in the liver during chronic hepatitis B virus infection. *Hepatology*, **2**, 557–61
26. Poitrine, A., Chousterman, S., Chousterman, M., Naveau, S., Thang, M. N. and Chaput, J. C. (1985). Lack of in vivo activation of the interferon system in HBsAg positive chronic active hepatitis. *Hepatology*, **5**, 171–4
27. Onji, M., Lever, A. and Thomas, H. C. (1989). Hepatitis B virus reduces the sensitivity of cells to interferon. *Hepatology* (in press)
28. Fowler, M. J. F., Greenfield, C., Chu, C.-M., Karayiannis, P., Dunk, A., Lok, A. S. F., Lai, C. L., Yeoh, E. K., Menjardino, J., Wankya, B. M. and Thomas, H. C. (1986). Integration of HBV-DNA may not be a prerequisite for the maintenance of the state of malignant transformation. An analysis of 110 liver biopsies. *J. Hepatol.*, **2**, 218–29
29. Shafritz, D. A. (1982). Hepatitis B virus DNA molecules in the liver of HBsAg carriers: mechanistic considerations in the pathogenesis of hepatocellular carcinoma. *Hepatology*, **2**, 35S–41S
29a. Carman, W., Jaiyna, M., Hadziyannis, S., McGarvey, M., Mabris, A. and Thomas, H. C. (1989). Mutation preventing formation of hepatitis B e antigen in patients with chronic hepatitis B infection. *Lancet*, **2**, 588–590
30. Scullard, G. H., Smith, C. I., Merigan, T. C., Robinson, W. S. and Gregory, P.B (1981). Effects of immunosuppressive therapy on viral markers in chronic active hepatitis B. *Gastroenterology*, **81**, 987–91
31. Weller, I. V. D., Bassendine, M. F., Murray, A. K. Craxi, A., Thomas, H. C. and Sherlock, S. (1982a). Successful treatment of HBs and HBeAg positive chronic liver disease: prolonged inhibition of viral replication by highly soluble adenine arabinoside 5′-monophosphate (ARA-MP). *Gut*, **23**, 717–23
32. Weller, I. V. D., Bassendine, M. F., Murray, A. K., Craxi, A., Thomas, H. C. and Sherlock, S. (1982b). The effects of prednisolone/azathioprine in chronic hepatitis B viral infection. *Gut*, **23**, 650–5
33. Bassendine, M. F., Chadwick, R. E., Salmeron, J., Shipton, V., Thomas, H. C. and Sherlock, S. (1981). Adenine arabinoside therapy for HBS Ag-positive chronic liver disease: a controlled study. *Gastroenterology*, **80**, 1016–22
34. Hoofnagle, J. H., Hansor, R. G., Minuk, G. Y., Pappas, C., Schafer, D. F., Dusheiko, G. M., Straus, S. E., Popper, H. and Jones, E. A. (1984). Randomised controlled trial of adenine arabinoside monophosphate for chronic type B hepatitis. *Gastroenterology*, **86**, 150–7
35. Weller, I. V. D., Lok, A. S. F., Minel, A., Karayiannis, P., Galpin, S., Menjardino, J., Sherlock, S. and Thomas, H. C. (1985). A randomised controlled trial of adenine arabinoside 5′-monophosphate (ARA-AMP) in chronic hepatitis B virus infection. *Gut*, **26**, 745–51
36. Trepo, C., Hantz, O., Ouzan, D., Chossegros, P., Chevallier, P., Berthillou, P. and Brette, R. (1984). Therapeutic efficacy of ARA-MP in symptomatic HBe Ag positive CAH: a randomised, placebo control study. *Hepatology*, **4**, 1055 (abstract 193)
37. Thomas, H. C. and Scully, L. J. (1986). Antiviral therapy in chronic hepatitis B virus infection. *Br. Med. Bull.*, **41**, 374–80
38. Weller, I. V. D., Carreno, V., Fowler, M.J.F., Menjardino, J., Makinen, D., Vurghese, Z., Dweny, P., Thomas, H. C. and Sherlock, S. (1983). Acyclovir in hepatitis B antigen-positive

chronic liver disease: inhibition of viral replication and transient renal impairment with i.v. bolus administration. *J. Antimicrob. Chemother.*, **11**, 223–31

39. Greenberg, H. B., Pollard, R. B., Lutwick, L. I., Gregory, P. B., Robinson, W. S. and Merigan, T. C. (1976). Effect of human leukocyte interferon on hepatitis B virus infection in patients with chronic active hepatitis. *N. Engl. J. Med.*, **295**, 517–22
40. Schalm, S. W. and Heijtink, R. A. (1982). Spontaneous disappearance viral replication and liver cell inflammation in HBs-Ag positive chronic active hepatitis: results of placebo vs. interferon trial. *Hepatology*, **2**, 791–4
41. Smith, C. I., Weissberg, J., Bernhardt, L., Gregory, P. B., Robinson, W. S. and Merigan, T. C. (1983). Acute Dane particle suppression with leukocyte recombinant interferon in chronic HBV infection. *J. Infect. Dis.*, **148**, 907–13
42. McDonald, J. A., Caruso, L., Karayiannis, P., Scully, L. J., Harris, J. R. W., Forster, G. and Thomas, H. C. (1987). Diminished responsiveness of male homosexual chronic HBV carriers with HIV antibodies to recombinant alpha interferon. *Hepatology*, **7**, 719–23
43. Brook, M. G., Petrovic, L., McDonald, J. A., Scheuer, P. J. and Thomas, H. C. (1989). Evidence of histological improvement following anti-viral treatment in chronic hepatitis B virus carriers and identification of histological features that predict response. *J. Hepatol.*, **8**, 218–25
44. Barbara, L., Mazzella, G. and Baraldini, M. (1986). A randomized controlled trial with human lymphoblastoid inferon vs. no therapy in chronic HBV infection. *J. Hepatol.*, **3** (Suppl. 2), S235–S238
45. Alexander, G. M., Brahm, J., Fagan, E. A., Eddlisten, A. and Williams, R. (1987). Loss of HBsAg with interferon therapy in chronic HBV infection. *Lancet*, **ii**, 66–9
46. Brook, M. G., Scully, L., Lever, A. and Thomas, H. C. (1989). A randomised controlled trial of lymphoblastoid interferon alpha in the therapy of Europid men with chronic HBV infection. *Br. Med. J.*, **299**, 652–6
47. Lok, A. S. F., Novick, D. M., Karayiannis, P., Dunk, A. A. and Sherlock, S. (1985). A randomised study of the effect of adenine arabinoside monophosphate (4 or 8 week courses) versus lymphoblastoid interferon on hepatitis B virus (HBV) replication. *Hepatology*, **5**, 1132–8
48. Scully, L. J., Shein, R., Karayiannis, P., McDonald, J. A. and Thomas, H. C. (1987). Lymphoblastoid interferon therapy of chronic HBV infection. A comparison of 12 v 24 weeks of thrice weekly treatment. *J. Hepatol.*, **5**, 51–8
49. Hoofnagle, J. H., Mullen, K. D., Jones, B., Rustki, V, Di-Bisceglie, A., Peters, M., Waggener, J. G., Yoon Park, R. N. and Jones, E. A. (1986). Treatment of chronic non-A, non-B hepatitis with recombinant human alpha interferon. *N. Engl. J. Med.*, **315**, 1575–8
50. Perrillo, R. P., Regerstein, F. G., Bodicky, C. J., Campbell, C., Sanders, G. E. and Sunwoo, Y. C. (1985). Comparative efficacy of ARA-MP in prednisolone withdrawal followed by ARA-MP in treatment of HBV induced CAH. *Gastroenterology*, 780–6
51. Yokosuka, O., Ometa, M., Imazeki, F., Hirota, K., Mori, J., Uchiumi, K., Ito, Y and Okuda, K. (1985). Combination of short term prednisolone and adenine arabinoside in the treatment of chronic hepatitis B: a controlled study. *Gastroenterology*, **89**, 246–51
52. Schalm, S. W., Heijtink, R. A., Van Buuren, H. R. and de Man, R. A. (1985). Acyclovir enhances the antiviral effect of interferon in chronic hepatitis B. *Lancet*, **ii**, 358–60
53. Pignatelli, M., Waters, J., Brown, D., Lever, A. M. L., Iwarson, S., Schaff, Z., Gerety, R. and Thomas, H. C. (1986). HLA Class I antigens on hepatocyte membrane: increased expression during interferon therapy of chronic hepatitis B. *Hepatology*, **6**, 349–53
54. Chen, G., Karayianis, P., McGarvey, M. J., Lever, A. M. C., McDonald, J. A., Scully, L. J., Kanatakis, S. and Thomas, H. C. (1989). Subclasses of anti-HBe in chronic HBV carriers: changes during treatment with interferon and predictors of response. *Gut*, **30**, 1123–8
55. Davis, G. L. and Hoofnagle, J. H. (1985). Reactivation of chronic type B presenting as acute hepatitis. *Ann. Intern. Med.*, **102**, 762–5
56. Scully, L. J., Lever, A. M. L., Yap, I., Pignatelli, M. and Thomas, H. C. (1986). Identification of factors influencing response rate to antiviral therapy of chronic HBV infection. *J. Hepatol.*, **3** (Suppl. 2), S291–S299

Section I: Basic Mechanisms in Liver Infections

3
Liver reaction patterns in infections

V. J. DESMET

INTRODUCTION

This review is written from the point of view of the histopathologist, whose task it is to distill specific, if possible aetiologic, diagnoses out of the morphological tissue reaction patterns observed in liver biopsies, but also with some interest in pathogenetic mechanisms.

Like most organs, the liver disposes of only a limited number of reaction patterns in infections. The reaction patterns are determined by the intrinsic properties of the constituent cell populations of the organ; they are modulated by numerous extrahepatic and systemic factors which influence the course of defence reactions (amongst others, the immunological, haematological and endocrine state of the patient), and are further dependent to a variable extent on the nature of the offending agent. Although not entirely agent-specific, these various patterns often allow the pathologist to suspect or to recognize a particular aetiology on liver biopsy.

In spite of some overlap, liver reaction patterns in infections can be schematically categorized under a few general headings.

MAIN REACTION PATTERNS OF THE LIVER IN INFECTIONS

Immunological pattern

The immunological reaction pattern is observed in several conditions, in which cell-mediated and humoral immune mechanisms appear to play a predominant role. The prototype examples of this category are acute and chronic hepatitis due to hepatotropic viruses (A, B, non-A, non-B and D). However, a similar or analogous reaction pattern also occurs in non-infectious immune-mediated liver diseases, as exemplified by autoimmune hepatitis and some forms of drug-induced hepatitis. This overlap explains the difficulty in differentiating between viral, drug-induced and autoimmune hepatitis on purely histopathological grounds.

The immunological reaction pattern is morphologically characterized by involvement of immunologically competent cells: various subsets of lymphocytes and accessory cells, and damage to epithelial cells (hepatocytes and bile duct cells).

The basic necro-inflammatory lesions of the immunological reaction pattern comprise focal or spotty necrosis, piecemeal necrosis, confluent lytic necrosis, and occasionally bile duct lesions.

Focal necrosis

The histopathological picture of focal or spotty necrosis is a simple one: a local accumulation of a few mononuclear cells, including lymphocytes, around one or a few liver parenchymal cells which appear necrotic or are missing altogether[1] (Figure 1). In contrast to the simple histology, the immunopathological mechanisms underlying these focal reaction patterns are quite complicated, and still incompletely resolved.

The accumulating lymphocytes are mainly of the CD8 phenotype (presumably suppressor/cytotoxic lymphocytes[2], admixed with non-lymphoid mononuclear cells which probably function as accessory or antigen-presenting cells[3]. The antigen to which the lymphocytes are sensitized depends on the nature of the disease: self-antigen in autoimmune hepatitis; drug or drug–metabolite induced neo-antigen in drug-induced hepatitis, or viral antigens in case of viral hepatitis. In chronic viral hepatitis type B the target antigen appears to correspond to components of the viral nucleocapsid (HBcAg and HBeAg)[4–7].

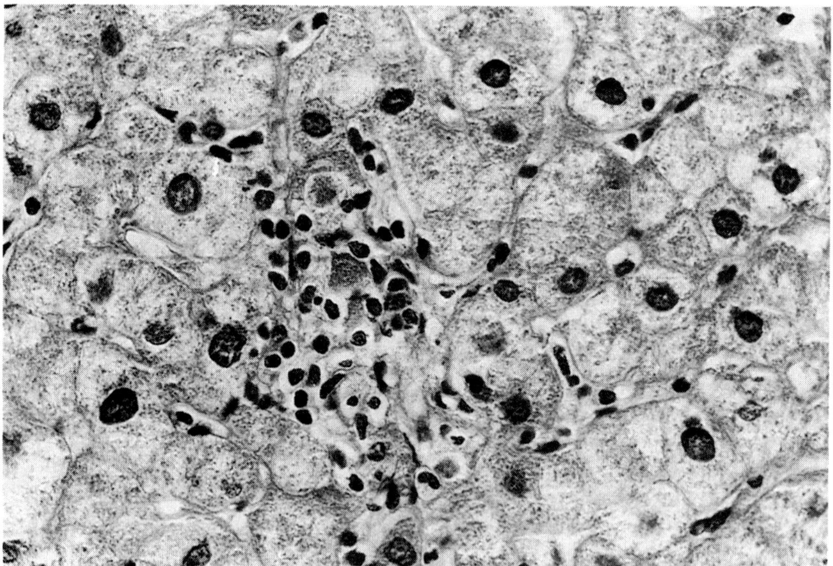

Figure 1 Focal (or spotty) necrosis in chronic viral hepatitis B. A focal accumulation of lymphocytes and mononuclear cells is seen in an area with partial interruption of liver cell plates. An acidophil body (apoptotic body) lies in the middle of the infiltrate (Haematoxylin and eosin, ×540)

The focal accumulation of mononuclear cells indicates that they have extravasated from the vascular compartment, and are retained in that particular tissue area.

Recently, more information was obtained on the mechanisms involved in extravasation and local retention of migrating lymphocytes. In normal conditions the circulating population of lymphocytes extravasates under control of appropriate signals at 'routine' exits from the blood stream, represented by the high endothelial venules of secondary lymphoid tissues (lymph nodes, Peyer's patches, etc.)[8]. In case of damage or invasion of offending agents in a tissue, lymphocytes have to extravasate at 'emergency' exits to fulfil their role *loco dolenti.*

Lymphocytes 'stick' to vascular endothelium and – after extravasation – to target cells because of the expression on their surface of special signal molecules which interact with specific ligands expressed on endothelial cells and target cells.

Activated lymphocytes acquire their adhesive properties by the expression of molecules which are members of the 'integrin family' of adhesion receptors[9]. Important members of this group are lymphoid cell surface molecules known as 'accessory' molecules, which are fundamental in antigen-independent intercellular adhesion, and facilitate immune interactions by strengthening cell–cell conjugate formation. Such accessory molecules include leucocyte function associated antigen 1 (LFA-1), the sheep erythrocyte receptor on T cells (CD2), and CD4 and CD8 markers[10–14]. The ligands for the integrin molecules constitute a large number of structurally distinct molecules with a broad tissue distribution. The ligand for LFA-1 is the intercellular adhesion molecule 1 (ICAM-1), whereas the specific ligand for CD2 is leucocyte function associated antigen 3 (LFA-3)[13].

Cytokines, including interleukin-1, tumor necrosis factor α, and interferon γ, are capable of upgrading or inducing *de novo* the expression of adhesion molecules on vascular endothelial cells and some epithelial cells, in coordination with upgraded or *de novo* expression of MHC class I and class II molecules[14].

In areas of focal necrosis in the liver, parenchymal cells have been shown to express MHC class I and class II antigens[2], in association with *de novo* expression of thrombospondin receptor, ICAM-1 and LFA-3. The lymphocytes 'sticking' in the foci of spotty necrosis express CD8, LFA-1 and CD2[15].

ICAM-1 and other adhesion molecules expressed on sinusoidal lining cells and hepatocytes thus also seem to play a major role in the 'emergency' exit of lymphocytes from the blood into the liver at sites of tissue injury, since the ICAM-1 response is dormant in normal liver, and only induced as part of the tissue response to pathogens and other forms of tissue damage[15], comparable to what happens, for instance, in inflammatory skin reactions[16].

What is recognized by the pathologist as a focal necrosis (a focal inflammatory response) in the liver, is based on active participation of liver parenchymal cells by their cytokine-induced expression of ICAM-1 and other adhesion molecules, which play a central role in recruitment, activation and regulation of lymphoid cells[14].

The mode of cell death of the hepatocytes involved in 'spotty necrosis' is apoptosis[17], which is the mode of cell death of target cells under immunological attack by cytotoxic T lymphocytes, killer and natural killer cells[18].

Under the light microscope, apoptotic parenchymal cells are not very conspicuous; they consist of portions of intensely eosinophilic-staining cytoplasm, sometimes containing small, densely basophilic (pyknotic) nuclear fragments[17]. Since apoptotic bodies are rapidly phagocytosed by neighbouring macrophages and parenchymal cells, many foci of 'spotty necrosis' can be observed, which are only composed of a cluster of mononuclear and lymphoid cells without remaining visible remnants of apoptotic parenchymal cells.

Piecemeal necrosis

Piecemeal necrosis is a feature of several, mainly chronic and immunologically mediated liver diseases, including chronic active hepatitis (whether of viral, autoimmune or drug-induced origin), primary biliary cirrhosis and primary sclerosing cholangitis[19–22]. Morphologically, piecemeal necrosis represents an interphase hepatitis, that is: mononuclear leucocyte infiltration associated with liver cell necrosis at the interphase between connective tissue stroma (portal tracts and fibrous septa) and parenchyma. The slow destruction of hepatocytes leads to irregular erosion of the limiting plate and an imprecise delineation of the portal perimeter (Figure 2); the lesion thus resembles a lichenoid tissue reaction in the skin[23]. The most important cell types participating in periportal piecemeal necrosis are antigen-presenting reticulum cells[24] and T lymphocytes[19]. CD4 helper/inducer lymphocytes predominate in the central part of the portal area, whereas CD8 suppressor/cytotoxic lymphocytes are located mainly in the peripheral connective tissue–parenchymal interphase[19]. The mechanism of cell death in piecemeal necrosis is apoptosis[25].

Authentic piecemeal necrosis must be differentiated from other types of periportal hepatocellular necrosis[22].

The pathogenesis of piecemeal necrosis is not well understood. Most of the available evidence suggests an antibody-dependent cellular cytotoxicity reaction. The target antigen may be autoantigens of the LSP (liver specific protein) or LMAg (liver membrane antigen complex[26,27]). On the other hand, immunohistochemical studies revealed strong expression of HLA class I molecules on hepatocytes, and HLA class I and class II molecules on sinusoidal lining cells in periportal areas of piecemeal necrosis[28]. Furthermore, as in focal necrosis, endothelial cells show upregulated, and hepatocytes display *de novo*, expression of ICAM-1 and LFA-3, whereas the infiltrating lymphocytes express the corresponding adhesion receptors LFA-1 and CD2[15]. The phenotype of (presumably professional antigen-presenting) dendritic cells corresponds to that of dendritic reticulum cells in the central part of the portal tract, and to that of interdigitating reticulum cells in the peripheral areas of piecemeal necrosis[3].

Although these data are helpful in elucidating some mechanisms of

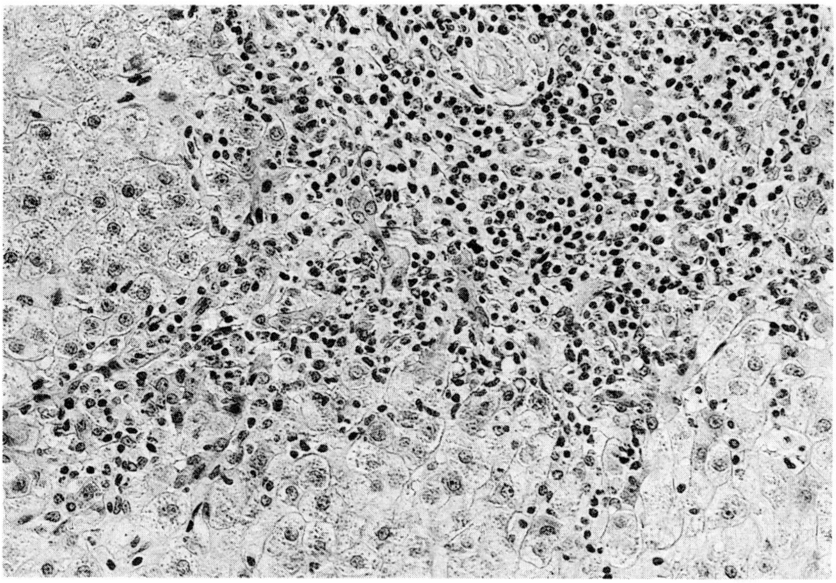

Figure 2 Periportal piecemeal necrosis in chronic active hepatitis. The portal tract (upper right half) is densely infiltrated by mononuclear cells which extend beyond the portal–parenchymal interface; the periportal infiltration is associated with focal loss of parenchymal cells, creating an irregular and imprecise borderline between portal tract and parenchyma (Haematoxylin and eosin, × 270)

lymphocyte retention and local inflammation, they fail to reveal the basic immunological mechanism.

The antigen involved in lymphocyte stimulation remains uncertain, and the CD4 or CD8 phenotype of T lymphocytes is no guaranteed indicator of their helper/inducer or suppressor/cytotoxic function respectively[23,29]. As for inflammatory skin diseases, it remains to be seen whether piecemeal necrosis represents predominantly a cytotoxic, a tolerogenic or a pro-inflammatory tissue response[16], depending on the predominant type of antigen-presenting cells (professional or epithelial), the role of cytokines involved (interferon γ, tumor necrosis factor) and the surface molecules expressed (ratios of ICAM-1 versus HLA-DR or MHC class II antigen expression)[16].

Confluent lytic necrosis

A more severe component of necro-inflammatory change in immunological liver reaction patterns is confluent lytic necrosis[30].

Ballooning or hydropic swelling of hepatocytes is thought to be a precursor stage of lytic necrosis of these cells. The mechanism of this type of cell damage and death is not established, but there is reason to assume that the primary damage is at the level of the cell membrane[31].

Lytic necrosis of hepatocytes is a rapid event: the cells disappear in a very short time. It follows that lytic necrosis is recognized histologically as absence of cells, often described as 'drop-out of liver cells', and resulting in denudation of the reticulin framework. Lytic necrosis usually affects groups of hepatocytes, leading to the disappearance of confluent areas of parenchyma; hence the term 'confluent lytic necrosis'.

Confluent lytic necrosis may affect smaller or larger parenchymal territories. These do not display a random topography, but tend to occur in well-defined territories which correspond to the microcirculatory periphery of simple or complex parenchymal units. The anatomical distribution of confluent necrosis is best explained on the basis of the acinar concept of liver architecture, resulting in various patterns of so-called 'bridging hepatic necrosis'[7,30,32,33] (Figure 3).

The pathogenetic mechanisms of confluent lytic necrosis remain unknown. The predilection of the lesion to occur in peripheral areas of the microcirculation, its topographic relationship to the angio-architecture of the liver, and the relative scarcity of lymphocytes in the denuded areas are features which suggest that in this mode of necrosis other mechanisms are involved than those operating in focal necrosis and piecemeal necrosis. The most plausible mechanism is a humoral one[7,33,34]. Activation of the complement system by circulating endotoxins due to Kupffer cell failure[35] or a Schwarzman-like reaction to the liver[36] have been suggested as possible mechanisms.

An experimental rat model has been proposed in which acute, massive

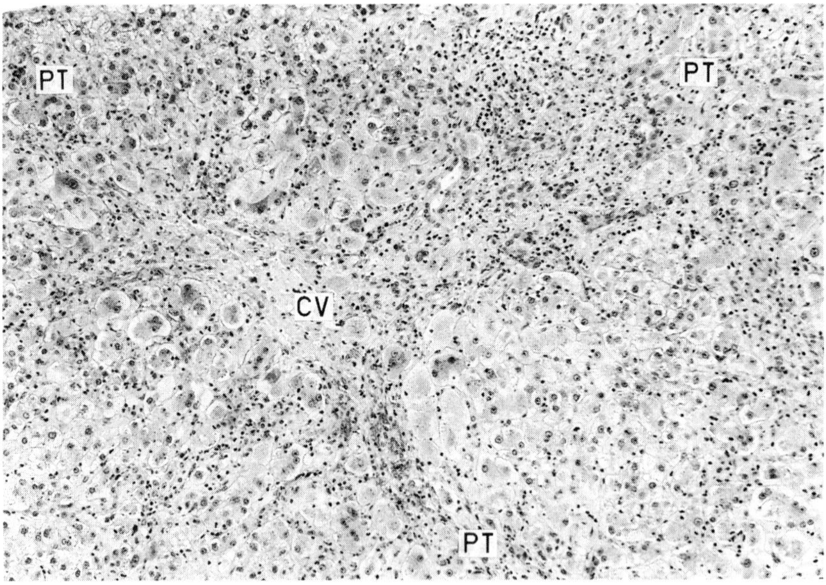

Figure 3 Chronic hepatitis with bridging hepatic necrosis. A terminal hepatic venule (central vein (CV) is surrounded by a star-shaped area which extends into surrounding portal tracts (PT). The star-shaped area is characterized by disappearance of parenchymal cells (confluent lytic necrosis) and beginning collapse of the reticulin framework. Example of portal–central bridging hepatic necrosis (haematoxylin and eosin, × 100)

hepatic necrosis was produced by intravenous injection of a monoclonal antibody to a liver cell membrane antigen[37,38].

Massive hepatic necrosis developed extremely fast, within 1 h, without associated cellular reaction or lymphocyte infiltration. Induction of liver cell lysis was also achieved *in vitro* with purified antibody and complement, without addition of lymphocytes[38]. Complement components have been shown to cause a lytic type of cell necrosis, since they behave like a membrane-piercing protein[39,40]. Piercing of the cell membrane causes rapid deregulation of ionic pumps, rapid influx of calcium ions and immediate cell lysis[41].

At present the clinical relevance of this antibody–complement model remains unclear, but it is of interest in this respect that in fulminant viral hepatitis B the antibody response is greatly enhanced as shown by the early appearance of anti-HBsAg and anti-HBeAg, and accelerated plasma clearance of HBsAg[42,43].

In another experimental model[44] a monoclonal antibody directed against a 43 kDa organ-specific liver membrane antigen in rabbits produced considerable hepatocellular damage *in vivo* and *in vitro.* In this study the role of complement activation and complement-mediated lysis of the hepatocytes was neither proven nor ruled out.

Further, in hepatitis B, increased antibody production has been linked to increased amounts of circulating immune complexes which may induce an Arthus reaction in the sinusoids[45,46].

The experimental antibody–(complement) models[37,38,44] urge reassessment of the role of antigen–antibody reactions in causing hepatocyte lysis in case of confluent lytic necrosis in severe human acute and chronic hepatitis.

Bile duct lesion

In acute and chronic viral hepatitis a minority of cases reveal bile duct lesions which usually affect smaller portal ducts[47]. The hepatitis is usually, but not invariably, due to non-A, non-B hepatitis virus[48].

The damage may involve the whole or only part of the circumference of the affected duct. These segmental changes comprise swelling and vacuolation together with stratification of the bile duct lining cells, with mononuclear leucocytes infiltrating between the bile duct epithelium. The affected duct segments are seen within dense lymphoid infiltrates in the portal tract (Figure 4). The basement membrane is not ruptured, and no evidence of duct destruction has been obtained. On occasion this hepatitic bile duct lesion may resemble the changes observed in primary biliary cirrhosis[49].

Increased expression of MHC class I molecules and *de novo* display of MHC class II antigens has been demonstrated on the bile ducts with 'hepatitic' bile duct changes[50], but the pathogenesis of the lesion remains unknown[51].

Exudative pattern

The exudative pattern refers to the classical acute inflammatory reaction, characterized by vasodilatation, increased vascular permeability with for-

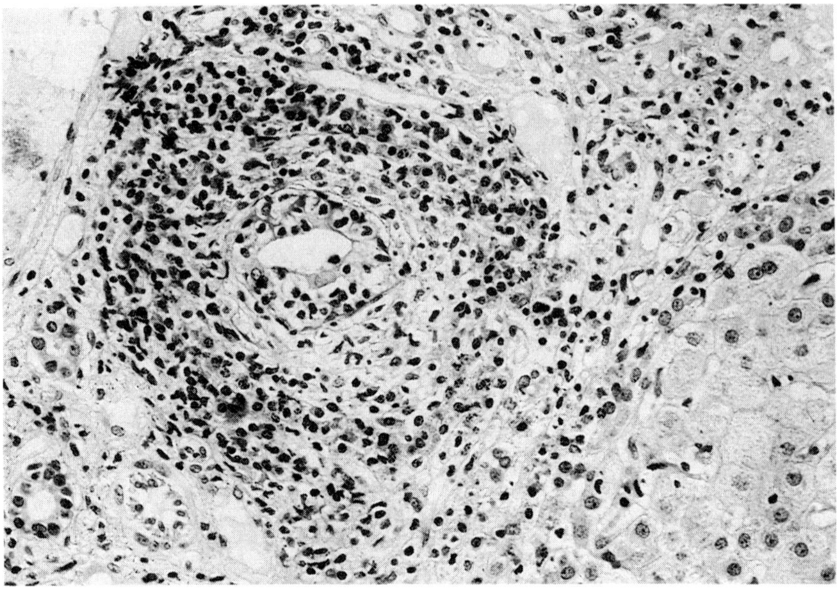

Figure 4 Hepatitic bile duct lesion in chronic active hepatitis. The picture shows a portal tract with dense lymphoplasmocytic infiltrate. The centre is occupied by an interlobular bile duct which shows stratification and vacuolization of its lining cells, permeated by some lymphocytes and mononuclear cells (Haematoxylin and eosin, × 270)

mation of fluid exudate (oedema), and emigration of neutrophil polymorphonuclear leucocytes from the bloodstream into the interstitium[52].

This type of liver tissue reaction pattern is mainly observed in bacterial infections of the bile ducts (cholangitis), of the portal vein (pylephlebitis) and of the systemic circulation (septicaemia). A vigorous bile ductular reaction accompanies the inflammatory changes in most cases. Focal intralobular granulocytic exudates are found in some specific conditions mentioned below.

Cholangitis

Acute suppurative cholangitis is usually due to bacterial infection complicating an obstructive biliary lesion, in most cases extrahepatic[53] but it may also be of haematogenic origin[49,54]. The portal tracts appear oedematous, and are infiltrated with neutrophil polymorphs. The latter inflammatory cells are also found in the lumen and between the lining epithelial cells of portal bile ducts (Figure 5). Ruptured and completely destroyed bile ducts may be seen in severe cases, and result in the formation of cholangitic abscesses.

The portal inflammatory reaction may extend beyond the limits of the portal tract, destroy the limiting plate and cause periportal parenchymal necrosis of variable extent.

The suppurative cholangitis in so-called 'toxic shock syndrome', associated with tampon use by menstruating women, appears to be a haematogenic toxaemic complication of a local staphylococcal infection[55,56]. Oriental

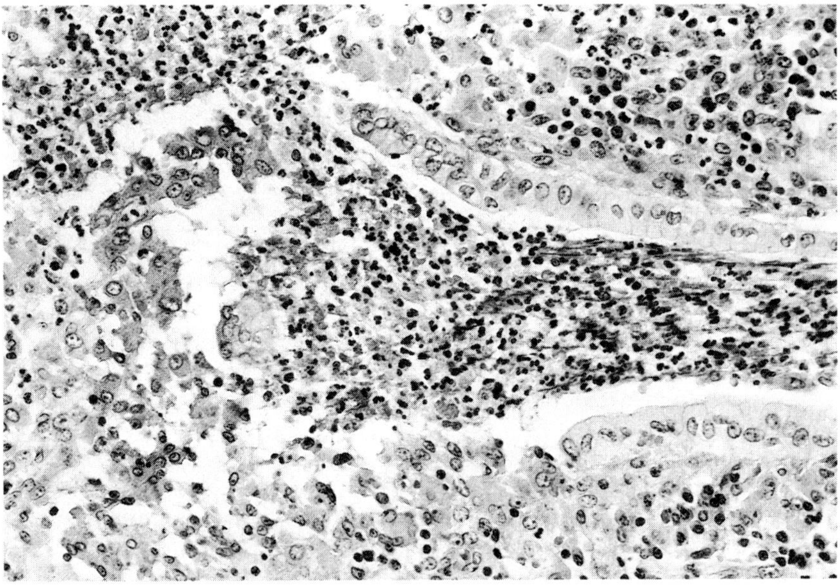

Figure 5 Purulent or suppurative cholangitis. The picture shows a larger interlobular bile duct, filled with neutrophil polymorphs and pyocytes. The epithelium lining the duct is ruptured (left side of picture); the surrounding portal connective tissue is infiltrated by various inflammatory cells, including neutrophils, macrophages, lymphocytes and plasmocytes (Haematoxylin and eosin, × 270)

recurrent pyogenic cholangitis remains ill-defined in its aetiology and pathogenesis[57].

Pylephlebitis

The incidence of pylephlebitis has been greatly reduced since the introduction of antibiotic therapy. Suppurative pylephlebitis is usually associated with thrombosis of the portal vein or its tributaries, and is related to purulent hepatitis and hepatic abscesses[58].

The source of infection is an organ drained by the portal system (appendix, colon, pancreas) which results in portal pyaemia, septic portal thrombophlebitis and multiple abscesses.

Intrahepatic portal vein branches show partial or complete thrombosis, with infiltration of the thrombus, the vessel wall and the surrounding portal tracts by neutrophil polymorphs. Suppuration may lead to formation of multiple abscesses.

Septicaemia

Septicaemia may cause cholestasis and sinusoidal congestion in acinar zone 3.

A peculiar cholangiolitis develops in some cases. Whereas the portal bile ducts show little or no change, a marked increase in ductular profiles is observed at the interphase between portal tracts and parenchyma. The ductules show a variably dilated lumen, filled with inspissated, bile-stained concrements; the ductular lining cells are flattened and may display degenerative changes or necrosis. Neutrophil polymorphs infiltrate in and around the proliferated ductules (Figure 6). The lesion has been related to the 'cholangitis lenta' from the older literature. It represents an ominous feature with dismal prognosis[59,60].

Bile inspissation in the ductules is thought to be due to paralysis of the normal bicarbonate-rich fluid secretion and flushing function of the ductular cells by circulating endotoxin and bacterial products.

Intralobular granulocytic necroses

Focal accumulations of neutrophil polymorphs in circumscribed areas of the liver parenchyma are observed in several infectious and non-infectious conditions[31].

In cytomegalovirus hepatitis some infected cells are surrounded by clusters of polymorphs, apparently associated with lysis of the affected hepatocyte[61] (Figure 7). Neutrophil polymorphs accumulate around degenerating hepatocytes in foci of so-called surgical necrosis, caused by manipulation of the liver during surgical intervention[62] (Figure 8).

In alcoholic hepatitis, Mallory-body containing hepatocytes may be surrounded by more or less numerous neutrophil polymorphs, a feature known as 'satellitosis'[1].

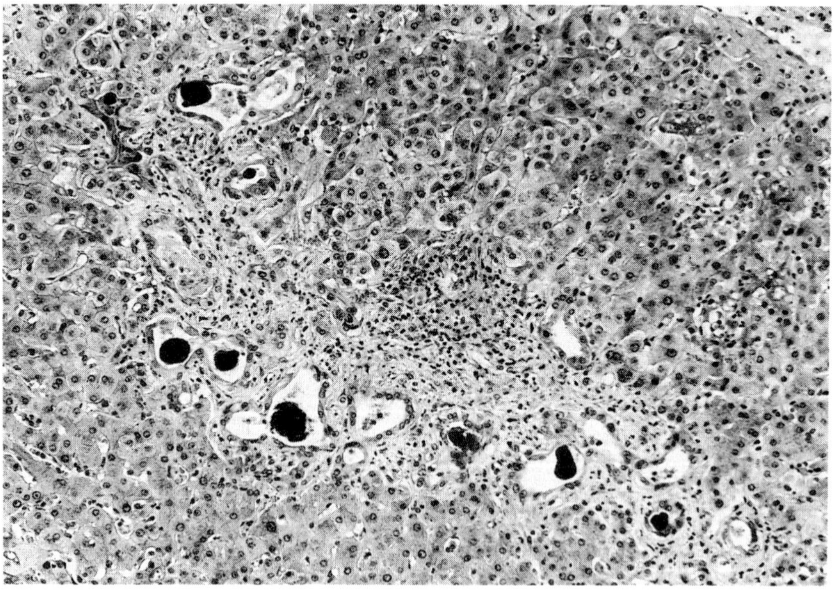

Figure 6 Liver biopsy from patient with candida sepsis. A portal tract is bordered by a series of greatly dilated ductules containing inspissated bile concrements and surrounded by oedematous stroma sprinkled with inflammatory cells (Haematoxylin and eosin, × 100)

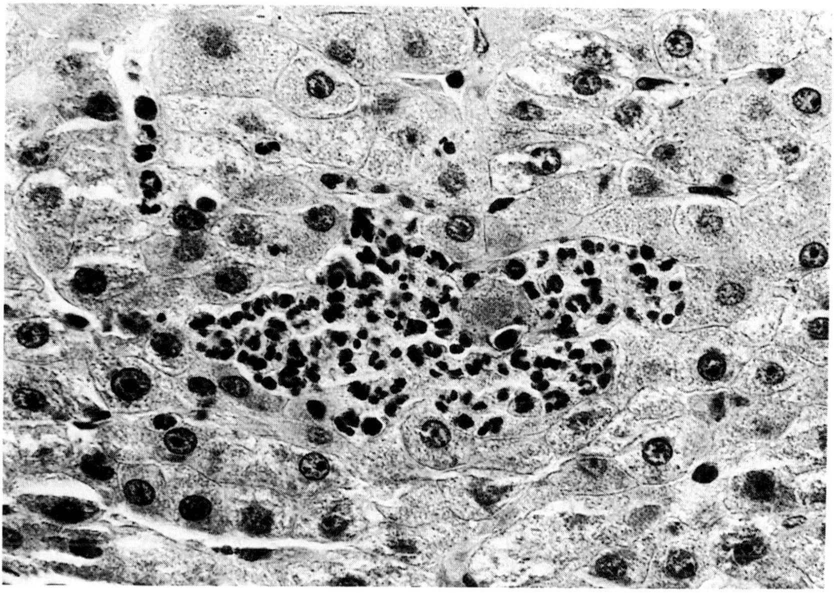

Figure 7 Cytomegalovirus hepatitis. A cluster of polymorphonuclear leucocytes surrounds an infected hepatocyte. The latter is characterized by cytoplasmic basophilia, and the presence in its nucleus of a cytomegalo-inclusion surrounded by a clear halo (Haematoxylin and eosin, × 540)

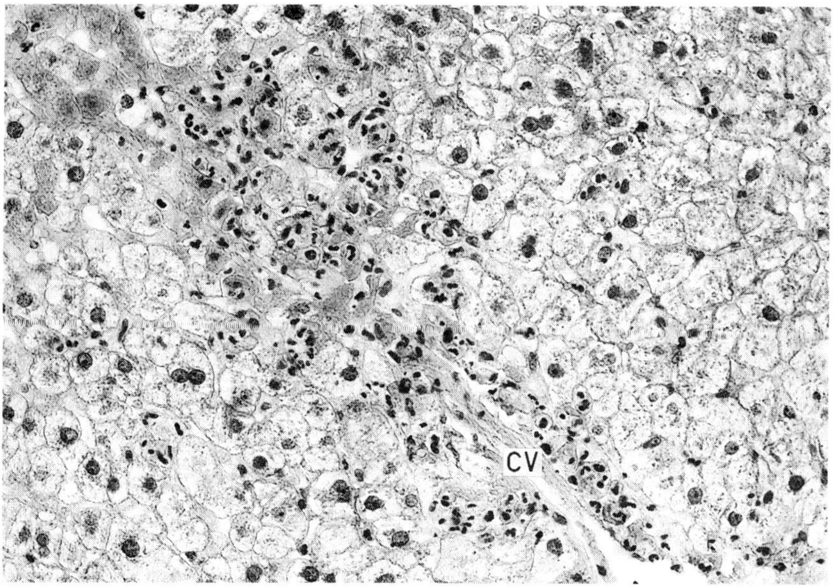

Figure 8 'Surgical necrosis' in surgical wedge biopsy from the liver. Several hepatocytes near a terminal hepatic venule (central vein) (CV) show acidophil condensation or necrosis and infiltration by neutrophil polymorphonuclear leucocytes (Haematoxylin and eosin, × 270)

In neonatal giant cell hepatitis, multinucleated parenchymal giant cells with degenerative features may be surrounded and infiltrated by neutrophil polymorphs[54].

Granulomatous pattern

Granulomas can be defined as localized, chronic inflammatory reactions to persistent irritants[63]. They can be divided into immunological, cell-mediated and non-immunological, foreign-body types[64]; in this classification, hypersensitivity-type granulomas[65], such as those that occur in tuberculosis and sarcoidosis, are of the immunological type[64].

Typical granulomas contain epithelioid cells, which are a particular subset of histiocytes belonging to the mononuclear phagocyte system. They are induced by substances that are poorly soluble and difficult to eliminate, and also by cell-mediated immunological mechanisms. Their function is unclear; they show no evidence of ongoing phagocytic activity, but appear to have important secretory functions[66]. Their origin, either from freshly recruited monocytes or from transformed stationary cells, is still under debate[66].

Multinucleated giant cells are often found between the epithelioid components. These giant cells are also of monocyte/macrophage origin[67], and result from fusion of young and mature monocyte-derived cells under the influence of lymphokines secreted by activated T lymphocytes[68].

Fully developed epithelioid granulomas display an architectural organization. The centre is occupied by giant cells and epithelioid cells which express MHC class II molecules, admixed with CD4 and CD8 T lymphocytes. The relative predominance of CD4 and CD8 lymphocytes, as well as their spatial distribution, may vary depending on the aetiology and the evolutionary stage, or both, of the granuloma. A perigranulomatous cuff of B lymphocytes and accessory cells forms the periphery of the lesion[69,70] (Figure 9).

The multinucleated giant cells may function as antigen-processing and -presenting accessory cells, whereas activated T cells, of either the helper or suppressor type, may be operative in delayed-type hypersensitivity reactions. However, the finer rules of the cellular interplay in this ordered set-up of cellular interactions remain to be deciphered[69,70].

In the liver, granulomatous patterns of tissue reaction occur in numerous infectious and non-infectious diseases. The size, the cellular composition, the epithelioid differentiation and other characteristics of the granulomas vary in different disorders, so that some orientation towards a specific aetiology may be obtained. In many cases, however, the confirmation of the aetiologic agent depends on further clinical and laboratory investigations.

Excellent descriptions and exhaustive tabulations of granulomatous reaction patterns in the liver can be found in several reviews and textbooks[53,54,57,71–74].

Special patterns

Some reaction patterns of the liver in particular infections can hardly be included in the aforementioned categories. Some are quite typical for the

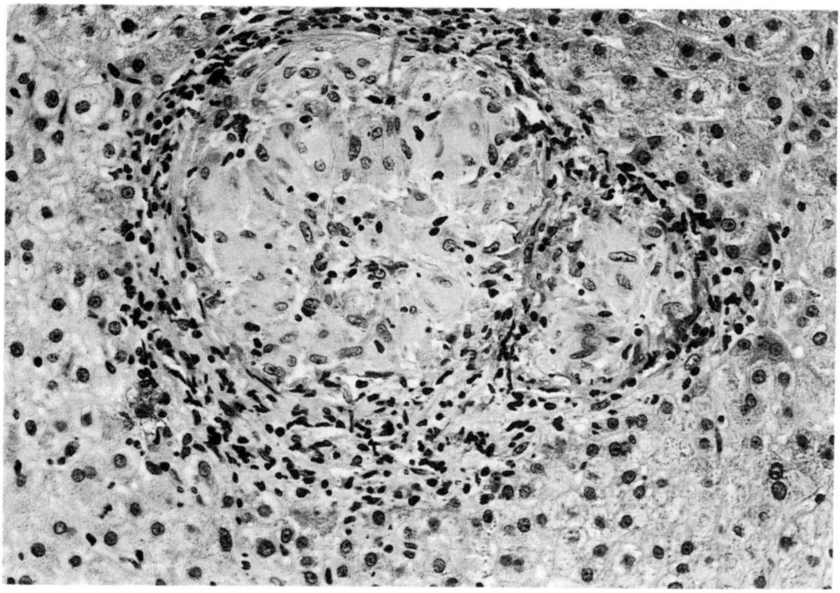

Figure 9 Liver biopsy from patient with sarcoidosis. The picture shows a granuloma composed of epithelioid cells and surrounded by a rim of lymphocytes (Haematoxylin and eosin, × 270)

offending agent and helpful in establishing an aetiological diagnosis.

Storage of infectious agents in reticuloendothelial cells, identifiable with special stains, allows recognition of the aetiological agent in liver tissue sections. This is the case for bacteria (e.g. the PAS-D positive bacteria of Whipple's disease), mycobacteria (e.g. *Mycobacterium avium intracellulare*, demonstrable with the Ziehl–Nielsen stain), fungi (e.g. *Histoplasma capsulatum*), and protozoal organisms (e.g. *Toxoplasma gondii, Leishmania donovani*, using the Giemsa stain)[72].

Malaria and schistosomiasis can be suspected on the finding of black, finely granular, iron-negative and birefringent pigment granules in Kupffer cells and macrophages[72]. Leptospirosis (Weil's disease) causes a marked dissociation of liver parenchymal cells. This change, which may not entirely be due to tissue autolysis, suggests that rupture of intercellular junctions may be a primary and basic lesion. It is associated with cholestasis and high numbers of liver cell mitoses[75] (Figure 10).

Non-specific reactive hepatitis

The term non-specific reactive hepatitis was first proposed by Popper and Schaffner[58], when they described a morphological entity which represents a hepatic response to a variety of extrahepatic diseases, especially febrile illnesses and inflammation elsewhere in the splanchnic bed.

The changes tend to be focal, with not all portal tracts involved and parenchymal changes of non-uniform distribution.

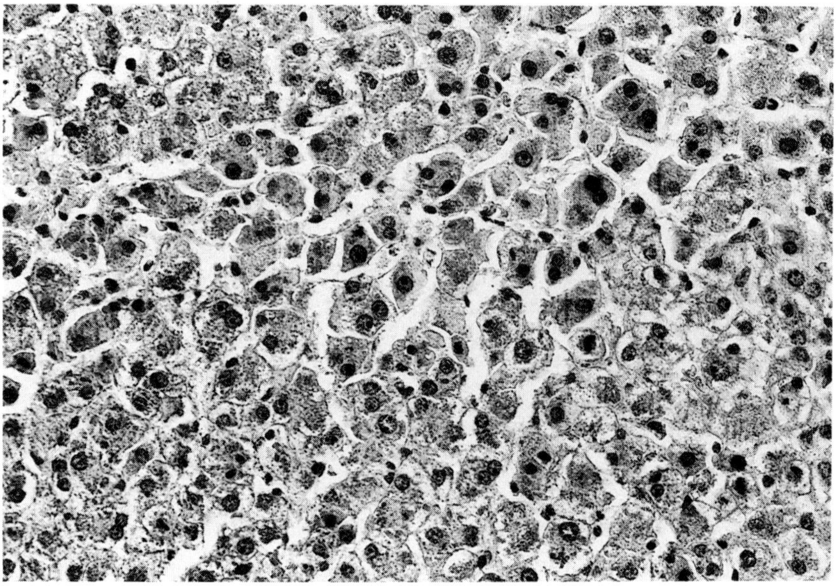

Figure 10 Liver specimen from patient with leptospirosis. The centrolobular parenchyma is characterized by cholestasis, liver cell mitoses, and dissociation of parenchymal cells (Haematoxylin and eosin, × 270)

The portal changes affect medium-sized and smaller portal tracts, and consist of mild mononuclear cell infiltration, mainly lymphocytes and occasional macrophages. The parenchymal changes comprise foci of 'focal' or 'spotty' necrosis, Kupffer cell prominence and lipofuscinosis of hepatocytes.

Non-specific reactive hepatitis may be difficult to differentiate from residua of healing acute hepatitis and from chronic, persistent hepatitis[57,58,76].

Fibrosis

Fibrosis is an unavoidable sequel of most inflammatory reaction patterns of longer duration. It may occur in various patterns, dependent on the nature and extent of the initial lesion and the duration of the reactive process. It follows that fibrosis is an integral component of the morphological changes in the liver in most forms of chronic infection of the liver by various aetiological agents.

REFERENCES

1. Bianchi, L. (1983). Liver biopsy interpretation in hepatitis. Part I. Presentation of critical morphologic features used in diagnosis (glossary). *Pathol. Res. Pract.*, **178**, 2–19
2. Van den Oord, J. J., De Vos, R. and Desmet, V. J. (1986). In situ distribution of major histocompatibility complex products and viral antigens in chronic hepatitis B virus infection: evidence that HBc-containing hepatocytes may express HLA-DR antigen. *Hepatology*, **6**, 981–9

3. Van den Oord, J. J. and Desmet, V. J. (1989). Non-lymphoid, accessory cells in chronic HBV infection. (In preparation)
4. Alberti, A., Trevisan, A., Fattovich, G. and Realdi, G. (1984). The role of hepatitis B virus replication and hepatocyte membrane expression in the pathogenesis of HBV-related hepatic damage. In Chisari, F. V. (ed.), *Advances in Hepatitis Research*, pp. 134–43 (New York: Masson)
5. Mondelli, M., Naumov, N. and Eddleston, A. L. W. F. (1984). The immunopathogenesis of liver cell damage in chronic hepatitis B virus infection. In Chisari, F. V. (ed.), *Advances in Hepatitis Research*, pp. 144–51 (New York: Masson)
6. Thomas, H. C., Pignatelli, M., Goodall, A., Waters, J., Karayiannis, P. and Brown, D. (1984). Immunologic mechanisms of cell lysis in hepatitis B virus infection. In Vyas, G. N., Dienstag, J. L. and Hoofnagle, J. H. (eds), *Viral Hepatitis and Liver Disease*, pp. 167–77 (Orlando: Grune & Stratton)
7. Desmet, V. J. (1988). Liver lesions in hepatitis B viral infection. *Yale J. Biol. Med.*, **61**, 61–83
8. Berg, E. L., Goldstein, L. A., Jutila, M. A., Nakache, M., Picker, L. J., Streeter, P. R., Wu, N. W., Zhou, D. and Butcher, E. C. (1989). Homing receptors and vascular addressins: cell adhesion molecules that direct lymphocyte traffic. *Immunol. Rev.*, **108**, 5–18
9. Hynes, R. O. (1987). Integrins: a family of cell surface receptors. *Cell*, **48**, 549–54
10. Doyle, C. and Strominger, J. (1987). Interaction between CD4 and class II MHC molecules mediates cell adhesion. *Nature*, **330**, 256–9
11. Martz, E. (1987). LFA-1 and other accessory molecules functioning in adhesion of T and B lymphocytes. *Hum. Immunol.*, **18**, 3–37
12. Norment, A., Salter, R., Parham, P., Engelhard, V. and Littman, D. (1988). Cell–cell adhesion mediated by CD8 and MHC class I molecules. *Nature*, **336**, 79–81
13. Springer, T. A., Dustin, M. L., Kishimoto, T. K. and Marlin, S. D. (1987). The lymphocyte function-associated LFA-1, CD2 and LFA-3 molecules: cell adhesion receptors of the immune system. *Ann. Rev. Immunol.*, **5**, 223–52
14. Wawryk, S. O., Novotny, J. R., Wickx, I. P., Wilkinson, D., Maher, D., Salvaris, E., Welch, K., Fecondo, J. and Boyd, A. W. (1989). The role of the LFA-1/ICAM-1 interaction in human leucocyte homing and adhesion. *Immunol. Rev.*, **108**, 135–61
15. Volpes, R., Van den Oord, J. J. and Desmet, V. J. (1989). Expression of adhesion molecules in liver inflammation. (In preparation).
16. Nickoloff, B. J. (1988). Role of interferon-γ in cutaneous trafficking of lymphocytes with emphasis on molecular and cellular adhesion events. *Arch. Dermatol.*, **124**, 1835–43
17. Searle, J., Harmon, B. V., Bishop, C. J. and Kerr, J. F. R. (1987). The significance of cell death by apoptosis in hepatobiliary disease. *J. Gastroenterol. Hepatol.*, **2**, 77–96
18. Stacey, N. H., Bishop, C. J., Halliday, J. W., Halliday, W. J., Cooksley, W. G., Powell, L. W. and Kerr, J. F. (1985). Apoptosis as the mode of cell death in antibody-dependent lymphocytotoxicity. *J. Cell Sci.*, **74**, 169–79
19. Desmet, V. J. (1985). New aspects of piecemeal necrosis. In Bianchi, L., Gerok, W. and Popper, H. (eds), *Trends in Hepatology*, pp. 183–200. (Lancaster: MTP Press)
20. Popper, H. (1983). Changing concepts of the evolution of chronic hepatitis and the role of piecemeal necrosis. *Hepatology*, **3**: 758–62
21. Popper, H. (1986). General pathology of the liver: light microscopic aspects serving diagnosis and interpretation. *Semin. Liver Dis.*, **6**, 175–84
22. Baptista, A., Bianchi, L., De Groote, J., Desmet, V. J., Ishak, K. G., Korb, G., MacSween, R. N. M., Popper, H., Poulsen, H., Scheuer, P. J., Schmid, M. and Thaler, H. (1988). The diagnostic significance of periportal hepatic necrosis and inflammation. *Histopathology*, **12**, 569–79
23. Shiohara, T. (1988). Lichenoid tissue reaction: an immunological perspective. *Am. J. Dermatopathol.*, **10**, 252–6
24. Bardadin, K. A. and Desmet, V. J. (1984) Interdigitating and dendritic reticulum cells in chronic active hepatitis. *Histopathology*, **8**, 657–67
25. Kerr, J. F. R., Cooksley, W. G. E., Searle, J., Halliday, J. W., Halliday, W. J., Holder, L., Roberts, I. and Burnett, W. (1979). The nature of piecemeal necrosis in chronic active hepatitis. *Lancet*, **2**, 827–8
26. Bianchi, L. (1986). Necroinflammatory liver diseases. *Semin. Liver Dis.*, **6**, 185–98

27. Montano, L., Aranguibel, F., Boffill, M., Goodall, A. H., Janossy, G. and Thomas, H. L. (1983). An analysis of the composition of the inflammatory infiltrate in autoimmune and hepatitis B virus-induced chronic liver disease. *Hepatology*, **3**, 292–6
28. Van den Oord, J. J. and Desmet, V. J. (1984). Verteilungsmuster der Histokompatibilitäts-Hauptantigene in normalen und pathologischen Lebergewebe. *Leber Magen Darm*, **14**, 244–54
29. Swain, S. L., Dennert, G., Wormsley, S. and Dutton, R. W. (1981). The Lyt phenotype of a long-term allospecific T cell line. Both helper and killer activities to Ia are mediated by Ly-1 cells. *Eur. J. Immunol.*, **11**, 175–80
30. International Group (1977). Acute and chronic hepatitis revisited. *Lancet*, **2**, 914–19
31. Desmet, V. J. and De Vos, R. (1984). Structural analysis of acute liver injury. In Keppler, D., Bianchi, L. and Reutter, W. (eds), *Mechanisms of Hepatocyte Injury and Death*, pp. 11–30. (Lancaster: MTP Press)
32. Boyer, J. L. and Klatskin, G. (1970). Pattern of necrosis in acute viral hepatitis. Prognostic value of bridging (subacute hepatic necrosis). *N. Engl. J. Med.*, **283**, 1063–71
33. Desmet, V. J. (1989). Acute viral hepatitis. Hepatitis B. In Gitnick, G. (ed.), *Modern Concept of Acute and Chronic Hepatitis*, pp. 87–111. (New York: Plenum)
34. Desmet, V. J. (1978). Die Morphogenese der chronischen Hepatitis. *Münch. Med. Wochenschr.*, **120**, 1523–30
35. Liehr, H. and Grun, M. (1979). Endotoxins in liver disease. *Prog. Liver Dis.*, **6**, 313–16
36. Mori, W., Shiga, J. and Irie, H. (1986). Schwarzman reaction as a pathogenetic mechanism in fulminant hepatitis. *Semin. Liver Dis.*, **6**, 267–76
37. Sato, K., Ikeda, K., Katami, K. and Ogawa, H. (1985). Preparation of monoclonal antibody to hepatocellular membrane and its application to induction of liver cell membrane damage. *Acta Pathol. Jpn.*, **35**, 1375–83
38. Sato, K., Ikeda, T., Kawai, F. and Osada, Y. (1987). Isolation and purification of a rat liver-specific antigen from hepatocyte membrane. *J. Biochem.*, **102**, 933–8
39. Bhakdi, S. and Tranum-Jensen, J. (1983). Membrane damage by channel-forming proteins. *Trends Biochem. Sci.*, **8**, 134–6
40. Tranum-Jensen, J. and Bhakdi, S. (1983). Freeze–fracture analysis of the membrane lesion of human complement. *J. Cell Biol.*, **87**, 618–26
41. Trump, B. F., Berezesky, I. K. and Cowley, R. A. (1982). The cellular and subcellular characteristics of acute and chronic injury with emphasis on the role of calcium. In Cowley, R. A. and Trump, B. F. (eds), *Pathophysiology of Shock, Anoxia and Ischemia*, pp. 6–46. (Baltimore: Williams & Wilkins)
42. Trepo, C. G., Robert, D., Motin, J., Trepo, D., Sepetjian, M. and Prince, A. M. (1976). Hepatitis B antigen (HBsAg) and/or antibodies (anti-HBs and anti-HBc) in fulminant hepatitis: pathogenic and prognostic significance. *Gut*, **17**, 10–13
43. Okuda, K. (1989). Acute massive necrosis of the liver induced by antibody/complement, not by T-cells. *Hepatology*, **10**, 118–19
44. Poralla, T., Ramadori, G., Dienes, H. P., Manns, M., Gerken, G., Dippold, W., Hütteroth, T. H. and Meyer zum Büschenfelde, K.-H. (1987). Liver cell damage caused by monoclonal antibody against an organic-specific membrane antigen in vivo and in vitro. *J. Hepatol.*, **4**, 373–80
45. Canalese, J., Wyke, R. J., Vergani, D., Eddleston, A. L. and Williams, R. (1981). Circulating immune complexes in patients with fulminant hepatic failure. *Gut*, **22**, 845–8
46. Tabor, E., Krugman, S., Weiss, E. G. and Gerety, R. J. (1981). Disappearance of hepatitis B surface antigen during an unusual case of fulminant hepatitis B. *J. Med. Virol.*, **8**, 277–82
47. Poulsen, H. and Christoffersen, P. (1972). Abnormal bile duct epithelium in chronic aggressive hepatitis and cirrhosis. A review of morphology and clinical, biochemical and immunologic features. *Hum. Pathol.*, **3**, 217–25
48. Schmid, M., Pirovino, M., Altorfer, J., Gudat, F. and Bianchi, L. (1982). Acute hepatitis non-A, non-B; are there any specific light microscopic features? *Liver*, **2**, 61–7
49. International Group (1983). Histopathology of the intrahepatic biliary tree. *Liver*, **3**, 161–75
50. Van den Oord, J. J., Sciot, R. and Desmet, V. J. (1986). Expression of MHC products by normal and abnormal bile duct epithelium. *J. Hepatol.*, **3**, 310–17

51. Desmet, V. J. (1987). Cholangiopathies: past, present and future. *Semin. Liver Dis.*, **7**, 67–76
52. Walter, J. B. and Israel, M. S. (1979). *General Pathology*, 5th edn. (Edinburgh: Churchill Livingstone)
53. Patrick, R. S. and McGee, J. O'D. (1988). *Biopsy Pathology of the Liver*, 2nd edn. (London: Chapman & Hall)
54. Thaler, H. (1987). *Leberkrankheiten*, 2nd edn. (Berlin: Springer-Verlag)
55. Ishak, K. G. and Rogers, W. A. (1981). Cryptogenic acute cholangitis. Association with toxic shock syndrome. *Am. J. Clin. Pathol.*, **76**, 619–26
56. Paris, A. L., Herwaldt, L. A., Blum, D., Schmid, G. P., Shands, K. N. and Broome, C. V. (1982). Pathologic findings in twelve fatal cases of toxic shock syndrome. *Ann. Intern. Med.*, **96**, 852–7
57. MacSween, R. N. M., Anthony, P. P. and Scheuer, P. J. (1987). *Pathology of the Liver*, 2nd edn. (Edinburgh: Churchill Livingstone)
58. Popper, H. and Schaffner, F. (1957). *Liver: Structure and Function.* (New York: McGraw-Hill)
59. Lefkowitch, J. H. (1982). Bile ductular cholestasis: an ominous histopathologic sign related to sepsis and 'cholangitis lenta'. *Hum. Pathol.*, **13**, 19–24
60. Vyberg, M. and Poulsen, H. (1984). Abnormal bile duct epithelium accompanying septicemia. *Virchows Arch. Pathol. Anat.*, **402**, 451–8
61. Vanstapel, M. J. and Desmet, V. J. (1983). Cytomegalovirus hepatitis: a histological and immunohistochemical study. *Appl. Pathol.*, **1**, 41–9
62. Christoffersen, P., Poulsen, H. and Skeie, E. (1970). Focal liver cell necrosis accompanied by infiltration of granulocytes arising during operation. *Acta Hepato-Splenol.*, **17**, 240–5
63. Boros, D. L. (1980). The granulomatous inflammatory response: an overview. In Boros, D. L. and Takeshi, Y. (eds), *Basic and Clinical Aspects of Granulomatous Diseases*, p. 1. (New York: Elsevier–North Holland)
64. Warren, K. S. (1976). A functional classification of granulomatous inflammation. *Ann. N.Y. Acad. Sci.*, **278**, 7–18
65. Epstein, W. L. (1967). Granulomatous hypersensitivity. *Prog. Allergy*, **11**, 36–88
66. Turk, J. L. and Narayanan, R. B. (1982). The origin, morphology and function of epithelioid cells. *Immunobiology*, **161**, 274–82
67. Adams, D. O. (1976). The granulomatous inflammatory response. *Am. J. Pathol.*, **84**, 164–91
68. David, J. R. and Remold, H. G. (1979). The activation of macrophages by lymphokines. In Cohen, S., Pick, E. and Oppenheim, J. (eds), *Biology of the Lymphokines*, p. 121. (New York: Academic Press)
69. Van den Oord, J. J., De Wolf-Peeters, C., Facchetti, F. and Desmet, V. J. (1984). Cellular composition of hypersensitivity-type granulomas: immunohistochemical analysis of tuberculous and sarcoid lymphadenitis. *Hum. Pathol.*, **15**, 559–65
70. Van den Oord, J. J., De Wolf-Peeters, C. and Desmet, V. J. (1985). Cellular composition of suppurative granulomas: an immunohistochemical study of suppurative granulomatous lymphadenitis. *Hum. Pathol.*, **16**, 1009–14
71. Ishak, K. G. (1983). Liver granulomas. In Ioachim, H. L. (ed.), *Pathology of Granulomas*, pp. 307–69. (New York: Raven Press)
72. Ishak, K. G. (1987). New developments in diagnositc liver pathology. In Farber, E., Phillips, M. J. and Kaufman, N. (eds), *Pathogenesis of Liver Diseases*, pp. 223–373. (Baltimore: Williams & Wilkins)
73. Scheuer, P. J. (1988). *Liver Biopsy Interpretation*, 4th edn. (London: Baillière Tindall)
74. James, D. G. (1985). Hepatic granulomas. In Brunner, H. and Thaler, H. (eds), *Hepatology, a Festschrift for Hans Popper*, pp. 269–80. (New York: Raven Press)
75. Arean, V. M. (1962). The pathologic anatomy and pathogenesis of fatal human leptospirosis (Weil's disease). *Am. J. Pathol.*, **40**, 393–423
76. Bianchi, L. (1983). Liver biopsy interpretation in hepatitis. Part II: Histopathology and classification of acute and chronic viral hepatitis/differential diagnosis. *Pathol. Res. Pract.*, **178**, 180–213

4
The macrophages and their signal products

K. DECKER

INTRODUCTION

The macrophages belonging to the mononuclear phagocyte system are part of the body's defensive machinery. Their major functions include phagocytosis, presentation of antigens, unspecific immune response (immunomodulation), and biochemical attack. Macrophages are recruited from the bone marrow, but may in some instances, e.g. in the liver, propagate at the site of their final destination. The latter also seems to influence their differentiation and to endow each type with particular metabolic and structural features. We can clearly recognize specific capabilities in the mobile blood-borne macrophages (monocytes), in the singly moving but sequestered (peritoneal and alveolar) macrophages and in the various sessile macrophages such as those residing in the bone marrow, the spleen, the brain, the skin, and the liver[1,2].

Antigen presentation and the process of phagocytosis *per se* will not be covered in this contribution; it is also impossible to deal with the species and organ specificities of the various macrophages. But a brief account of the presently known signal substances of macrophages in general will be given, and their elicitation and function as well as the regulation of their synthesis and action discussed.

ELICITATION OF SIGNAL PRODUCTION AND RELEASE

Receptor-mediated phagocytosis

It has been known for some time that the process of phagocytosis in macrophages is accompanied by the release of specific molecules. The contact between a suitable particle and its receptor elicits the production of signals that include reactive oxygen species (ROIs) and arachidonate metabolites (eicosanoids); however, depending on the kind of receptor engaged, different transduction paths may be activated in a given cell so that not all the possible signals are realized at the same time. In recent years it has become increasingly clear that the particle-stimulated synthesis and release of signal substances does not require the internalization, but only the close contact, of the particle to be phagocytosed with a specific receptor or binding site; perhaps lateral contacts of several of these interacting molecules are necessary for signal transduction[3]. It was found[4] that rat Kupffer cells exposed to immunocomplex-coated latex particles produce superoxide even when the cells were pretreated with cytochalasin B[4] that prevents the formation of coated pits and phagosomes. In fact, substantial O_2^- release into the medium occurred only in the pretreated cells, indicating that the majority of the superoxide formed remained within the boundaries of the coated vesicles.

This example also illustrates the presence of F_c receptors on Kupffer cells, which are well known on other macrophages and instrumental in the binding and uptake of immunocomplexes (Table 1). Besides these F_c receptors, specific binding sites have been identified for glycoproteins carrying terminal mannose or fucose[5], galactose or *N*-acetylgalactosamine[6] residues, unopsonized erythrocytes[2] or senescent advanced glycosylated end-products (AGE)[7], e.g. glycosylated albumin. Furthermore, receptors for the complement component C3[3], Mac-1 (cell adhesion molecules)[8], and modified low-density lipoprotein (LDL) ('scavenger receptor')[9] were observed on macrophages. These receptors are involved in phagocytosis. In addition, the receptors for interleukin-6 (IL-6)[10] and interferon-γ[11] deserve particular interest; the former belong to the immunoglobulin superfamily, are found on T cells and mitogen-activated B cells, but mainly (about 80%) on hepatocytes[12]; the latter convey the message of interferon-γ that is considered as one of the most potent activators of cells of the monocyte macrophage lineage[13].

Activators and immunomodulators

Besides the elicitation of signal production by phagocytosis of particles, a great number of soluble substances is able to activate or stimulate macrophages

Table 1 Receptors and binding sites on macrophages

Involved in phagocytosis
F_c (several)
Mannose/fucose
Galactose/*N*-acetyl-galactosamine
AGE (advanced glycosylated end-products)
Modified LDL ('scavenger')
C3
Mac-1 (cell adhesion molecules)
E_R (unopsonized erythrocytes)
Others
Interleukin-6
Interferon-γ
PGE_2
Apolipoprotein B
Fibronectin
Insulin
Glucagon

(Table 2). They are also known as 'biological response modifiers' (BRMs)[14]. They may bind to specific receptors or sites on the plasma membrane such as the peptide factors C5a, f-Met-Leu-Phe, interferon-γ or nucleotide triphosphates; or in the cytosol, e.g. lipopolysaccharides (LPS) or phorbol esters (PMA).

Their binding leads to the release of mediators or signal molecules and also in some instances confers the ability to kill foreign cells, e.g. tumour cells, by a mechanism different from that of phagocytosis[15]. Full activation of macrophages including the cytotoxic capability is a two-stage process and appears to require a cytokine, e.g. interferon-γ, and an elicitor, e.g. LPS. It should be noted that apparently closely related macrophages such as mouse and rat Kupffer cells may behave differently towards activators. While the former require the two-stage activation in order to become cytotoxic and to release eicosanoids, the latter are in the 'primed' state already (even when obtained by the same procedure from germ-free rats) and need the elicitor only[16]; the cytokine has just a small stimulatory effect with rat Kupffer cells[17]. In general, however, it is safe to consider interferon-γ as *the* 'macrophage activating factor' (Table 3).

Lipopolysaccharides, the endotoxins of Gram-negative intestinal bacteria, play a prominent role as immunomodulators. Their interaction with macrophages is probably one of the most important features of inflammation or shock following bacterial invasion. Kupffer cells have been identified as the first and most avid scavenger cells for LPS coming in through the portal vein[18]. Detoxification by partial degradation and clearance[19,20] of LPS occurs mainly in the liver macrophage, but the spleen has also been confirmed as a site of LPS uptake and modification. LPS is assumed to be taken up by receptor-mediated endocytosis and bound by an intracellular binding protein, but up to now neither a specific receptor nor mechanisms of endocytosis and signal transduction have been identified. Myristoylation of certain proteins in LPS-exposed cells has been associated with the intracellular action of endotoxin[21].

It will be discussed later that LPS is the major inducer of peptide mediators such as TNF-α, IL-6 or IL-1. It triggers in some macrophages the production

Table 2 Activators and immunomodulators of macrophages

Interferon-γ (INF-γ) = macrophage activating factor (MAF)
Lipopolysaccharide (endotoxin, LPS)
Tumour necrosis factor-α (TNF-α)
Viruses (Sendai, Newcastle disease)
Colony-stimulating factors (GM-CSF, M-CSF)
Macrophage migration inhibitory factor (MIF, = INF-γ?)
Macrophage deactivation factor
Transforming growth factor-β
Complement component C5a
Chemotactic peptide (*N*-formyl-Met-Leu-Phe)
Platelet-activating factor (PAF)
Muramyl dipeptide
Nucleotide tri- and diphosphates
Phorbol myristate acetate (PMA)
Ionophores changing the intracellular H^+ and Ca^{2+} concentrations

Table 3 Effects of interferon-γ

Cellular level
Antiviral activity (first detected effect)
Increase of NK cell activity together with IL-2 (against some but not all cells)
Antiproliferative + antitumour activity
Increase of number of F_c receptors
Molecular level
Induction of oligoadenylate synthesis, P1/elF-2α protein kinase (activated by double-stranded RNA)
Induction of guanylate-binding proteins
Induction of MHC class II antigens
Enhancement of lymphotoxin production and effects
Activation of the Na^+/H^+ exchanger, Ca^{2+} efflux
Enhanced production of superoxide (in some macrophages)
Induction of IL-1 and TNF production (in some macrophages)
No change in arachidonate release

of reactive oxygen species[22], in others it acts as an enhancer of stimuli[23] while in some, e.g. rat Kupffer cells (unpublished), it cannot elicit ROI production. LPS is also able to stimulate the release of eicosanoids, although at a very slow rate as compared to the effects of PMA or of zymosan phagocytosis[24]. Nevertheless, the prostaglandin E_2 (PGE_2) production of LPS-exposed liver macrophages seems to have great relevance in the response to endotoxins (see 'Regulation'). Again, LPS priming further enhances the stimulated metabolism of arachidonate in some, e.g. peritoneal macrophages[23], while it is without this effect in others (Kupffer cells). A very interesting observation connects LPS with the modulation of c-fos and c-myc proto-oncogenes in macrophages[25]: LPS increases temporarily the mRNA levels up to 20-fold.

Of special interest is the recently described[26] ability of extracellular nucleotide tri- or diphosphates to stimulate liver macrophages to release eicosanoids. The source of the extracellular nucleotides is not yet sufficiently established (they may originate from activated platelets or synaptic transmission); several effects of these nucleotides have been reported in recent years[27]. It is assumed that purinergic and perhaps pyrimidinergic receptors are involved in these stimulations.

SIGNAL PATHS

Activators or immunomodulators require peri- or intracellular binding sites in order to elicit specific actions in target cells (Table 4). The responses which may be of rather complex nature, such as modulation of growth or differentiation, can be traced to activation/inactivation and induction/repression, respectively, of enzymes or functional proteins. 'Fast' and 'slow' signal realization is quite often connected with these different mechanisms.

The binding site of the effector and the protein or structure to be modified are usually topologically separated; a possible exception may be PMA that is thought to interact directly with proteinkinase C leading to its activation.

Table 4 General scheme of signal transduction in macrophages

1. Interaction of ligand and receptor
2. Signal transduction, e.g. by G proteins
3. Generation of second messengers
4. Action of second messengers:
(a) in the cytosol, e.g. activation/inactivation of enzymes by phosphorylation/dephosphorylation
(b) in the genome, e.g. by induction/repression of protein synthesis

In most cases, however, the signal received at the receptor has to be transduced to the locus of realization.

A dominant role in signal transduction from plasma membrane-associated ligand–receptor interactions is attributed to guanylate-binding proteins, G proteins[28]. They are a family of membrane-integrated heterotrimeric proteins (subunits α, β, γ) that transduce the receptor–ligand interaction into enzymatic activities on the cytosolic side of the plasma membrane. The activation is associated with the binding of GTP, hydrolysis to and dissociation of GDP from the receptor–ligand complex. The total number of different G proteins in a given cell is not yet known, but individual G proteins are connected with specific receptors as well as target enzymes. The α-subunit becomes ADP-ribosylated in the presence of certain bacterial toxins, e.g. from *V. cholerae* or *B. pertussis.* Enzymes known to be regulated by G proteins include adenylate cyclase, stimulated by G_s and inhibited by G_i, and phospholipase(s) C hydrolysing phosphatidyl-inositol polyphosphates to inositol polyphosphate (IP_n) and diacylglycerol (DAG) (Figure 1). There is also evidence that G proteins are involved in the regulation of ion channels; whether they act directly on channel proteins or are mediating an activation–deactivation process (e.g. through proteinkinase/phosphoprotein phosphatase action) remains to be seen. All the G protein-mediated signal transduction paths are of relevance to the elicitation of macrophages by activators or immunomodulators.

Adenylate cyclase activation followed by a rise of intracellular cAMP levels has been observed after PGE_2 and LPS treatment of macrophages[29]. A very short spike of cAMP was also seen after contact of these macrophages with zymosan particles[30]; this agrees with reports of a cAMP rise subsequent to ligation of $F_{c\gamma 2a}$ receptors of P388D1 macrophage-like cells[31]. cAMP-mediated reactions seem to participate in interferon-α-induced anti-growth activity of a murine macrophage cell line[32].

Regulation of phospholipase C appears to be a major process in signal transduction in macrophages. Its enhanced activity may lead to activation of proteinkinase C (through the DAG formed), to Ca^{2+} mobilization from the endoplasmic reticulum (through IP_3) and possibly to Ca^{2+} influx from outside (through IP_4). Thus, a key proteinkinase and a second messenger (Ca^{2+}) are directly mobilized while cleavage of arachidonate from DAG and phospholipase A_2 (PLA_2) activation by Ca^{2+}/calmodulin are secondary effects leading to the release of important signal molecules, the eicosanoids.

Phospholipase C is coupled to a G protein, designated G_p, but not yet fully identified. The latter appears to be closely related or even identical with

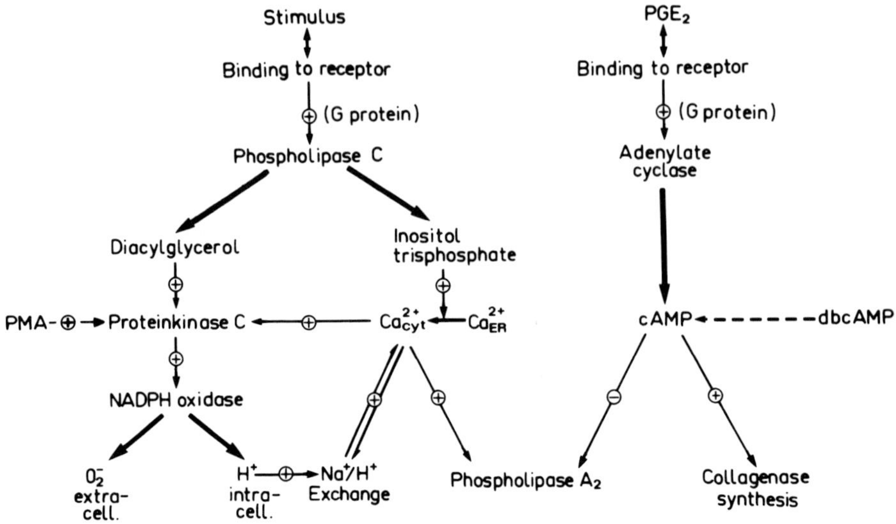

Figure 1 Known signal paths in rat Kupffer cells. ⊕ and ⊖ indicate stimulatory and inhibitory influences, respectively. PMA, phorbol myristate acetate; dbcAMP, dibutyryl cyclic AMP.

the product of the ras oncogene[33]. Phosphatidylinositol-4,5-bisphosphate interacts with components of the cytoskeleton, e.g. actin[34]; it may be instrumental in the changes of macrophage morphology such as occur during phagocytosis or movement. The two-pronged signal transduction through DAG and IP_3 opens particularly intriguing aspects of regulation as the targets of both interact[35]: Ca^{2+} is required for binding to the plasma membrane and activation of proteinkinase C, while the proteins phosphorylated by proteinkinase C may influence Ca^{2+} movement and binding within the cell. Experiments with rat Kupffer cells indicate that proteinkinase C is involved in the activation of the NADPH ('respiratory burst') oxidase and the Na^+/H^+ antiporter while Ca^{2+} is necessary for PLA_2 activation and eicosanoid synthesis[36]. Phorbol esters are thought to mimic DAG in creating the lipid environment for membrane anchorage of proteinkinase C.

Ca^{2+} is a well-established second messenger of cellular regulation[37]. It binds to specific modulator molecules, e.g. calmodulin, or directly to effector proteins such as PLA_2. The very low intracellular basal level of the free ion ($<0.2\,\mu$mol/l) can be changed by the IP_3-stimulated influx from the storage sites (mainly endoplasmic reticulum, but to some extent also mitochondria), the net uptake from the outside by activation of Ca^{2+} channels or antiporters ($2\,Na^+/Ca^{2+}$), or by modulation of the activity of the ATP-driven Ca^{2+} pump. The intracellular Ca^{2+} level is also related to the internal pH; activation of the Na^+/H^+ antiporter, e.g. after zymosan addition, in macrophages is connected with a transcellular Ca^{2+} influx[38,39].

Inorganic signals

Macrophages are able to respond to certain stimuli with the secretion of inorganic compounds (simple ion fluxes not considered). It is a matter of definition whether the active oxygen intermediates are considered signals or – preferably – chemical weapons for immediate use. They do not act in specific ways (through receptors or binding sites) but exploit their chemical reactivity on any suitable compounds with which they collide. Unless the O_2^- produced by phagocytosing macrophages comes in contact with myeloperoxidase from granulocytes forming the powerful hydroxyl radicals, its activity is mainly restricted to attacking phagocytosed material sequestered in coated pits or coated vesicles.

A specific inorganic signal molecule that macrophages synthesize and excrete is nitric oxide (NO). It has been identified as an endothelium-derived relaxing factor, a powerful agent in adjusting the blood pressure in small vessels[40]. NO is synthesized by LPS-activated rat Kupffer cells from arginine (unpublished), evidently by the mechanism found in other macrophages[41] (Figure 2). It can be assumed that nitric oxide originating within the liver plays a role in the regulation of hepatic blood flow.

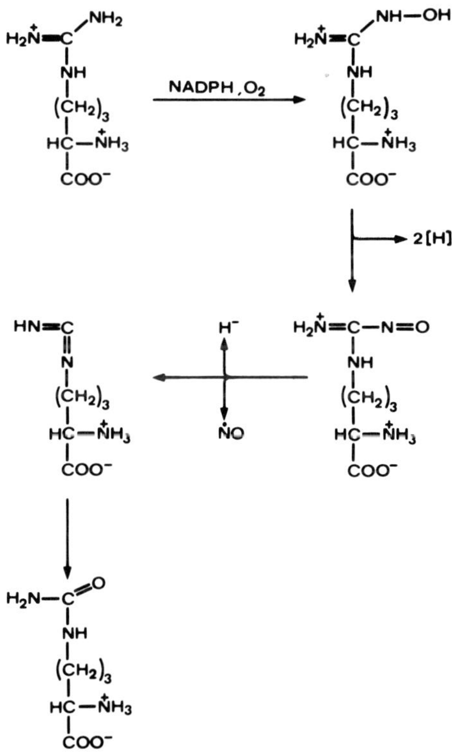

Figure 2 Formation of nitric oxide (NO) from L-arginine

Peptidic signals

Work in many laboratories has identified more than 50 compounds of peptidic nature that are secreted from stimulated macrophages. They include numerous enzymes, mainly hydrolases of various specificities. A functional significance, however, can be attributed to enzyme release only if leakiness of the activated (and sometimes damaged) cells is excluded[42]. It is questionable whether macrophages – in contrast to polymorphonuclear neutrophils! – secrete lysosomal enzymes actively. Some of them produce and secrete collagenase, fibronectin, and a cytolytic protease that is instrumental in tumour cytotoxicity. Further polypeptides identified by various investigators as products of macrophages are listed in Table 5.

Of particular interest among the typical signal polypeptides are the *cytokines* of which interleukins 1 (IL-1) and 6 (IL-6), tumour necrosis factor-α (cachectin) and interferon-α/β are well-defined products of macrophages. Research on these mediators has been greatly enhanced by the availability of the recombinant molecules from several species, as well as of monoclonal antibodies against them. Of course, one should bear in mind that recombinant cytokines lack the carbohydrate side chains present on some native molecules and may possess somewhat different affinities to enzymes and receptors.

IL-1, formerly also known as lymphocyte-activating factor (LAF) or as endogenous pyrogen is mainly produced by blood monocytes[43], but sessile macrophages and astrocytes[44] were also shown to synthesize and secrete this mediator of inflammation and pain. It is most abundantly elicited by lipopolysaccharides. The molecular mass of the mature compound is 14 kDa[45]; it arises from a precursor by removal of four amino acid residues from the N-terminus catalysed by a peptidyl aminopeptidase[46]. IL-1 stimulates IL-2 production by T cells; it affects and finally destroys the insulin-producing B cells of the pancreas[47].

IL-6 was formerly known as INF-β2, BSF-2 or HSF; this points to the numerous physiological functions which must be attributed to this cytokine (Table 6). (For a recent review see ref. 10).

Table 5 Peptides released from activated macrophages

Interleukin-1
Interleukin-6
Interferon α/β
Tumor necrosis factor-α (cachectin)
Macrophage colony-stimulating factor
Granulocyte/macrophage colony-stimulating factor
Collagenase
Apolipoprotein E
Clotting factors
Complement components 1–5
Erythropoietin
Fibronectin
α_2-Macroglobulin
Plasminogen activator
Plasminogen activator inhibitor

Table 6 Effects of interleukin-6

Induction of terminal B cell maturation
Stimulation of activated B cells to secrete IgM, IgG and IgA
Induction of acute-phase protein synthesis in hepatocytes
Enhancement of proliferation of haemopoietic progenitor cells (together with IL-3, M-CSF or GM-GSF)
Induction of cellular differentiation in PC12 nerve cells
Release of ACTH from cultured pituitary cells

The mature, sometimes N-glycosylated IL-6 has a molecular mass of 26 kDa[48]; it arises from a precursor with a 26 amino acid extension (signal sequence). IL-6 is synthesized upon inflammatory stimulation (e.g. LPS, TNF-α, IL-1) or viruses by a variety of cells including fibroblasts, endothelial cells, monocytes, macrophages and also some tumours. The level of IL-6 in normal human serum is 50 HGF units/ml[10]; it rises during inflammation up to 100-fold dependent on the severity of the condition. IL-6 is considered as a sensitive indicator of meningitis, graft rejection and rheumatoid arthritis.

As Kupffer cells are located in close proximity to hepatocytes their capacity to release IL-6 is of particular interest. Exposure to 1 ng LPS/ml stimulates the liver macrophages to an IL-6 secretion of 300–400 pg per 10^6 cells[49]. It can be measured by the B cell hybridoma growth test[50]. Dexamethasone at 1 μmol/l completely suppresses the LPS-elicited IL-6 synthesis. PGE_2 that also inhibits TNF-α release was without effect on IL-6 production. Besides LPS and TNF-α some viruses (Sendai, Newcastle disease) elicited rat Kupffer cells to produce IL-6 (Figure 3). TNF-α also induces IL-6 production in fibroblasts.

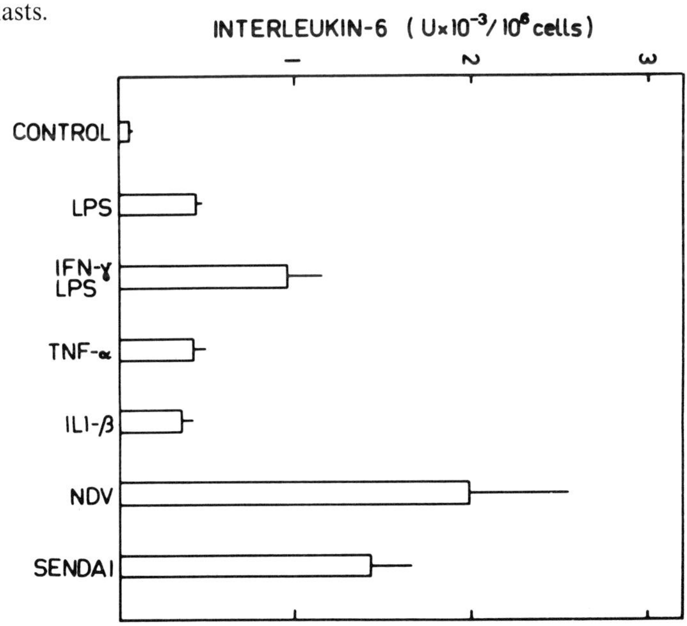

Figure 3 Stimulated synthesis of interleukin-6 by rat Kupffer cells in primary culture. NDV, Newcastle disease virus.

Interferon-α/β

The interferons (INF) comprise a group of molecules that have initially been defined by their antiviral activity (for review see ref. 51). At present two major families of interferons with overlapping activities but unrelated structures are known: the interferon-γ mentioned already as stimulator of macrophages and the closely related interferon-α and -β. The former was first described as a product of peripheral leukocytes, the latter as a product of fibroblasts. Because of their structural and functional similarities INF-α and INF-β are usually considered as an operational entity. They have also been observed in supernatants of activated macrophages[52]. INF-α/β secreted by murine Kupffer cells[53] augments the liver-associated natural killer activity[54]. In general, viruses and double-stranded RNA have proven to be the most efficient inducers of INF-α/β expression. Besides their antiviral property these cytokines inhibit tumour growth, modulate cell differentiation, induce the expression of class I MHC antigens including β_2-microglobulin and of F_c receptors. In some cases they antagonize INF-γ, e.g. in the down-regulation of the mannosyl fucosyl receptor.

Both interferons appear to be produced in several variants, their molecular mass ranging from 16 to 27 kDa for human INF-α and around 20 kDa for the β-form. Murine INF-β was obtained as a 26 and a 35 kDa species. Both INF-α and -β are predominantly found in glycosylated forms.

Specific receptors for INF-α/β are present on susceptible cells which are down-regulated by an excess of the ligand.

Tumour necrosis factor-α (cachectin)

A very important component of the group of signal molecules produced by macrophages after inflammatory stimulation is the tumour necrosis factor-α (TNF-α) also known as cachectin (for review see ref. 55). It was originally described independently as a mediator of tumour necrosis seen after inflammations, and as the agent responsible for the anorexia in chronic neoplastic or inflammatory diseases. Molecular cloning of the respective compounds brought definite proof of their identity[56]. Major producers are the blood monocytes and the macrophages. In the rat the Kupffer cells seem to be the most abundant source of this cytokine[17]. TNF-α synthesis and release is strongly stimulated after exposure of macrophages or monocytes to LPS (+ interferon-γ) or to some viruses, e.g. Sendai or Newcastle disease virus. The cytokine is synthesized as a precursor having an N-terminal extension of 76 (man) and 79 (mouse) amino acids, respectively[55]. It can be obtained as soluble polypeptide from the extracellular space consisting of 157 (man) or 156 (mouse) amino acids.

TNF-α released from the producing macrophage binds to plasma membrane receptors of target cells. These receptors, whose mass was estimated as about 300 kDa, appear to be widely distributed in the animal body. The mechanisms of signal transduction from the liganded receptor to the various intracellular effector systems are not yet understood.

The overall effects of TNF-α are manifold; those seen in rat liver are listed in Table 7. This cytokine is now thought to mediate most if not all the consequences of endotoxin exposure in sensitive animals. It was shown to be the endogenous pyrogen of rabbits; the action of administered LPS can be suppressed by antibodies raised against TNF-α. Anaemia is produced by this cytokine through reduction of erythrocyte synthesis and lifespan[55]. Fever is the result of the TNF-α-mediated stimulation of PGE_2 synthesis in the hypothalamus as well as of interleukin-1 induction in peripheral cells[55].

Vascular endothelial cells respond to TNF-α by up-regulation of class I MHC antigens and of intercellular adhesion molecules. These, as well as the sinusoidal endothelial cells of rat liver[57], are binding TNF-α and eliciting the adherence of granulocytes concomitantly with their activation (release of hydrolytic enzymes and reactive oxygen intermediates). Furthermore, the cytokine induces procoagulant activity and IL-1 production. It is obvious that these effects are able to contribute to the pathological changes seen after LPS administration or in endotoxin shock.

TNF-α is one of the signal molecules able to trigger the cells that produced it (autostimulation). It activates macrophages to become cytotoxic and to produce IL-1, IL-6 and PGE_2[58,59]. This eicosanoid is also released together with collagenase by TNF-α-treated fibroblasts and synovial cells. Together with IL-1, TNF-α constitutes the osteoclast-activating factor bringing about the mobilization of Ca^{2+} from the bone and the breakdown of proteoglycans.

A number of malignantly transformed cells are lyzed by TNF-α-producing macrophages. The mechanism of this cytotoxic action of the cytokine is not yet understood, but the involvement of a cytolytic proteinase activated in stimulated macrophages is widely assumed[15]. A membrane-associated form of TNF-α having a mass similar to that of its precursor may function in conferring the cytotoxic properties[60]. The anorexia often observed in malignant or inflammatory states appears to result from biochemical events in adipocytes elicited by TNF-α leading to a preferentially lipolytic, catabolic state of this tissue[55]. It has been shown that the expression of lipoprotein lipase, the fatty acid-binding protein, glycerol-3-phosphate dehydrogenase and probably also of some enzymes of triglyceride synthesis from acetate, is suppressed while the hormone-sensitive lipase of the fat cells is activated[55].

Another cytokine has been identified in the circulation of man and other mammalian species, whose physiological activities are very much like those of TNF-α. It is called *lymphotoxin*[55] or TNF-β. It is structurally related to

Table 7 Tumour necrosis factor-α of rat liver

Is synthesized by Kupffer cells, not by hepatocytes or sinusoidal endothelial cells
Synthesis is elicited by endotoxin (LPS) and viruses, not by phagocytosis, phorbol ester or Ca^{2+} ionophore
Synthesis is instantly suppressed by dexamethasone or PGE_2
Increases preferentially rate of PGE_2 synthesis (like LPS)
Mediates most (if not all) effects of endotoxin
Replaces LPS in the galactosamine-enhanced cytotoxicity
Elicits sticking of granulocytes to sinusoidal endothelial cells
Fails to trigger superoxide production in Kupffer cells
Fails to induce acute-phase reaction in hepatocytes

TNF-α (28% sequence homology) and encoded on the same gene. It differs, however, with regard to the source and the elicitors. While TNF-α is synthesized mainly by macrophages in response to endotoxin or viruses, lymphotoxin is produced by challenged T cells or lymphoblastoid cell lines[61].

Angiogenesis factor(s)

Macrophages are able to produce a factor that promotes the migration of vascular endothelial cells into areas of inflammation and tumour growth[62]. It can be differentiated from various other growth factors by its lack of binding to heparin sepharose. The factor has not yet been presented as a purified protein allowing definite identification.

LIPIDIC SIGNALS

With regard to their chemical nature we may differentiate two major groups of lipidic signal substances produced by macrophages: the derivatives of arachidonic acid collectively called eicosanoids and the 1-alkyl-2-acetyl-glycero-3-phosphocholines known as platelet-activating factors (PAF).

Arachidonic acid and its metabolites

Arachidonic acid, eicosa-6,9,12,15-all-cis-tetraenoic acid ($C_{20:4}$, n-6), is formed from the essential fatty acid, linoleic acid, by chain elongation and desaturation. Deficiency of essential fatty acid or feeding with unsaturated fatty acids, such as triene- or pentaene-C_{20} acids, prevents conversion to biologically active products, and has a profound effect on processes thought to involve the arachidonic acid cascade.

The intracellular concentration of the free acid is extremely low; almost all of the cellular content is esterified to the 2-position of phosphatides (Figure 4). In the extracellular space, arachidonic acid is non-covalently bound to serum albumin or phosphatide-bound in lipoproteins. In most cells, specifically in macrophages, arachidonic acid is subject to a rapid turnover employing the enzymes PLA_2 for removal of the acid from the phosphatide, long-chain acyl-CoA synthetase for activation and acyltransferase for reintegration into the phospholipid. Exchange with the albumin-associated arachidonate seems to be rapid and efficient[63]. The direct influence of these enzymes on the availability of free arachidonic acid makes them participants in the regulatory network of eicosanoid metabolism and likely targets for pharmacological interference.

The most important signal substances are made from arachidonate by two pathways, one involving cyclo-oxygenase (prostaglandin H synthase) the other 5-lipoxygenase (Figure 5). The main products of the former are the prostaglandins, prostacyclin and thromboxane. The 5-lipoxygenase pathway produces 5-hydroperoxy-6,8,11,14-eicosatetraenoic acid (5-HPETE), 5-hydr-

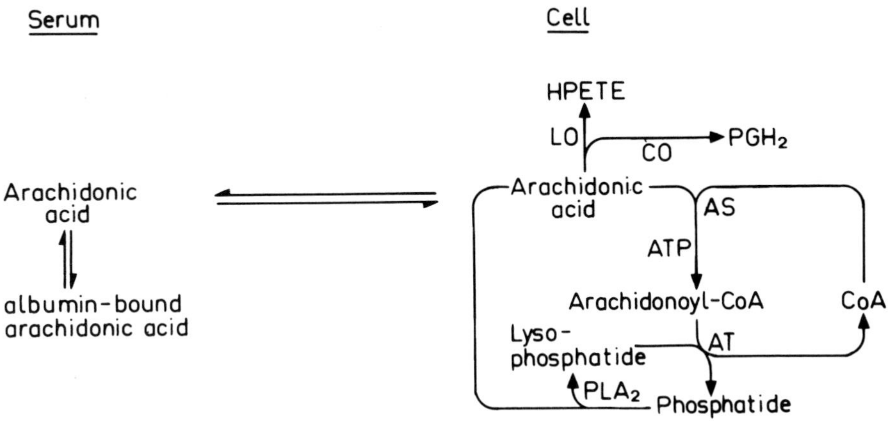

Figure 4 Metabolism of arachidonic acid. AS, arachidonoyl-CoA synthetase; AT, arachidonoyl transferase; CO, cyclo-oxygenase; LO, lipoxygenase

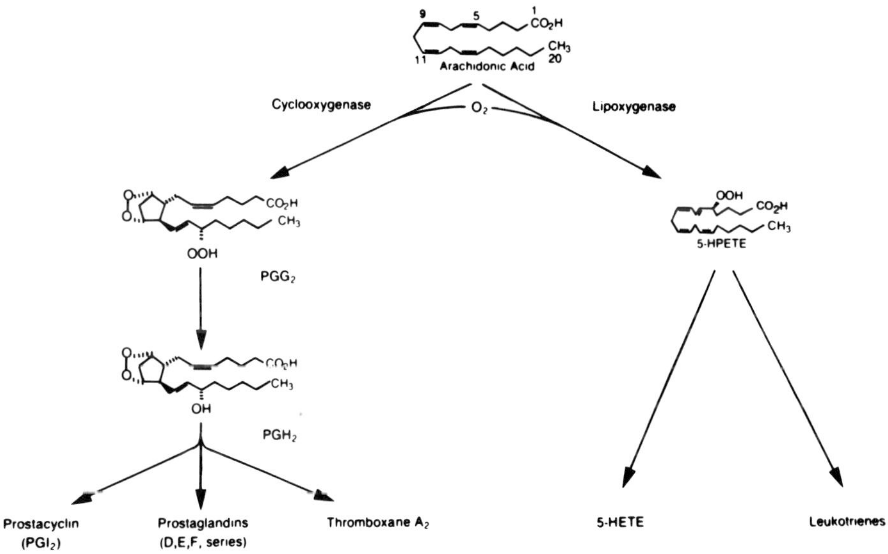

Figure 5 Scheme of mediator synthesis from arachidonic acid

oxy-eicosatetraenoic acid (5-HETE), LTB_4, the lipoxins, and the peptido-leukotrienes. Both mechanisms have been found to be operative in macrophages, though the extent and the resulting pattern differ depending not only on the kind of stimulation of the cells but also on the type of macrophage and the species from which they are derived. In the liver the major producers of eicosanoids are the Kupffer cells[64]. A small contribution, mainly of thromboxane, prostacyclin and PGE_2, comes from the sinusoidal endothelial cells; hepatocytes do not produce substantial amounts of eicosanoids. None of the eicosanoids has been found to accumulate or to be stored within a macrophage. Furthermore, their half-life in the circulation is short, ranging from seconds for TXA_2 and PGI_2 to minutes for some leukotrienes. Thus, the availability of these signal substances depends on their synthesis on demand.

The *cyclo-oxygenase* contains two separate activities: that of a prostaglandin endoperoxide (PGG_2) synthase and of a peroxidase converting PGG_2 to PGH_2. The enzyme is activated by hydroperoxides and inhibited by some non-steroidal anti-inflammatory drugs such as aspirin or indomethacin. PGH_2 can be converted to prostaglandins D_2, E_2 and $F_{2\alpha}$, to prostacyclin and to thromboxane A_2 by specific, well-characterized enzymes (Figure 6). A side-product of cyclo-oxygenase activity is hydroxy-heptatrienoic acid (HHT), whose formation is greatly augmented in the presence of heme compounds.

Synthesis of these compounds requires stimulation of the macrophage. In most instances, e.g. phagocytosis, phorbol ester or Ca^{2+} ionophore treatment, the regulated step seems to be the provision of substrate (arachidonate) rather than the conversion of arachidonate. This follows from the fact that a sufficient supply of free arachidonate leads to the same prostaglandins as zymosan stimulation. Lipopolysaccharides and some viruses, however, influence directly[65] the activity of the isomerase converting PGH_2 to PGE_2. Topological factors such as the proximity of enzymes providing and consuming certain intermediates may also lead to specific effects on individual steps of the cyclo-oxygenase pathway. In rat Kupffer cells stimulated by phagocytosis, intracellular Ca^{2+} elevation or phorbol ester the major eicosanoid formed is PGD_2, but thromboxane and PGE_2 are also seen[65]. In the presence of free arachidonate the prostaglandins are still formed, but

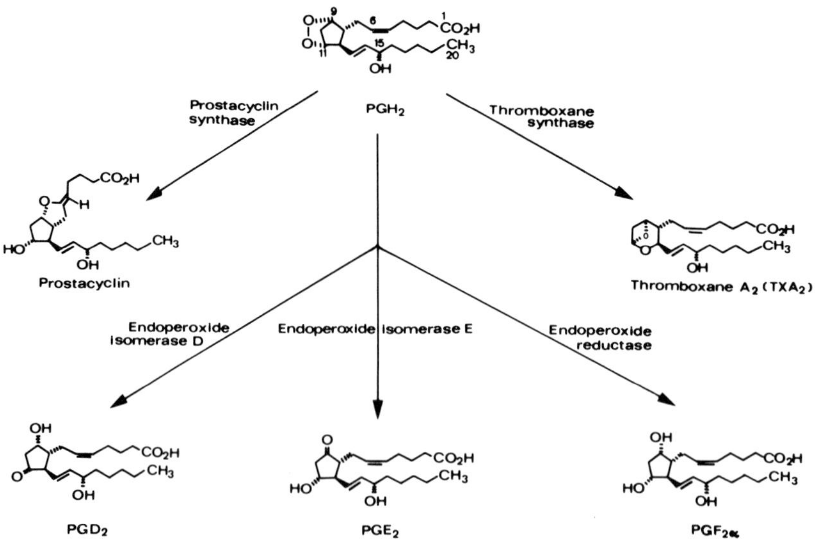

Figure 6 Conversion of PGH_2 to metabolically active prostanoids

thromboxane is absent from the released products[63]. Exposure to LPS, on the other hand, increases dramatically the amount of PGE_2 synthesized without affecting the rate of PGD_2 and thromboxane production[17].

The effects of the prostanoids are manifold. They are mediated by specific receptors on target cells and reflect the kind of signal-transducing path and the responsive enzyme outfit of the recipient cell rather than the prostanoid itself. With regard to macrophages, the self-stimulation with PGE_2 deserves attention. This prostaglandin elicits in rat Kupffer cells the stimulated production of cAMP followed, e.g., by an increased collagenase synthesis[29]. It also inhibits quite specifically the LPS-induced synthesis of TNF-α[66]. In hepatocytes it increases the glycogenolytic activity, though not as much as thromboxane A_2 which was shown to be responsible for about 80% of the PMA-triggered effect in the perfused liver[67]. Prostaglandins are also produced in the brain; PGD_2 was identified as a potent sleep-evoking substance antagonizing PGE_2 and thereby participating in the sleep/wake cycle[68].

The second route of arachidonate metabolism is initiated by peroxidation catalysed by lipoxygenases (for review see ref. 69). Various C-atoms of the unsaturated fatty acid can be targets of the position-specific enzymes, e.g. the 5-, 11-, 12-, 13-, or 15-position. The most important of these reaction products are those synthesized by the ATP- and Ca^{2+}-dependent 5-lipoxygenase (Figure 7). This enzyme is most abundant in leucocytes and neutrophils, but is also present in monocytes and macrophages such as peritoneal macrophages. It may be isolated from the cytosolic compartment of the cells but gains its full activity only after attachment to membrane components. The first product of the enzyme, 5-HPETE, can be converted to three different products:

1. reduction by glutathione leads to 5-HETE, which is a powerful chemoattractant and a typical product of neutrophilic granulocytes.
2. using 15-HPETE as a substrate 5-lipoxygenase can introduce another hydroperoxy group that finally rearranges to 5,6,15- or 5,14,15-trihydroxy-eicosatetraenoic acids, called *lipoxins* (A_4 and B_4, respectively). Alveolar macrophages[70] have been shown as source of these compounds that are able to trigger superoxide formation and degranulation in human neutrophils.
3. 5-Lipoxygenase may convert 5-HPETE to the 5,6-epoxy derivative, leukotriene A_4. This compound is either converted by a specific hydrolase to leukotriene B_4 (LTB_4), a strong chemotactic and adhesions-promoting factor of granulocytes and macrophages, or to leukotriene C_4 (LTC_4) by the transferase-catalysed reaction with glutathione. The latter process occurs readily in stimulated mast cells, leucocytes and monocytes. Peritoneal and some other macrophages are also able to synthesize significant amounts of peptido-leukotrienes[71].

γ-Glutamyl transferase rapidly converts LTC_4 to LTD_4; a peptidase may further split off the glycine residue to form LTE_4. *N*-acetylation of that compound is a common though not necessary step in the inactivation and removal of the peptido-leukotrienes; it occurs in hepatocytes and allows the elimination of a substantial part of these mediators through the bile[72].

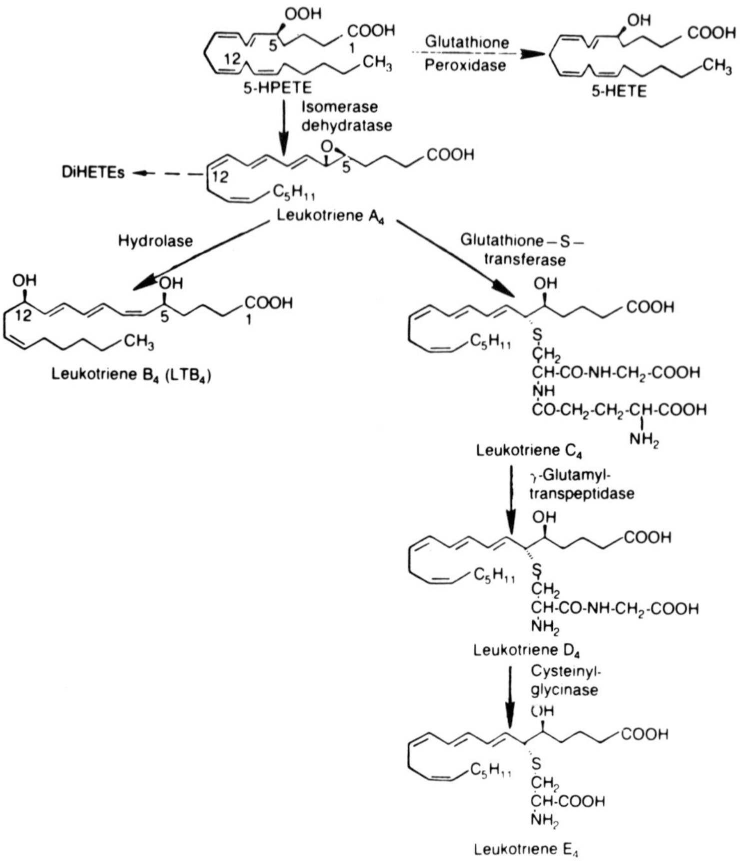

Figure 7 The 5-lipoxygenase pathway

The peptido-leukotrienes were first recognized as the 'slow-reacting substance' of anaphylaxis. More recently they were shown to be important secondary mediators of endotoxin-triggered shock[73,74]. Vaso- and bronchoconstriction, enhanced vascular permeability and the activation of leucocytes, granulocytes and macrophages are prominent features of their action spectrum. Receptors for LTC_4 and LTD_4 have been identified on many supposed target cells; receptor antagonists such as FPL 55712 or MK 886[75] proved very helpful in elucidating the role of these signal molecules.

The platelet-activating factor (PAF)

Activation and aggregation of thrombocytes under the influence of products from activated leucocytes was first reported in 1971. It turned out that the active agent was a lipid of the phosphoglyceride class (for review see ref. 76); its characteristics are the ether bond between the 1-position and a long-chain (C_{13}–C_{18}) alkyl residue, the short-chain (usually acetyl) fatty acid esterified to the 2-position and a phosphodiester bond with phosphorylcholine on C_3 of the glycerol backbone (Figure 8).

Neutrophils stimulated sequentially with cytochalasin B and the Ca^{2+} ionophore A 23187 or *N*-formyl-Met-Leu-Phe seem to be the best source of PAF. But basophils, endothelial cells, platelets and macrophages were also shown to produce this lipid mediator upon stimulation. Macrophages are known to contain relatively large amounts of plasmalogens. PAF synthesis appears to follow mainly the route from plasmalogens (1-alkyl-2-(long-chain)acyl phosphorylcholine through PLA_2-catalysed lyso-PAF formation and reacylation of the 2-position with acetyl-CoA by a specific Ca^{2+}-dependent lyso-PAF acetyltransferase.

The biological activity of PAF is most likely mediated by cell surface-integrated receptors; however, isolation and physicochemical characterization has not yet been reported. PAF elicits the release of vasoactive amines from thrombocytes and the aggregation of platelets with themselves and also with endothelial cells. The strong lytic activity of lyso-PAF may take part in these events. PAF was also shown to induce the degranulation of neutrophils and the activation of macrophages to produce superoxide and eicosanoids. Livers perfused with PAF respond with increased release of glucose and an enhanced turnover of phosphoinositides. Hepatocytes, however, do not respond with increased glucose production to PAF; it is likely that the hepatic action of PAF is mediated by the Kupffer cells that have been shown to produce the signal substances required to elicit the observed effects on hepatocytes.

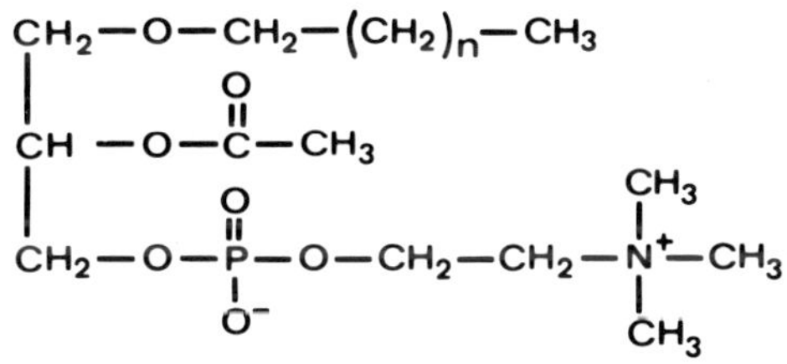

Figure 8 Structure of the platelet-activating factor (PAF)

REGULATION

The fine-tuning of signal action occurs on several levels:

1. regulation of synthesis, of secretion and transport, and of inactivation of the signal;
2. regulation by self-activation or self-destruction of enzymes;
3. regulation of receptor availability (up- or down-regulation) involving synthesis, internalization, degradation and recycling of receptor structures;
4. regulation of the signal transduction paths including G proteins, second messengers, and activation/deactivation of target molecules;

5. regulation of the cell–cell interaction, e.g. signal transmission or autostimulation.

The regulation of the cytokine/prostaglandin signal system may serve as an example: TNF-α and other cytokines are produced by macrophages after exposure to lipopolysaccharides and interferon-γ. Although gene expression following stimulation increases only about threefold, mRNA levels may reach up to 1% of all messenger RNAs and the extracellular cytokine will become the major secreted protein[55]. On the other hand, macrophages from LPS-resistant mice can form high levels of mRNA after LPS but hardly secrete any TNF-α. Their synthesis is controlled partly at the post-transcriptional level involving an untranslated, U,A-rich extension of the mRNA at the 3′-end[77]. This region is thought to shorten the half-life of the mRNA; as a corollary to this instability one would expect that activation of the cells that leads to a rapid onset of cytokine production should also remove or suppress this element. The finding[15] that inhibitors of the elicited TNF-α synthesis in rat Kupffer cells such as dexamethasone prevent cytokine formation even when given simultaneously with LPS point in the same direction. PGE_2 suppresses the synthesis of TNF-α but not that of IL-6[50]. It is remarkable that PGE_2 production in Kupffer cells is stimulated by LPS and by TNF-α[59] to the same extent; the PGE_2 level after exposure to LPS is several times higher than that after zymosan or PMA stimulation, indicating a regulated event at the level of the PGH_2 metabolizing enzymes[65]. Furthermore, PGE_2 inhibits its own production in LPS- but not in TNF-α-elicited cells. It is evident that the intricate interaction of TNF-α and PGE_2 forms a self-limiting regulatory cycle (Figure 9) that may explain the kinetics of both the TNF-α and PGE_2 production.

The key enzymes of the arachidonate cascade, prostaglandin H synthase and lipoxygenase, serve as examples of regulation by self-activation and self-destruction, respectively (for review see ref. 69). Hydroperoxides, including initial products of the cyclo-oxygenase reaction, act as activators of the reaction. The phenomenon can be seen in the acceleration of the initial sluggish reaction to its maximal velocity; the latter can be obtained immediately if hydroperoxy fatty acids are added to the reaction mixture. Inversely, the highly reactive intermediates of the lipoxygenase reaction – the same is true for the thromboxane synthase – inactivate the enzyme by oxidation of some of its amino acid side chains (such as methionine)[78].

Regulation at the receptor level has been documented quite clearly for the IL-6 receptor (for review see ref. 10). IL-6 is the most potent stimulator known for the elicitation of acute-phase protein synthesis in hepatocytes. Little mRNA for this receptor is found in quiescent parenchymal cells; however, after exposure to glucocorticoid hormones its intracellular level is greatly enhanced. This observation seems to explain the permissive effect of these hormones in the acute-phase response. IL-6 receptors are also found on blood monocytes; their synthesis is repressed by LPS that induces IL-6 formation and also down-regulated by IL-6 and IL-1; thus, self-stimulation of the monocytes by their own products is prevented. In the normal situation IL-6 receptors are present on monocytes and on hepatocytes, but in the

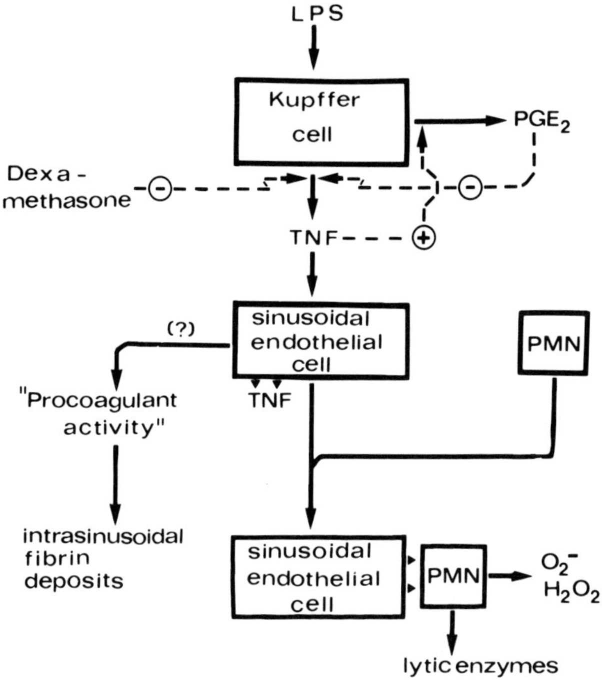

Figure 9 Regulation of TNF and PGE_2 action in rat Kupffer cells

inflammatory state they are low in monocytes and high in hepatocytes (and also in B cells). A case of positive autocrine cooperation was observed in multiple myeloma cells: here, IL-6 is a growth factor for the cells which produce at the same time the IL-6 receptor.

Most of the regulatory phenomena in the world of signal transmission involve more than one cell type, although autocrine stimulations and inhibitions are also known. In a compact organ such as the liver, the interplay of parenchymal and non-parenchymal cells can be expected to be an important event in the functional regulation of the whole organ. As an example the various influences between liver macrophages and hepatocytes may be mentioned. IL-6 that is produced upon exposure to inflammatory substances (LPS, viruses) by the Kupffer cells in the neighbourhood of the parenchymal cells elicits the production of the anti-inflammatory acute-phase proteins[79]. At the same time, thromboxane and PGE_2 triggered by the same stimuli increase the rate of glycogenolysis, thereby supplying the hepatocytes and other cells with the energy-providing substrate, glucose.

On the other hand, hepatocytes do not produce hormones and mediators but respond to many of them; they also inactivate most of these substances and serve in this way the signal character of the mediators. This became clearly evident when it was found that in the liver eicosanoids are synthesized by the non-parenchymal sinus-lining cells, mainly by the Kupffer cells, while the inactivation, degradation and elimination (into bile) is almost exclusively done by the hepatocytes[80]. There are also strong indications for an important interaction between Kupffer cells and fat-storing (Ito) cells in their transformation into collagen-producing fibroblast-like cells in the course of liver fibrosis[81].

References

1. Walker, W. S. (1976). Functional heterogeneity of macrophages. In Nelson, S. W. (ed.), *Immunobiology of the Macrophage*, pp. 91–111. (New York, San Francisco, London: Academic Press)
2. Gordon, S., Crocker, P. R., Morris, L., Lee, S. H., Perry, V. H. and Hume, D. A. (1986). Localisation and function of tissue macrophages. In Ciba Foundation Symposium 118, *Biochemistry of Macrophages*, pp. 54–67. (London: Pitman)
3. Ezekowitz, R. A. B. and Gordon, S. (1986). Interaction and regulation of macrophage receptors. In Ciba Foundation Symposium 118, *Biochemistry of Macrophages*, pp. 127–36. (London: Pitman)
4. Latocha, G., Dieter, P., Schulze-Specking, A. and Decker, K. (1989). F_c receptors mediate prostaglandin and superoxide synthesis in cultured rat Kupffer cells. *Biol. Chem. Hoppe-Seyler*, **370**, 1055–61
5. Stahl, P. and Gordon, S. (1982). Expression of a mannosyl–fucosyl receptor for endocytosis on cultured primary macrophages and their hybrids. *J. Cell Biol.*, **93**, 49–56
6. Kolb, H. and Kolb-Bachofen, V. (1978). A lectin-like receptor on mammalian macrophages. *Biochem. Biophys. Res. Commun.*, **85**, 678–83
7. Vlassara, H. and Brownlee, M., as quoted by Marx, J. L. (1988). Cytokines are two-edged swords in disease. *Science*, **239**, 257–8
8. Springer, T. A. and Anderson, D. C. (1986). The importance of the Mac-1, LFA-1 glycoprotein family in monocyte and granulocyte adherence, chemotaxis, and migration into inflammatory sites: insights from an experiment of nature. In Ciba Foundation Symposium 118, *Biochemistry of Macrophages*, pp. 102–26. (London: Pitman)
9. Nathan, C. F. (1986). General discussion. In Ciba Foundation Symposium 118, *Biochemistry of Macrophages*, p. 232. (London: Pitman)
10. Bauer, J. (1989). Interleukin-6 and its receptor during homeostasis, inflammation and tumor growth. *Klin. Wochenschr.*, **67**, 697–706
11. Celada, A., Gray, P. W., Rinderknecht, E. and Schreiber, R. D. (1984). Evidence for a gamma-interferon receptor that regulates macrophage tumoricidal activity. *J. Exp. Med.*, **160**, 55–74
12. Kishimoto, T. (1987). B-cell stimulatory factors (BSFs). Molecular structure, biological function, and regulation of expression. *J. Clin. Immunol.*, **7**, 343–55
13. Russell, S. W. and Pace, J. L. (1987). The effects of interferons on macrophages and their precursors. *Vet. Immunol. Imunopathol.*, **15**, 129–65
14. Oldham, R. K. (1983). Biological response modifiers. *J. Natl. Canc. Inst.*, **70**, 789–96
15. Adams, D. O. and Hamilton, T. A. (1984). The cell biology of macrophage activation. *Ann. Rev. Immunol.*, **2**, 283–318
16. Decker, T., Lohmann-Matthes, M.-L., Karck, U., Peters, T. and Decker, K. (1989). Cytotoxicity, tumor necrosis factor, and prostaglandin release after stimulation: an interspecies comparison of rat Kupffer cells, murine Kupffer cells and murine inflammatory liver macrophages. *J. Leukocyte Biol.*, **45**, 139–47
17. Karck, U., Peters, T. and Decker, K. (1988). The release of tumor necrosis factor from endotoxin-stimulated rat Kupffer cells is regulated by prostaglandin E_2 and dexamethasone. *J. Hepatol.*, **7**, 352–61
18. Freudenberg, M. A., Freudenberg, N. and Galanos, C. (1982). Time course of cellular distribution of endotoxin in liver, lungs and kidneys of rats. *Br. J. Exp. Pathol.*, **63**, 56–65
19. Freudenberg, M. A. and Galanos, C. (1985). Alterations in rats *in vivo* of the chemical structure of lipopolysaccharide from *Salmonella abortus equi*. *Eur. J. Biochem.*, **152**, 353–9

20. Fox, E. S., Thomas, P. and Broitman, S. A. (1989). Clearance of gut-derived endotoxins by the liver. Release and modification of ^{3}H, ^{14}C-lipopolysaccharide by isolated rat Kupffer cells. *Gastroenterology*, **96**, 456–61
21. Aderem, A. A. (1988). Protein myristoylation as an intermediate step during signal transduction in macrophages: its role in arachidonic acid metabolism and in responses to interferon gamma. *J. Cell Sci. Suppl.*, **9**, 151–67
22. Nathan, C. F. and Tsunawaki, S. (1986). Secretion of toxic oxygen products by macrophages: regulatory cytokines and their effects on the oxidase. In Ciba Foundation Symposium 118, *Biochemistry of Macrophages*, pp. 211–30. (London: Pitman)
23. Aderem, A. A. and Cohn, Z. A. (1986). Bacterial lipopolysaccharides modify signal transduction in the arachidonic acid cascade of macrophages. In Ciba Foundation Symposium 118, *Biochemistry of Macrophages*, pp. 196–210. (London: Pitman)
24. Birmelin, M., Karck, U., Dieter, P., Freudenberg, N. and Decker, K. (1986). Distribution of endotoxin and endotoxin-stimulated prostanoid production in primary cultures of rat Kupffer cells. In Kirn, A., Knook, D. L. and Wisse, E. (eds), *Cells of the Hepatic Sinusoid*, Vol. 1, pp. 295–300 (Rijswijk: Kupffer Cell Foundation).
25. Introna, M., Hamilton, T. A., Kaufman, R. E., Adams, D. O. and Bast, R. C. (1986). Treatment of murine peritoneal macrophages with bacterial lipopolysaccharide alters expression of c-fos and c-myc oncogenes. *J. Immunol.*, **137**, 2711–15
26. Tran-Thi, T.-A., Häussinger, D., Gyufko, K. and Decker, K. (1988). Stimulation of prostaglandin release by Ca^{2+}-mobilizing agents from the perfused rat liver. A comparative study of the action of ATP, UTP, phenylephrine, vasopressin and nerve stimulation. *Biol. Chem. Hoppe-Seyler*, **369**, 65–8
27. Gordon, J. L. (1986). Extracellular ATP: effects, sources, fate. *Biochem. J.*, **233**, 309–19
28. Gilman, A. G. (1987). G proteins: transducers of receptor-generated signals. *Ann. Rev. Biochem.*, **56**, 615–49
29. Bhatnagar, R., Schade, U., Rietschel, Th. E. and Decker, K. (1982). Involvement of prostaglandin E and cyclic adenosine 3′,5′-monophosphate in lipopolysaccharide-stimulated collagenase release by rat Kupffer cells. *Eur. J. Biochem.*, **125**, 125–130
30. Birmelin, M. and Decker, K. (1984). Synthesis of prostanoids and cyclic nucleotides by phagocytosing rat Kupffer cells. *Eur. J. Biochem.*, **142**, 219–25
31. Nitta, T., Saito-Taki, T. and Suzuki, T. (1984). Phospholipase A_2 activity of $F_{c\gamma 2b}$ receptors of thioglycollate-elicited murine peritoneal macrophages. *J. Leukocyte Biol.*, **36**, 493–504
32. Nagata, Y., Rosen, O. M., Makman, M. H. and Bloom, B. R. (1984). Biochemical analysis of mutants of a macrophage cell line resistant to the growth-inhibitory activity of interferon. *J. Cell Biol.*, **98**, 1342–7
33. Wakelam, M. J. O., Davies, S. A., Houslay, M. D., McKay, I., Marshall, C. J. and Hall, A. (1986). Normal $p21^{N-ras}$ couples bombesin and other growth factor receptors to inositol phosphate production. *Nature (Lond.)*, **323**, 173–6
34. Lassing, I. and Lindberg, U. (1985). Specific interaction between phosphatidylinositol 4,5-biphosphate and profilactin. *Nature (Lond.)*, **314**, 472–4
35. Berridge, M. J. (1987). Inositol trisphosphate and diacylglycerol: two interacting second messengers. *Ann. Rev. Biochem.*, **56**, 159–93
36. Dieter, P., Schulze-Specking, A. and Decker, K. (1988). Ca^{2+} requirement for prostanoid but not for superoxide production by rat Kupffer cells. *Eur. J. Biochem.*, **177**, 61–7
37. Carafoli, E. (1987). Intracellular calcium homeostasis. *Ann. Rev. Biochem.*, **56**, 395–433
38. Birmelin, M. and Decker, K. (1983). Ca^{2+} flux as an initial event in phagocytosis by rat Kupffer cells. *Eur. J. Biochem.*, **131**, 539–43
39. Dieter, P., Schulze-Specking, A., Karck, U. and Decker, K. (1987). Prostaglandin release but not superoxide production by rat Kupffer cells in vitro depends on Na^{+}/H^{+} exchange. *Eur. J. Biochem.*, **170**, 201–6
40. Palmer, R. M., Ferrige, A. G. and Moncada, S. (1987). Nitric oxide accounts for the biological activity of endothelium-derived relaxing factor. *Nature (Lond.)*, **327**, 524–6
41. Marletta, M. A., Yoon, P. S., Iyengar, R., Leaf, C. D. and Wishnock, J. S. (1988). Macrophage oxidation of L-arginine to nitrite and nitrate: nitric oxide is an intermediate. *Biochemistry*, **27**, 8706–11
42. Dieter, P., Schulze-Specking, A., Karck, U. and Decker, K. (1988). Release of lysosomal enzymes is not correlated with superoxide and prostaglandin production by stimulated rat

Kupffer cells in primary culture. *J. Hepatol.*, **6**, 167–74
43. Dinarello, C. A. (1984) Interleukin-1 and the pathogenesis of the acute-phase response. *N. Engl. J. Med.*, **311**, 1413–18
44. Fontana, A., McAdam, K. P. W. J., Kristensen, F. and Weber, E. (1983). Biological and biochemical characterization of an interleukin 1-like factor from rat C_6 glioma cells. *Eur. J. Immunol.*, **13**, 685–9
45. Mizel, S. B. and Mizel, D. (1981). Purification to apparent homogeneity of murine interleukin 1. *J. Immunol.*, **126**, 834–7
46. Dalboge, H., Bayne, S., Christensen, T. and Hejnaes, K. R. (1989) Cloning and expression of an interleukin-1β precursor and its conversion to interleukin-1β. *FEBS Lett.*, **246**, 89–93
47. Spinas, G. A., Hansen, B. S., Linde, S., Kastern, W., Molvig, J., Mandrup-Poulsen, Dinarello, C. A., Nielsen, J. H. and Nerup, J. (1987). Interleukin 1 dose-dependently affects the biosynthesis of (pro)insulin in isolated rat islets of Langerhans. *Diabetologia*, **30**, 474–80
48. Bauer, J., Ganter, U., Geiger, T., Jacobshagen, U., Hirano, T., Matsuda, T., Kishimoto, T., Andus, T., Acs, G., Gerok, W. and Ciliberto, G. (1988). Regulation of interleukin-6 expression in cultured human blood monocytes and monocyte-derived macrophages. *Blood*, **72**, 1134–40
49. Busam, K., Bauer, T., Bauer, J., Gerok, W. and Decker, K. (1989). Regulation of interleukin-6 secretion by rat Kupffer cells. *J. Hepatol.*, **9** (Suppl. 1), S13
50. Aarden, L., Lansdorp, P. and De Groot, E. (1985). A growth factor for B cell hybridomas produced by human monocytes. *Lymphokines*, **10**, 175–85
51. Pestka, S. and Langer, J. A. (1987). Interferons and their action. *Ann. Rev. Biochem.*, **56**, 727–77
52. Havell, E. A. and Spitalny, G. L. (1983). Endotoxin-induced interferon synthesis in macrophage cultures. *J. Reticuloendothel. Soc.*, **33**, 369–76
53. Kirn, A., Koehren, F. and Steffan, M. A. (1982). Interferon synthesis in primary cultures of Kupffer and endothelial cells from the rat liver. *Hepatology*, **2**, 670–9
54. Werner-Wasik, M., von Muenchhausen, W., Nolan, J. P. and Cohen. S. A. (1989). Endogeneous interferon α/β produced by murine Kupffer cells augments liver-associated natural killing activity. *Cancer Immunol. Immunother.*, **28**, 107–15
55. Beutler, B. and Cerami, A. (1988). Cachectin (tumor necrosis factor): a macrophage hormone governing cellular metabolism and inflammatory response. *Endocrine Rev.*, **9**, 57–66
56. Beutler, B., Greenwald, D., Hulmes, J. D., Chang, M., Pan, Y.-C. E., Mathison, J., Ulevich, R. and Cerami, A. (1985). Identity of tumor necrosis factor and the macrophage-secreted cachectin. *Nature* (*Lond.*), **316**, 552–4
57. Schlayer, H. J., Laaf, H., Peters, T., Woort-Menker, M., Estler, C., Karck, U., Schaefer, H. E. and Decker, K. (1988). Involvement of tumor necrosis factor in endotoxin-triggered neutrophil adherence to sinusoidal endothelial cells and its modulation in acute phase. *J. Hepatol.*, **7**, 239–49
58. Bachwich, P. R., Chensue, S. W., Larrick, J. W. and Kunkel, S. L. (1986). Tumor necrosis factor stimulates interleukin-1 and prostaglandin E_2 production in resting macrophages. *Biochem. Biophys. Res. Commun.*, **136**, 94–101
59. Peters, T. and Decker, K. (1989). Recombinant mouse tumor necrosis factor alpha induces prostaglandin E_2 synthesis in rat Kupffer cells. In Wisse, E., Knook, D. L. and Decker, K. (eds), *Cells of the Hepatic Sinusoid*, Vol. II, pp. 182–5. (Rijswijk: Kupffer Cell Foundation)
60. Decker, T., Lohmann-Matthes, M.-L. and Gifford, G. E. (1987). Cell-associated tumor necrosis factor (TNF) as a killing mechanism of activated cytotoxic macrophages. *J. Immunol.*, **138**, 957–62
61. Ruddle, N. H., Powell, M. B. and Conta, B. S. (1983). Lymphotoxin, a biologically relevant model lymphokine. *Lymphokine Res.*, **2**, 23–9
62. Knighton, D. R., Hunt, T. K., Scheuenstuhl, H., Halliday, B. J., Werb, Z. and Banda, M. J. (1983). Oxygen tension regulates the expression of angiogenesis factor by macrophages. *Science* (*Wash DC*), **221**, 1283–5
63. Dieter, P., Peters, T., Schulze-Specking, A. and Decker, K. (1989). Independent regulation of thromboxane and prostaglandin synthesis in liver macrophages. *Biochem. Pharmacol.*, **38**, 1577–81
64. Decker, K. (1987). Eicosanoids as signal molecules between hepatocytes and sinusoidal

cells. In Reutter, W., Popper, H., Arias, I. M., Heinrich, P. C., Keppler, D. and Landmann, L. (eds), *Modulation of Liver Cell Expression*, pp. 397–409. (Lancaster: MTP Press)

65. Grewe, M., to be published
66. Kunkel, S. L., Spengler, M., May, M. A., Spengler, R., Larrick, J. and Remick, D. (1988). Prostaglandin E_2 regulates macrophage-derived tumor necrosis factor gene expression. *J. Biol. Chem.*, **263**, 5380–4
67. Tran-Thi, T.-A., Gyufko, K., Reinke, M. and Decker, K. (1988). Output and effects of thromboxane produced by the liver perfused with phorbol myristate acetate. *Biol. Chem. Hoppe-Seyler*, **369**, 1179–84
68. Hayaishi, O. (1988). Sleep–wake regulation by prostaglandins D_2 and E_2. *J. Biol. Chem.*, **263**, 14593–6
69. Needleman, P., Turk, J., Jakschik, B. A., Morrison, A. R. and Lefkowith, J. B. (1986). Arachidonic acid metabolism. *Ann. Rev. Biochem.*, **55**, 69–102
70. Kim, S. J. (1988). Formation of lipoxins by alveolar macrophages. *Biochem. Biophys. Res. Commun.*, **150**, 870–6
71. Lüderitz, T., Schade, U. and Rietschel, E. Th. (1986). Formation and metabolism of leukotriene C_4 in macrophages exposed to lipopolysaccharide. *Eur. J. Biochem.*, **155**, 377–82
72. Hagmann, W., Denzlinger, C., Rapp, S., Weckbecker, G. and Keppler, D. (1986). Identification of the major endogenous leukotriene metabolite in the bile of rats as *N*-acetyl leukotriene E_4. *Prostaglandins*, **31**, 239–51
73. Leffer, A. M. (1986). Leukotrienes as mediators of ischemia and shock. *Biochem. Pharmacol.*, **33**, 123–7
74. Keppler, D., Hagmann, W. and Rupp, S. (1987). Role of leukotrienes in endotoxin action in vivo. *Rev. Infect. Dis.*, **9**, S580–4
75. Gillard, J., Ford-Hutchinson, A. W., Chan, C., Charleson, S., Denis, D., Foster, A., Fortin, R., Leger, S., McFarlane, C. S., Morton, H., Piechuta, H., Riendeau, D., Rouzer, C., Rokach, J., Young, R., MacIntyre, D. E., Peterson, L., Bach, T., Eiermann, G., Hopple, S., Humes, J., Hupe, L., Luell, S., Metzger, J., Meurer, R., Miller, D. K., Opas, E. and Pacholok, S. (1989). MK 886 (3-1-(4-chlorobenzyl)-3-*t*-butyl-thio-5-isopropylindol-2-yl-2,2-dimethylpropanoic acid), a novel, orally active leukotriene biosynthesis inhibitor. *Canad. J. Physiol. Pharmacol.*, **67**, 456–64
76. Hanahan, D. J., (1986). Platelet activating factor: a biologically active phosphoglyceride. *Ann. Rev. Biochem.*, **55**, 483–509
77. Caput, D., Beutler, B., Hartog, K., Brown-Shimer, S. and Cerami, A. (1986). Identification of a common nucleotide sequence in the 3′-untranslated region of mRNA molecules specifying inflammatory mediators. *Proc. Natl. Acad. Sci. USA*, **83**, 1670–4
78. Rapoport, S., Härtel, B. and Hausdorf, G. (1984). Methionine sulfoxide formation: the cause of self-inactivation of reticulocyte lipoxygenase. *Eur. J. Biochem.*, **139**, 573–6
79. Andus, T., Geiger, T., Hirano, T., Kishimoto, T., Tran-Thi, T.-A., Decker, K. and Heinrich, P. C. (1988). Regulation of synthesis and secretion of major rat acute-phase proteins by recombinant human interleukin-6 in hepatocyte primary cultures. *Eur. J. Biochem.*, **173**, 287–93
80. Tran-Thi, T.-A., Gyufko, K., Henninger, H. P., Busse, R. and Decker, K. (1987). Studies in synthesis and degradation of eicosanoids by rat hepatocytes in primary culture. *J. Hepatol.*, **5**, 322–31
81. Tanaka, M. and Ishikawa, E. (1986). Histochemical study on the correlation between fat-storing cells, macrophages and lymphocytes in fibrotic lesion occurring after fulminant hepatitis. In Kirn, A., Knook, D. E. and Wisse, E. (eds), *Cells of the Hepatic Sinusoid*, Vol. I, pp. 259–62. (Rijswijk: Kupffer Cell Foundation)

5
The humoral immune response and the complement system in infections of the liver

H. C. THOMAS

As well as the specific humoral immune response to the agent infecting the liver, there are changes in the humoral immune system that occur as a result of acute or chronic liver damage. Hyperglobulinaemia[1–3] and depressed cell-mediated immunity[2–4] are common to most forms of chronic liver disease and it seems probable that these changes are a result of liver damage. This is supported by the observation that some of the changes can be induced in animals when they are rendered cirrhotic.

INFLUENCE OF LIVER DISEASE ON THE HUMORAL IMMUNE RESPONSE

Phagocytic function is markedly altered in patients with hepatic cirrhosis[3,5,6]. This results in changes in antigen distribution[5], which is a major factor in determining the characteristics of the ensuing humoral and cellular immune responses[6].

Antigens enter the circulation from the gastrointestinal tract, the larger ones via the mesenteric lymphatics and the smaller ones via the mesenteric venous circulation[2]. The liver, which is an important phagocytic organ, may therefore receive intestinally derived antigen either directly, via the portal circulation, when it acts as a filter interposed 'in series' with the rest of the body, or it may receive antigen from the systemic circulation via its arterial supply and in this situation acts as a filter 'in parallel'. The hepatic phagocytes render antigens non-immunogenic[5], while splenic and lymph node-derived macrophages serve to enhance immunogenicity. The distribution of antigen between liver and spleen (and other lymphoid organs) will therefore influence the magnitude of the immune response. Diversion of antigen from the liver to the spleen will enhance the immune response[2]. Changes in the phagocytic function of the liver have an effect on both portal and systemic routes of immunization.

Immune complexes are cleared from the portal and systemic blood by the hepatic sinusoidal phagocytes. Large complexes that fix complement are avidly cleared by the liver, whereas smaller complexes, which do not fix complement, are cleared by the spleen[6]. In hepatic cirrhosis these functions are impaired, and complexes accumulate in the plasma. In most cases[7] these complexes do not result in significant activation of C3 and do not cause tissue damage. The composition of such complexes is unknown, but it is likely that they contain food and bacterial antigens derived from the gut.

Endotoxins are phagocytosed and detoxified by the liver: they can be demonstrated in portal blood but not in systemic blood in normal subjects[8]. Endotoxinaemia has been demonstrated during fulminant hepatic failure[9] and in some subjects with established cirrhosis[10], presumably as a result of impaired hepatic clearance of this substance. It is suggested that it plays a significant role in the renal malfunction that often accompanies these diseases[9].

The altered handling of antigen in subjects with hepatic cirrhosis has a significant effect on the humoral immune response[3,5,11]. This is seen most clearly in the response to putative thymus-independent antigens[3,12,13], which are not influenced by changes in cell-mediated immunity that accompany the development of chronic liver disease. It seems probable that the increased *E. coli* titres found in patients with alcohol-induced cirrhosis[12], chronic active liver disease[14] and primary biliary cirrhosis[13] are the result of this phenomenon.

The response to thymus-dependent antigens is more complex, involving the cooperation not only of antigen presenting cells and B lymphocytes but also T lymphocytes. When patients with alcohol-induced cirrhosis, chronic active liver disease or primary biliary cirrhosis were immunized intravenously with the bacteriophage ϕX174, a thymus-dependent antigen, the primary and secondary responses were significantly decreased when compared with the responses of normal subjects[2,15]. In the presence of increased responses to thymus-independent antigens, this implies that the cooperating functions of T cells are reduced so that B cells challenged with thymus-dependent antigens cannot respond to the increased antigenic stimulus.

In addition to the quantitative changes in the humoral response of subjects with hepatic cirrhosis, there are also qualitative changes. In normal subjects, during a secondary response, more than 90% of the antibody is IgG, whereas in patients with primary biliary cirrhosis, chronic active hepatitis and alcohol-induced cirrhosis the percentage of IgM antibody is much increased[2,15]. This relative failure to change from IgM to IgG antibody production during the evolution of the immune response is also compatible with a defect in T cell function.

The relationship of the increased viral antibody titres, which have been described in chronic liver disease[16–20], to altered mononuclear phagocytic function, is more vexed. Small increases in titre to lipoprotein-coated viruses such as herpes simplex, cytomegalovirus and influenza A, are seen in HBsAg-positive and HBsAg-negative chronic active hepatitis[18], alcohol-induced cirrhosis[18] and primary biliary cirrhosis[18], but the 6-fold increase in titre to measles and rubella viruses, seen in lupoid chronic active liver disease, is peculiar to this disease[18]. It seems probable that the 1–2-fold increase in titre to several viruses, which occurs in any type of chronic liver disease, is a reflection of the altered immune function which often occurs after liver injury, but that the specific association of a high titre response to measles and rubella with lupoid chronic active liver disease, is an indication of the presence of an additional diathesis in the immune system of these patients[7].

The cumulative effect of these increased humoral responses is readily seen in the hypergammaglobulinaemia that accompanies any form of experimental[2] or natural chronic liver disease! The fact that this change is probably secondary to alterations in the mononuclear phagocytic system of the liver should not be allowed to direct attention away from the increased IgM of primary biliary cirrhosis, and IgA of alcohol-related disease[21,22] – changes specific to these diseases that may therefore give further clues to their pathogenesis.

An enterohepatic circulation of dimeric IgA, dependent on a receptor (secretory piece) on the hepatocyte membrane, has been described in lower mammals[23]. This mechanism returns dimeric IgA class antibodies to the intestinal microbial flora, back to the upper intestine via the biliary tree and may be important in preventing ascending infection of the lower biliary tract. In man a similar hepatic mechanism is operative[24] but it is the bile ductular cells, and not the hepatocytes, which bear secretory piece and are responsible for this function.

During hepatocyte necrosis and cholestasis, dimeric IgA and secretory IgA, respectively, reflux back into the blood[25,26]. This disruption of the enterohepatic circulation may impair the defence of the biliary tree and upper small intestine.

HUMORAL MECHANISM OF LIVER CELL DAMAGE

Gell and Coombs have described four hypersensitivity reactions in which either a humoral or cell-mediated immune response results in tissue damage[27]. The first three of these involve antibody.

Type I hypersensitivity reactions

These involve the patient developing IgE class antibody which may be beneficial or detrimental to the host. This type of humoral response is common in parasitic infections of the liver. The IgE antibody binds to the surface of platelets, eosinophils and mast cells and then, when the individual is rechallenged, the antigen binds to the IgE antibody fixed to the cell, resulting in degranulation of that cell releasing a variety of molecular mediators. In schistosomiasis, most cells sensitized with IgE anti-schistosome antibody release eosinophil chemotactic factor (ECF) following contact with antigen. The arriving eosinophils attach to the antibody-coated worm via their Fc receptors and act as important effectors in damaging the parasite – a beneficial effect of type 1 hypersensitivity[28]. In other situations (rupture of a hydatid cyst) the degranulation of IgE-sensitized mast cells may release vasoactive factors systemically causing anaphylaxis[28] – a detrimental effect of type I reactivity.

Type II hypersensitivity reactions

These involve IgG class antibodies binding to antigen fixed to cell membranes. Subsequent fixation of either complement or activation of killer cells causes cell damage. These types of response are seen in autoimmune liver disease[29] and also potentially in virus-induced liver disease. In the latter case it is argued that complement fixing IgM or IgG class antibodies binding to viral proteins displayed on the liver cell membrane will activate complement and result in destruction of infected liver cells. The evidence for the involvement of this type of process is limited. Metabolism of C3 has been studied in acute HBV infection and found to be increased[30]. However, the metabolism of albumin is also increased in these patients[30] and it is currently unclear whether the increased consumption of the components of the classical pathway of complement is due to immune fixation of these proteins or to hypercatabolism of all the serum proteins. This problem can be sorted out by examining sera for activation products such as C3b and C3d. This has not been done in either acute HBV or HAV infections. Changes in serum concentrations of complement are insufficient to incriminate activation of the complement system in tissue damage because these are also influenced by changes in synthesis. Many of these proteins are produced in the liver and will fall, therefore, as a consequence of acute or chronic reduction in liver cell mass[31].

Fixation of antibody to infected liver cell membranes may also result in the activation of killer lymphocytes. These cells, which bear Fc receptors, bind to and destroy cells coated in IgG immunoglobulin. This mechanism has been proposed to be operative in autoimmune chronic hepatitis where liver membrane antibodies activate K cells[29]. It is unclear at the present time whether this mechanism has any role in the clearance of virus-infected liver cells. Examination of the inflammatory infiltrate in the livers of patients with acute HBV infection reveals that although the majority of the infiltrating cells are cytotoxic T cells, 15–20% are of the NK/K cell phenotype[32]. These cells may kill infected hepatocytes either directly without antibody coating (non-specific killer (NK) cells) or may bind by interaction with immunoglobulin (K cells). Similar studies have not been done in other acute viral infections of the liver.

Type III hypersensitivity reactions

These occur when antibody and antigen interact, and result in activation of complement in the circulation and in the blood vessel wall. Serum complement normally functions to solubilize immune complexes to prevent their deposition in the vessel walls. In some patients complement deficiency will prevent this solubilization occurring, and under these circumstances immune complex damage may occur. Complement deficiencies have commonly been described in systemic lupus erythematosus, and also in lupoid chronic active hepatitis[31,32] but not in patients with infectious forms of liver disease[31].

Circulating viral or protozoan antigens may bind to antibody and activate complement. This may result in release of chemotactic fragments of complement (C3 and C5) which attract polymorphs and macrophages to the site of immune interaction. These cells then release toxic enzymes which damage the surrounding tissues. It has been proposed that type III hypersensitivity reactions may be involved in the causation of polyarteritis nodosum and membranoproliferative glomerulonephritis associated with chronic HBV infection. In these patients it is argued that viral proteins associated with immunoglobulin deposits in the arterial or glomerular vessel walls, activate complement[30,31] and cause the vascular lesions associated with these diseases.

As far as polyarteritis nodosum is concerned, when this is associated with chronic HBV infection the patient is usually HBe antigen-positive with continuing viraemia. This complication has usually been seen in the first years after HBV infection. It is unclear at the present time whether the viral proteins found at the site of the arterial lesion are involved in the primary pathogenetic process or are deposited merely as a secondary phenomenon, following on from a change in the permeability of the endothelial surface because of some other primary event.

Membranoproliferative glomerulonephritis, when studied in Poland, was found to be specifically associated with chronic HBV infection, whereas proliferative and minimal change nephritis were rarely associated with this infection[35]. This suggested that the viral proteins of chronic HBV were involved in the mediation of the glomerular lesion. Examination of the glomerulae for viral proteins has suggested that HBe antigen is involved rather than the envelope proteins (HBsAg)[36]. The HBe antigen is of low molecular weight (13–17.5 kd) whereas the HBs antigen is usually in particulate form in serum. Early studies in animal models showed that immune complexes containing low molecular weight soluble protein antigens were more likely to be involved in type III hypersensitivity reactions than particulate material, and for this reason the HBe antigen is a strong candidate for involvement in the pathogenesis of these lesions. However, once again it is difficult to rule out the possibility that some other immune reaction is responsible for the initial lesion, and that the HBe antigen diffuses into the arteritic area because of its presence in high concentration in the serum at the time of the alteration in permeability of the endothelium of the arteritic vessels. Other workers have suggested that these lesions are not the result of deposition of a preformed immune complex, but result from deposition of viral proteins on the basement membranes of the glomerular vessels with the subsequent deposition of antibody and complement. The HBe protein is formed by cleavage of a larger molecule by proteases[37]. The aminoterminal end of the molecule forms the HBe antigen and the carboxyl terminus a residual fragment. Serological tests have been designed to detect the HBe antigen; attention has therefore been focused on this fragment of the pre-core/core protein. Assays are not available for the carboxyl fragment;

therefore its role in various disease processes is uncertain. The carboxyl terminus of core is a protamine-like molecule which would associate with the components of basement membranes, and it may be this protein which is deposited in glomerulae and then antibody reaction may follow, causing the glomerular lesion. The involvement of complement in the lesions in these patients is suggested by the demonstration that fractional catabolic rates of Clq and C3 are increased whereas albumin turnover, a measure of general protein catabolism, is normal[30,32]. The causative relationship of the lesions to chronic HBV infection is strongly supported by data showing that when the HBV infection is treated the arteritic process subsides[34].

The modulation of type IV hypersensitivity responses by antibody

Cytotoxic T-cells recognize degraded viral peptides transported to the surface of the infected cell with MHC class I proteins. The viral proteins which are involved in this reaction are usually internal rather than envelope structures. In addition, the epitopes recognized by the cell-mediated immune response are linear non-conformational epitopes, whereas those recognized by the humoral immune response are usually conformational. It is of some importance that these two limbs of the immune system recognize different epitopes so that the antibody response does not block the cytotoxic T cell killing process. In chronic HBV infection, experiments with autologous HBV-infected hepatocytes have shown that the nucleocapsid protein is a target of the cytotoxic T cell response and rather anomalously the antibodies to the nucleocapsid epitopes block the T cell killing process[38]. This may be the reason why these patients have developed chronic HBV infection. These results have been confirmed *in vivo* by the injection of monoclonal anti-HBc and anti-HBe into chimpanzees: on challenge these animals developed protracted HBV infection[38]. This appears to be the *in vivo* counterpart of the *in vitro* antibody blocking experiment.

SUMMARY

The humoral immune response is altered in patients with acute and chronic liver damage, probably because of changes in the phagocytic functions of Kupffer cells and because of an accumulation in serum of gut-derived molecules such as lipopolysaccharides. In addition there are specific humoral immune responses to the constituent proteins of microbial agents infecting the liver, and some examples of how these are involved either in protection against infection, or in mediation of liver damage, have been drawn from parasitic and viral infection of the liver.

References

1. Feizi, T. (1968). Immunoglobulins in chronic liver disease. *Gut*, **9**, 193
2. Thomas, H. C. (1977). The role of the liver in immunological disease. *Proc. Roy. Soc. Med.*, **70**, 521

3. Triger, D. *et al.* (1972). Bacterial and dietary antibodies in liver diseases. *Lancet*, **1**, 60
4. Thomas, H. C. *et al.* (1976). The immune response in cirrhotic rats: antigen distribution, humoral immunity, cell-mediated immunity and splenic suppressor cell activity. *Clin. Exp. Immunol.*, **26**, 574
5. Thomas, H. C. *et al.* (1973). The role of the liver in controlling the immunogenicity of commensal bacteria in the gut. *Lancet*, **1**, 1288
6. Thomas, H. C. and Vaez-Zadeh, F. (1974). A homeostatic mechanism for the removal of antigen from the portal circulation. *Immunology*, **26**, 375
7. Munoz, L. E. *et al.* (1982). Complement activation in chronic liver disease. *Clin. Exp. Immunol.*, **47**, 548
8. Braude, A. I. *et al.* (1955). Studies with radioactive endotoxin. 2. Correlation of physiological effects with distribution of radioactivity in rabbits injected with lethal doses of *E. coli* endotoxin labelled with radioactive sodium chromate. *J. Clin. Invest.*, **34**, 858
9. Wilkinson, S. P. *et al.* (1974). Relationship of renal impairment and haemorrhagic diathesis to endotoxemia in fulminant hepatic failure. *Lancet*, **1**, 521
10. Liehr, H. *et al.* (1975). Endotoxemia and liver cirrhosis, treatment with polymixin D. *Lancet*, **2**, 810
11. Souhami, R. L. (1972). The effect of colloidal carbon on the organ distribution of sheep red blood cells and the immune response. *Immunology*, **22**, 685
12. Bjorneboe, M. *et al.* (1972). Antibodies to intestinal microbes in serum of patients with cirrhosis of the liver. *Lancet*, **1**, 58
13. Simjee, A. E. *et al.* (1975). Antibodies *Escherichia coli* in chronic liver disease. *Gut*, **16**, 871
14. Triger, D. R. (1976). Bacterial, viral and autoantibodies in acute and chronic liver disease. *Ann. Clin. Res.*, **8**, 174
15. Thomas, H. C. *et al.* (1976). Immune response to × 174 in man. 5. Primary and secondary antibody production in primary biliary cirrhosis. *Gut*, **17**, 844.
16. Closs, O. (1973). High titres of antibodies against rubella and morbili virus in patients with chronic hepatitis. *Scand. J. Gastroenterol.*, **8**, 523
17. Closs, O. (1971). Raised antibody titres in chronic liver disease. *Lancet*, **2**, 1202.
18. Crimmins, F. B. *et al.* (1980). Viral antibody titres in HBs antigen positive and negative chronic active hepatitis. *Scand. J. Gastroenterol.*, **15**, 107–12
19. Triger, D. R. *et al.* (1972). Raised antibody titres to measles and rubella viruses in chronic active hepatitis. *Lancet*, **1**, 665
20. Thomas, H. C. *et al.* (1975). Measles, rubella and lymphocyte antibodies in chronic active hepatitis. *Clin. Sci. Med.*, **49**, 27
21. Morgan, M. Y. *et al.* (1980). HLA B8., viral antibodies, immunoglobulins and autoantibodies in alcohol related liver disease. *J. Clin. Pathol.*, **33**, 488–95
22. Bjorneboe, M. *et al.* (1970). Tetanus antitoxin production and gamma globulin levels in patients with cirrhosis of the liver. *Acta Med. Scand.*, **188**, 541
23. Orlans, E. *et al.* (1978). Rapid active transport of immunoglobulin A from blood to bile. *J. Exp. Med.*, **147**, 588–92
24. Dooley, J. S., Potter, B. J., Thomas, H. C. and Sherlock, S. (1982). A comparative study of the biliary secretion of human dimeric and monomeric IgA in the rat and in man. *Hepatology*, **2**, 323–7
25. Thompson, R. A., Carter, R., Stokes, R. P. *et al.* (1983). Serum immunoglobulins complement components and autoantibodies in liver disease. *Clin. Exp. Immunol.*, **14**, 335–46
26. Goldblum, R. M., Powell, G. K. and Sickle, G. V. (1980). Secretory IgA in the serum of infants with obstructive jaundice. *J. Paediatr.*, **97**, 33–6
27. Gell, P. G. H. and Coombs, R. (eds) 1968. *Clinical Aspects of Immunology*, Section IV: The allergic state is responsible for clinical hypersensitivity and disease. (Blackwell Scientific Publications, Oxford)
28. Roitt, I. M., Brostoff, J. and Male, D. K. (1986). Hypersensitivity-type 1. In Roitt, I. M. *et al.* (eds), ch. 19. (Churchill Livingstone, Edinburgh)
29. Klingenstein, R. J. and Wands, J. R. (1982). Immunologic effector mechanisms in hepatitis B negative chronic active hepatitis. In Thomas, H. C. (ed.) *Immunological Aspects of Liver Disease*, pp. 39–51. (Springer–Verlag, Berlin)
30. Thomas, H. C., Potter, B. J., Elias, E. and Sherlock, S. (1979). Metabolism of the third component of complement in acute type B Hepatitis, HBs antigen positive glomeru-

lonephritis, polyarteritis nodosum and HBs antigen positive and negative chronic active liver disease. *Gastroenterology*, **76**, 673–87

31. Munoz, L. E., de Villiers, D., Markham, D., Whaley, K. and Thomas, H. C. (1982). Complement activation in chronic liver diseases. *Clin. Exp. Immunol.*, **47**, 548–54
32. Potter, B. J., Elias, E., Thomas, H. C. and Sherlock, S. (1980). Complement metabolism in chronic liver disease: catabolism of Clq in chronic active liver disease and primary biliary cirrhosis. *Gastroenterology*, **78**, 1034–42
33. Eggink, H. F., Houthoff, H. J., Huitema, S., Gips, C. H. and Poppema, S. (1982). Cellular and humoral responses in chronic active liver disease. *Clin. Exp. Immunol.*, **50**, 17–24
34. Lisker-Melman, M., Webb, D., di Bisceglie, A. M., Kassianides, C., Martin, P., Rustgi, V., Waggoner, J. G., Park, Y. and Hoofnagle, J. H. (1979). Glomerulonephritis caused by chronic hepatitis B virus infection: treatment with recombinant human alpha-interferon. *Ann. Intern. Med.* **111**(6), 479
35. Brzosko, W. J., Krawczynski, K., Nazarewicz, T., Morzycka, M. and Nowoslawski, A. (1974). Glomerulonephritis associated with hepatitis-B surface antigen immune complexes in children. *Lancet*, **2**, 478–82
36. Ito, H., Hattori, S., Matsuda, I. *et al.* (1981). Hepatitis Be antigen-mediated membranous glomerulonephritis. Correlation of ultrastructural changes with HBeAg in the serum and glomeruli. *Lab. Invest.*, **44**, 214–20
37. Nassal, M., Galle, P. R. and Schaller, H. (1989). Protease like sequence in hepatitis B virus core antigen is not required for e antigen generation and may not be part of an aspartic acid-type protease. *J. Virol.*, 2598–2604
38. Pignatelli, M., Waters, J., Lever, A. M. L., Iwason, S., Gerety, R. and Thomas, H. C. (1987). Cytotoxic T-cell responses to the nucleocapsid proteins of HBV in chronic hepatitis. *J. Hepatol.*, **4**, 15–21

6
Cellular immune reactions in infections of the liver: an introduction

D. SHOUVAL AND E. GALUN

INTRODUCTION

Many aetiologic agents, such as viruses, bacteria, mycobacteria, spirochaetes, rickettsia, mycoplasma, fungi, and parasites, may infect the liver. There are, however, only a few instances in which the liver serves as a primary target organ for a particular infectious agent. More often, the liver is only one of several secondary sites which are affected by systemic or gastrointestinal infection. It should be emphasized that the cellular immune response against infection, and in particular against hepatic infection, is not an isolated event. The host immune response against infectious aetiologic agents comprises a co-ordinated interaction between the host and the invading agent, in which the cellular immune response is only one limb in a complex cascade. It is beyond the scope of this brief introduction to cover the many facets of the immune response in infections of the liver. We wish, however, to introduce to the non-immunologist several of the basic concepts of cellular immune reactions to infection. It is hoped that this information will assist the reader in understanding the various pathophysiological mechanisms involved in specific infections of the liver, which will be reviewed individually in the chapters following.

GENERAL PRINCIPLES OF CELLULAR IMMUNE REACTIONS

The host immune response to an infectious agent is dependent on recognition of its antigens by lymphocytes. Once recognition has been established, enhancement or suppression mechanisms are activated, leading to elimination of the infectious agent via a combination of humoral and cellular pathways. Failure of the immune response may lead to wide-spread infection and death, or, alternatively, to the development of persistent infection. Furthermore, one of the hallmarks of an intact immune response is the distinction between self and non-self antigens. If this distinction fails, an autoimmune disease process may evolve.

Cell-mediated immunity is usually activated once sensitized thymus-dependent T lymphocytes recognize micro-organism-derived antigens on antigen presenting cells, or on infected host cells.

Peripheral blood lymphocyte markers

Mammalian peripheral blood lymphocytes (PBL) possess cell surface glycoproteins, also called CD for cluster differentiation[1]. The CD molecules can be identified phenotypically in blood and tissues through interaction with monoclonal antibodies (Table 1). The CD2 and CD3 antigens are present on most mature T cells, the former being an erythrocyte-binding glycoprotein, while the latter is part of the antigen receptor complex. Two distinct glycoproteins, namely CD4 and CD8, have a particular role in the cellular immune response (Table 2). Previously, there seemed to be a clear functional distinction between CD4 and CD8 cells. Subsets of T cells which were CD4 were designated helper T cells, while cells expressing the CD8 phenotype were called suppressor or cytotoxic T cells according to their activity. It became clear, however, that CD4 and CD8 cells may have overlapping functional activities. For example, CD4 cells can now be divided into two subsets of help and suppression. Furthermore, both cells can stimulate various immune responses via lymphokine activation and secretion.

Table 1 Conventional peripheral blood lymphocytes cell surface markers

Cell type	*Common markers*
All T cells	CD2, CD3
Helper T cells	CD4
Suppressor and cytotoxic T cells	CD8
B cells	CD20, SmIg
NK cells	NKH1

CD, cluster differentiation antigens

Table 2 Subsets of peripheral mature T cells

	CD4	*CD8*
MW (kDa)	57	32
Lymphocyte (%)	50–65	25–35
Identified by MoAb	OKT 4 Anti-Leu3	OKT 8 Anti-Leu2
MHC restriction	Class II	Class I
Functions	B cell helper CD8 inducer (Cytotoxic TL)	CD4 suppressor Cytotoxic TL

MoAb, monoclonal antibody; MHC, major histocompatibility complex; TL, T lymphocytes

T cell activation

Recruitment of T cells and their activation is a unique and complex process (Table 3). The various steps include antigen uptake by antigen presenting cells (APC), intracellular processing of the antigen within the APC, presentation of the processed antigen in association with a major histocompatibility complex (MHC) antigen on the surface of the APC to the T cell receptor, followed by T cell activation into helper, suppressor or cytotoxic functions.

Antigen uptake by antigen presenting cells

Pathogens may penetrate into accessory APCs or into primary host target cells, using adhesion proteins[2]. Often, antigens which are present in infectious agents must be presented to the T cell by the APCs, such as macrophages, Kupffer cells, spleen or lymph node dendritic cells or skin Langerhans cells. Even B cells may act as APCs. The APCs are therefore accessory-intermediate hosts for a variety of infectious agents. Alternatively, other agents may penetrate directly into their primary target cells, for example hepatocytes where an infectious agent-derived antigen may be presented directly to the T cell. Before presenting an antigen to a T cell, it frequently has to be processed intracellularly in the APC[3].

Antigen processing within the APC

Once APCs have taken up an antigen, a process of intracellular proteolytic degradation occurs, in which large antigens are split into small fragments of 8–24 amino acids. Only then can the processed antigen be presented to the T cell, in association with an MHC antigen. In contrast, antibodies produced by B cells are able to recognize native antigens with a specific conformation without proteolytic degradation. Sometimes, two different domains on the same antigen are recognized separately by T and B cells. An example of this important distinction was provided by Millich[4] for helper T cells which interact with Pre-S and S proteins during hepatitis B virus (HBV) infection. The antigenic recognition sites for the corresponding antibodies were shown to be different compared with epitopes recognized by the activated T cells. In addition to intracellular processing of already existing antigens, there are occasions in which viral infection of a host cell may lead to synthesis of new

Table 3 Steps in T cell activation

Antigen uptake by antigen presenting cells (APC)	
Antigen processing within APCs	
Presentation of processed antigen in association with MHC molecules on the surface of APC or target cells	
Binding of processed antigen-MHC molecules to the T cell receptor (CD4 or CD8)	
Activation of T cells into:	helper function,
	suppressor function,
	cytotoxic function

viral or host antigens, which, in turn, can be presented to T cells and lead to their activation.

MHC-restricted dual presentation of processed antigens to T cells

Molecules encoded by the MHC genes bind peptide fragments derived from foreign processed antigens, and present these peptides to the T lymphocytes[5]. Dual presentation of processed antigen and MHC antigens on the APC surface or the infected cell surface is critical for binding of the antigen to the T cell receptor and its activation[6]. In APCs, these antigens are presented to T cells (usually CD4 cells) in association with MHC class II molecules, while other endogenous antigens are presented to cytolytic CD8 cells in association with MHC class I molecules.

In 1987, the three-dimensional structure of the extracellular portion of an MHC class I molecule was first deciphered[7], revealing a single potential antigen binding site. A groove was shown to exist between two helices located at the top of the molecule and supported by a sheet of β strands which form the potential binding site for the processed antigen[7].

MHC class I antigens are practically expressed on all cell types except for erythrocytes and trophoblasts. However, in hepatocytes and striated muscle cells, which are normally negative or weakly positive for MHC class I antigens, expression can be induced by inflammatory states and by interferons. MHC class II antigens, which are mainly expressed by APCs such as macrophages or Kupffer cells, can also be induced and augmented by inflammatory states.

Currently, most evidence suggests that recognition of both processed antigens and MHC molecules by the T cell involves a single T cell receptor[8].

Binding of processed antigen–MHC complex to the T cell receptor

The T cell receptor (TCR), also known as the TCR–CD3 complex, consists of six polypeptides[9]. Usually, the antigen binding site on T cells has two glycosylated α and β polypeptides linked together by a disulphide bond, which forms a heterodimer of 90 kDa. The antigen binding polypeptides are associated with the CD3 protein which consists of four polypeptide chains. The TCR and CD3 proteins are coexpressed, and once the processed antigens and the MHC antigens delivered by the APC are bound to the TCR, the CD3 polypeptide transduces the binding signal to the cytoplasm of the T cell, leading to T cell activation. The TCR is characterized by a tremendous diversity generated through rearrangements and recombinations of gene segments that code for the TCR α, β, γ, and δ chains[10]. Each peptide chain has a constant and a variable region, similar to the structure of immunoglobulins produced by B cells where the variable region provides antigen specificity.

T cell activation

Once all conditions for antigen presentation under MHC restriction are fulfilled, T cell activation may occur. This will result in proliferation of helper

T cells (CD4), suppressor cells (CD8), or a generation of cytotoxic T cells (mainly CD8 cells). This process involves a sequence of transcription, translation, and expression of various gene products on the activated T cell. The activation of T cells is further associated with secretion of lymphokines, such as IL-2, mainly by CD4 helper cells and by expression of a membrane receptor to IL-3 on the T cell. Stimulation of this receptor by IL-2 leads in turn to T cell proliferation. Other lymphokines, such as IL-1 and γ interferon are also activated during this process.

Target cell cytolysis

Both the humoral and the cellular limbs of the immune system have specialized mechanisms to lyse infected cells or invading micro-organisms. While the effector mechanisms of the humoral immune system consist of antibodies and complement, the cellular immune system uses the cytotoxic T lymphocytes (CTL) and the natural killer (NK) cells. NK cells possess receptors for the Fc portion of immunoglobulins, which enables them to bind to an antibody-coated target cell and lyse it (ADCC). In contrast, the activated T cell, usually a CD8+ CD4− cell, binds to its target through non-specific adhesion molecules. Recently, a pore forming protein, also called perforin, has been purified[11]. Perforin produces transmembrane channels in a Ca^{2+}-dependent polymerization process which, in turn, may lead to passage of degradative enzymes to the target cell, leading to its cytolysis. Other Ca-independent mechanisms may also be involved.

THE ROLE OF CELLULAR IMMUNE REACTIONS IN INFECTION OF THE LIVER

Cellular immunity to bacteria and fungi

Some bacteria, mycobacteria, spirochaetes, rickettsia, mycoplasma and fungi may invade the liver in the context of systemic infection. Only in relatively rare situations does the liver become the primary infected target organ by such micro-organisms, for example in the case of a liver abscess. The reasons for colonization of micro-organisms in the liver are multiple: haematogenous systemic dissemination; lymphatic spread from neighbouring organs; mechanical obstruction of the biliary drainage; and immunosuppression of the host. In chronic liver disease, and especially in portal hypertension, defective cellular and humoral immune functions may contribute to the emergence of localized hepatic infection. Involvement of the liver in infection usually manifests itself as mild to moderate portal or lobular inflammation, but can also lead to granulomata formation. The sequence of events leading to bacterial infection of the liver is similar to infections in other organs[12] and can be divided into seven distinct steps: (a) uptake of the pathogen; (b) adhesion of pathogens to host cells; (c) invasion of adequate niches; (d) colonization of these niches; (e) evasion of host defense mechanisms; (f) stable infection; (g) clinical disease. Often the host immune response is fully activated only at step (f). The type of pathogen may sometimes dictate which limb of the immune system will be activated. For example, extracellular micro-organisms preferentially reside in extracellular spaces and can be eliminated by macrophages via phagocytosis. Alternatively, the host may use opsonization and antibodies to eradicate such an infection. In contrast, intracellular pathogens enter and replicate in host cells, which turn into targets for cytolytic T cells. Often, a mixed reaction will develop in which CD4 helper cells will be activated by macrophages acting as APCs. Activated CD4 cells will, in turn, provide help for antibody production by B cells. The CD4 cells will, in addition, secrete interleukins, which in turn enhance activities of macrophages, monocytes and T cells. CD4 lymphocytes are a crucial element in immune protection against intracellular bacteria and fungi and provide the so-called acquired cellular resistance which is crucial for long-standing immunity after natural infection, as well as for development of immunity after vaccination. Alternatively, CD4 lymphocyte dysfunction may lead to the emergence of persistent infection. As for CD8+ T cells, their role in controlling intracellular bacterial infection has been established in several infections, for example, in mycobacteria tuberculosis. In the case of tuberculosis, the role of CD8 cells varies with the stage of the disease[13].

In general, the MHC class I restricted CD8 T cell has an advantage over the CD4, MHC class II restricted T lymphocyte in its antimicrobial activity, since almost all human cells, including hepatocytes, express class I antigens. In contrast, expression of the MHC class II glycoproteins is limited to macrophages, Kupffer cells and a few other specialized cells, thus restricting their potential role in resistance. Finally, too effective CD8 T cell cytoxicity may harm the host through the escape of intracelular pathogens following target-cell lysis. Aside from local inflammatory reactions which may be clinically symptomatic, such cytolysis can facilitate colonization of secondary tissue sites; therefore, target-cell lysis by cytotoxic T cells requires scrupulous regulation via suppressor mechanisms and through the CD4 helper function which may contribute to antibody-dependent elimination of microbial agents.

Cellular immunity to viruses

There are only a few occasions in which the liver serves as a primary target organ for infection. This is the case with viral hepatitis caused by hepatitis A virus (HAV), hepatitis B virus (HBV) and hepatitis C virus (HCV). As in other systemic infections, the immune system recognizes hepatitis virus antigens in association with MHC antigens, leading to T cell activation. The cellular and humoral limbs of the immune system act in concert to destroy the free virus. However, virus-induced immune responses may themselves result in an immunopathological process leading to autoimmune phenomena and chronic liver disease[14].

In acute HBV infection, viraemia precedes hepatocellular injury. Interferon-α secretion induced by the viral infection leads to increased display of HLA class I molecules on infected hepatocytes in association with viral antigens[15]. There is some evidence to suggest that Pre-S and S epitopes, present on the surface of infected liver cells during acute infection, serve as target molecules for activated T cells, leading to immune-mediated cytolysis of infected hepatocytes[16]. Furthermore, there is also evidence that T helper cells provide the stimulation to B cells for production of neutralizing antibodies to Pre-S proteins during acute HBV infection[17].

In chronic hepatitis B virus infection, HBcAg and, most probably, HBeAg are the crucial antigens presented to T cells by the infected hepatocytes in association with MHC class I molecules. It is still debated whether the nucleocapsid antigens are processed before display on the infected hepatocyte, change their conformation, or are presented with the same epitopes to T and B cells.

The reasons for the development of chronic persistent infection and chronic hepatitis in the infected adult are not completely understood. Genetically or virally induced interferon-α deficiency, which does not enable sufficient HLA class I display on infected liver cells, has been suggested as one possible reason for the emergence of persistent infection. Another hypothesis suggests that integration of HBV DNA sequences into the host genome shuts off expression of HBcAg, which is the trigger for immune clearance in long-standing infection. Therefore, hepatocytes with integrated HBV DNA may escape immune attack and continue to divide and, in some cases, also to secrete HBsAg[15,16].

There is one additional aspect of chronic HBV that deserves attention. Several studies have documented a decreased CD4/CD8 ratio, determined immunohistologically, in liver biopsies from patients with chronic HBV[18-20]. The decreased ratio is often the result of increased CD8 suppressor activity. Support for these observations came from studies in which mainly T cells, with the CD8 phenotype, were cloned from such biopsies with the help of IL-2[21]. These studies suggest that an immunoregulatory defect present in some patients with HBV leads to increased suppressor cell activity and a decreased humoral response to HBV antigens. This could also be a mechanism involved in development of chronic hepatitis.

The reasons for development of chronic hepatitis B following neonatal infection may be different, as compared with infection in adults. One hypothesis suggests that transplacental transfer of the nucleocapsid antibody to HBeAg leads, in association with anti-HBc, to tolerance to viral antigens, thus preventing T cell-mediated immune lysis of infected hepatocytes in the newborn. Some support for this explanation is derived from experiments where co-administration to chimpanzees of monoclonal anti-HBe and anti-HBc with the infectious inocculum of HBV leads to a protracted course of infection[22].

On the same lines, one can explain the occasional development of fulminant hepatitis B in the first months of life[16]. Transplacental maternal anti-HBc and anti-HBe may protect T cell activation by the infected hepatocytes. HBV infection will then continue to spread from cell to cell. Several months after birth, maternal anti-HBc and anti-HBe are degraded, leading to rapid sensitization of the child's T cells, followed by fulminant hepatitis B due to immune lysis of hepatocytes.

In comparison with hepatitis B, relatively little is known about the cellular immune response in acute hepatitis A virus infection. The HAV is not cytopathic, and immune-mediated lysis of infected hepatocytes is most probably the mechanism which leads to hepatocellular injury. However, the role of the different limbs of the cellular immune system is not defined in acute HAV. One report by Kurane and co-workers suggests that increased α-interferon activity, triggered by HAV, activates NK cells which, in turn, lead to cytolysis of infected liver cells[23].

Cellular immunity in parasitic infections

The complexity of the host immune response to parasites, in systemic as well as hepatic infections, is such that no brief summary can do it justice. The reader is therefore referred to an introduction to the immune response in parasitic diseases and two recent reviews[24–26]. There are, however, a few common immunological phenomena in parasitic infections that deserve attention. Many protozoa are intracellular parasites, often multiplying and surviving in macrophages, where they may be protected against immune attack. In contrast, nematodes do not usually replicate in the human host. However, an antigenic overload of worms may impose a tremendous burden on the immune system. Furthermore, parasites may undergo tremendous antigenic transformations in the various stages of their life cycle. Thus, acquired immunity to one form may provide little protection against the same species derived from another stage of the parasite's life cycle. A number of parasites have developed distinctive escape mechanisms, such as antigenic mimicry, antigenic depletion, antigenic variation, immunological indifference, immunological diversion and immunological subversion[24]. Not rarely, parasitic infections by themselves cause a significant immunosuppressive effect in the host. These mechanisms provide a partial explanation for the so-common failure of the immune system to clear a parasitic infection.

SUMMARY

In summary, this brief overview represents an attempt to review the general principles of the cellular immune response in infection with special emphasis on infections of the liver, which are discussed separately in the chapters following. The interested reader is referred to updated reviews cited in the bibliography.

References

1. Nossal, G. J. V. (1987). Current concepts in immunology: the basic components of the immune system. *N. Engl. J. Med.*, **316**, 1320–3
2. Shaw, S. and Shimizu, Y. (1988). Two molecular pathways of human T cell adhesion: establishment of receptor–ligand relationship. *Curr. Opin. Immunol.*, **1**, 92–7
3. Long, E. O. (1988). Processing requirements for presentation of antigens to T lymphocytes. *Curr. Opin. Immunol.*, **1**, 98–102

4. Millich, D. R. (1988). T and B cell recognition of hepatitis B viral antigens. *Immunol. Today*, **9**, 380–6
5. Long, E. O. and Kindt, T. J. (1988). Antigen recognition – overview. *Curr. Opin. Immunol.*, **1**, 71–2
6. Fox, B. S. (1988). Interaction of major histocompatibility complex molecules with immunogenic peptides. *Curr. Opin. Immunol.*, **1**, 103–6
7. Bjorkman, P. J., Saper, M. A., Samraoui, B., Bennet, W. S., Strominger, J. L. and Wiley, D. C. (1987). Structure of the human class I histocompatibility antigen, HLA-A2. *Nature (London)*, **329**, 506–12
8. Unanue, E. R., Beller, D. I., Lu, C. Y. and Allen, P. M. (1984). Antigen presentation: comments on its regulation and mechanism. *J. Immunol.*, **132**, 1–5
9. Ezquerra, A. and Coligan, J. E. (1988). T cell receptors: structure and genetics. *Curr. Opin. Immunol.*, **1**, 77–83
10. Matis, L. A. (1988). Diversity and antigen specificity of the T cell receptor. *Curr. Opin. Immunol.*, **1**, 84–7
11. Zychlinsky, A., Joag, S. and Young, J. D. E. (1988). Cytolytic mechanisms of the immune system. *Curr. Opin. Immunol.*, **1**, 63
12. Kaufmann, S. H. E. (1989). Immunity to bacteria and fungi. *Curr. Opin. Immunol.*, **1**, 431–40
13. Piessens, W. F. (1989). Introduction to the immunology of tuberculosis. *Rev. Inf. Dis.*, **11**, S436–S442
14. Zurbriggen, A. and Fujinami, R. S. (1989). Immunity to viruses. *Curr. Opin. Immunol.*, **1**, 427–30
15. Pignatelli, M., Waters, J., Brown, D., Lever, A., Iwarson, S., Schaff, S., Gerety, R. and Thomas, H. C. (1986). HLA class I antigens on the hepatocyte membrane during recovery from acute hepatitis B virus infection and during interferon therapy in chronic hepatitis B virus infection. *Hepatology*, **6**, 349–53
16. Thomas, H. C., Jacyna, M., Waters, J. and Main, J. (1988). Virus host interaction in chronic hepatitis B virus infection. *Semin. Liver Dis.*, **8**, 342–9
17. Vento, S., Ranier, S., Williams, R., Ronaldi, E. G., O'Brien, C. J. and Eddleston, A. L. W. F. (1987). Prospective study of cellular immunity to hepatitis B virus antigens from the early incubation phase of acute hepatitis B. *Lancet*, **2**, 119–22
18. Chisari, F. V., Castle, K. L., Xavier, C. and Anderson, D. S. (1981). Functional properties of lymphocyte subpopulations in hepatitis B virus infection. I. Suppressor cell control of T lymphocyte responsiveness. *J. Immunol.*, **126**, 38–49
19. Lemm, G., Salzer, K. and Warnatz, H. (1983). Studies on immunoregulatory mechanisms in acute and chronic hepatitis B. *Clin. Exp. Immunol.*, **52**, 250–8
20. Yang, P. M., Su, I. J., Lai, M. Y. and Sung, J. L. (1988). Immunohistochemical studies on intrahepatic lymphocyte infiltrates in chronic type B hepatitis with special emphasis on the activation status of the lymphocytes. *Am. J. Gastroenterol.*, **83**, 948–53
21. Hoffmann, R. M. Pape, G. R., Rieber, P., Eisenburg, J., Dohrmann, J., Zachoval, R., Paumgartner, G. and Riethmüller, G. (1986). Cytolytic T cell clones derived from liver tissue of patients with chronic hepatitis B. *Eur. J. Immunol.*, **16**, 1653–8
22. Pignatelli, M., Waters, J., Lever, A., Iwarson, S., Gerety, R. and Thomas, H. (1987). Cytotoxic T cell responses to the nucleocapsid proteins of HBV in chronic hepatitis. Evidence that antibody modulation may cause protracted infection. *J. Hepatol.*, **4**, 15–21
23. Kurane, I., Binn, L. N., Bancroft, W. H. and Ennis, F. A. (1985). Human lymphocyte responses to hepatitis A virus infected cells: Interferon production and lysis of infected cells. *J. Immunol.*, **135**, 2140–4
24. Keusch, G. T. (1982). Immune responses in parasitic disease. Part A: General concepts. *Rev. Infect. Dis.*, **4**, 751–5
25. Liew, F. Y. (1989). Immunity to protozoa. *Curr. Opin. Immunol.*, **1**, 441–7
26. Wakelin, D. (1989). Immunity to helminths. *Curr. Opin. Immunol.*, **1**, 448–53

7
Clinical implications of infections with respect to the liver

W. GEROK

If infectious agents invade the organism of the host, the liver may be affected in different ways. The clinical implications of interactions between the liver and infectious agents will be described and discussed under three headings:

1. the liver as target organ of infectious agents,
2. interactions between the liver and extrahepatic infections,
3. influence of pre-existing liver diseases on infections.

1. THE LIVER AS TARGET ORGAN OF INFECTIOUS AGENTS

The unspecific immune defence of the liver

The liver has its own unspecific immune system. The main cellular components are resident macrophages (Kupffer cells). The humoral components are summarized in Table 1.

The significance of the liver as an important organ of the unspecific immune system is underlined by the fact that 80–90% of the reticuloendothelial system (RES) is localized within the liver as Kupffer cells and sinusoidal cells[1]. Phagocytosis of circulating bacteria by the Kupffer cells is considered to be the most important defence mechanism against bacterial infections in the liver. About 50% of the monocytes circulating in the blood immigrate into

Table 1 Unspecific immune system of the liver

Cellular components
Macrophages (Kupffer cells)
Humoral components
Complement (alternative pathway)
Interferons
Acute-phase proteins
Enzymes (proteases, lysozyme, etc.)
Oxygen radicals

the liver and are transformed to Kupffer cells. Compared to resident macrophages in other tissues, the turnover of Kupffer cells is rapid (*ca.* 21 days)[2].

The unspecific immune system is very effective against bacteria. Their destruction or inactivation is performed by

1. phagocytosis mediated by the component C3b of the complement system,
2. the membrane attack complex of the complement system,
3. enzymatic degradation,
4. active oxygen radicals (oxidative burst).

These processes may take part in the general defence of the host against bacterial infections to various degrees.

Specific immune responses within the liver

In contrast to the unspecific immune system of the liver, the components of the specific immune system (Table 2) are not primarily localized in the liver. These components are of extrahepatic origin and derive from the lymphatic system. As a consequence of infection, T cells may immigrate into the liver. In addition B-cell-derived immunoglobulins are transported to the liver via the bloodstream.

The specific immune system is essential for the inactivation of virions and for the removal of virus-infected cells. Immunoglobulins are important for the removal of virions via immune complex formation and uptake by F_c-receptor bearing cells. The antibody response may be T cell-dependent. The removal of virus-infected cells is predominantly performed by cytotoxic T cells and only partially mediated by antibodies. These specific immune mechanisms leading to the removal of virions and virus-infected cells are supported by the unspecific immune system: components of the complement system are involved in the lysis of infected cells, macrophages in the presentation of antigens, interferons in the protection of cells against infection.

Clinical consequences

Bacterial infections of the liver and severe affections of the liver during bacterial septicaemia are rarely observed in the adult. In 1140 patients with septicaemia by Gram-negative bacteria, only in 0.6% could participation of

Table 2 Specific immune system

Cellular components
T-Lymphocytes
Humoral components
Immunoglobulins
Not primarily localized in the liver, migration or transport of the components to the liver
High efficiency against viral infection

the liver be demonstrated. In septicaemia with Gram-positive bacteria involvement of the liver is even more rare[3]. Jaundice in septicaemia with involvement of the liver is mostly moderate (5–10 mg/dl), the activities of transaminases are infrequently (30%) and only moderately increased. Histologically, the exudative reaction pattern is most common in bacterial infections of the liver. The rare or only weak involvement of the liver in bacterial infections is especially remarkable, since the blood from the intestine, including the colon with its intensive bacterial colonization, directly arrives at the liver. Therefore high-grade protection of the liver against bacterial infections must exist. This protection is based predominantly on the unspecific immune system within the liver.

A special variant of hepatic response is represented by the 'concomitant hepatitis' which occurs as a complication of bacterial enteritis (Table 3). This hepatitis is not caused by bacterial infection of the liver, but most likely is the effect of bacterial endotoxins or of a delayed hypersensitivity reaction.

In contrast to bacterial infections, viral infections of the liver are frequent. The liver can be a main target organ for viral infection, especially in the case of infections with the hepatitis virions A, B, C, D and E. In addition, a viral invasion into the liver may also occur during systemic viral infections (Table 4). Such 'concomitant hepatitides' can be frequently observed in systemic infection with EBV, CMV or with herpes simplex virus. More rarely they are caused by rubella, measles, coxsackie B or adenovirus infection. Histologically, the virus-induced hepatitis is characterized by a special 'immunological pattern' (cf. Chapter 3). The reason for the high frequency of viral infections of the liver may be the lack of a specific hepatic defence system against virions. An antiviral defence system becomes effective only as a subsequent, secondary event by the immigration of T cells and the influx of immunoglobulins into the liver. In line with this explanation is the observation that a severe hepatitis with a fulminant course can be caused by herpes simplex virus or varicella zoster virus in immunodeficient or

Table 3 'Hepatitis' in bacterial enteritis

Shigella species
E. coli species
Salmonella species
Yersinia species
Klebsiella
Providencia
Effect of endotoxin!
No bacterial invasion into the liver!

Table 4 Systemic viral infections involving the liver

Hepatitis virus A, B, C, D, E
Epstein–Barr virus (30–40%)
Cytomegalovirus (80%)
Herpes simplex virus
Coxsackie B virus
Adenovirus

immunosuppressed patients.

In parasitic infections the reaction of the liver is much more complex than after bacterial or viral infection. The reasons are the size of the parasites, their complex development and mode of infection, and the high variability and great number of their antigens. Both the unspecific as well as the specific immune system, with its humoral and cellular components, are involved in the defence against parasites. Corresponding with the variability of antigens and with the different defence mechanisms and histological reactions, the potential disturbances of liver function show a high variability (see part 3).

A special form of the hepatic reaction to infection is the formation of granulomas consisting of a focal accumulation of lymphocytes, macrophages, epithelioid cells and giant cells. Granulomas may be caused by a large variety of substances. In animal experiments, granulomas can be produced after sensibilization with a soluble antigen and a second application of the same antigen in an insoluble form. Granulomas may also arise as the consequence of the interaction of lymphocytes and macrophages with antigens, which cannot be removed by phagocytosis and enzymatic degradation. T_4 lymphocytes are significant for the recognition of antigens. Macrophages are subsequently attracted under the influence of lymphokines. They become activated and transformed to epithelioid cells, and possibly also to giant cells[4].

The most frequent infections in the aetiology of granulomas are tuberculosis, brucellosis, lepromatous leprosy, and typhoid fever.

Granulomas are a typical symptom in various diseases. Granulomas are typical reactions to intracellular, localized infectious agents (*Mycobacterium tuberculosis, Leishmania, Listeria monocytogenes*) or to other large and highly resistant agents, and their products (schistosomiasis). Granulomas are frequently a casual finding in liver biopsies. They are important for the diagnosis of the basic disease. Clinical symptoms exist only in cases with a very large number of granulomas in liver tissue ('granulomatosis hepatitis') or by special localization, for instance in the periportal field in schistosomiasis.

Summary of part 1

1. The liver is rarely the target organ of bacterial infections. This is due to the unspecific immune system present in the liver, which is highly effective against bacteria and their toxins.
2. Viral infections commonly affect the liver. The specific immune system eliminating the virus is secondarily activated after immigration of the cellular components into the liver.
3. Hepatitis accompanying bacterial enteritis is due to endotoxins.
4. Granuloma of the liver arises under special infectious conditions (intracellular agent resistant against degradation).

2. INTERACTION BETWEEN THE LIVER AND EXTRAHEPATIC INFECTIONS

The acute phase response

Any major extrahepatic infection induces the so-called acute phase response. This reaction is unspecific; it is the answer not only to infection, but also to tissue injury, neoplastic growth, trauma or immunological disorders. The aim of this reaction is to restore the disturbed physiological homeostasis. Within the acute phase response one can discriminate between a local reaction at the site of injury, and a systemic reaction (Figure 1). (For review, see refs 5 and 6).

The local reaction

The local reaction is characterized by the aggregation of platelets, immigration and activation of granulocytes and of mononuclear cells, and by the activation of different unspecific reaction systems: complement system, coagulation and fibrinolytic system, and kinin system. These reaction systems consist of proteolytic cascades. This means that an enzymatically inactive protein is transformed to a proteolytically active enzyme by splitting a peptide from the protein through limited proteolysis. The activated proteolytic enzyme can activate a second inactive protein by limited proteolysis with transformation of the inactive protein to an active protease. The repeated sequence from inactived to activated protein results in an amplification of a small primary effect within a short time interval. The end-products of the proteolytic

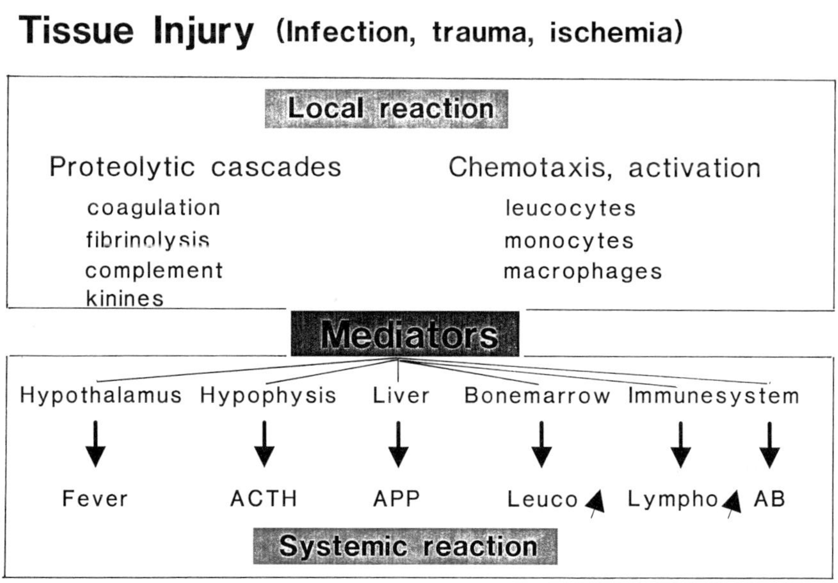

Figure 1 The acute-phase response

cascades are proteins or polypeptides with important biological functions:

1. Complement components form the membrane attack complex against bacteria. Other components such as C3a and C5a act as anaphylatoxins, which induce the degranulation of mast cells with release of histamine. In addition, anaphylatoxins induce the release of lysosomal proteases and eicosanoids. The same complement components have a chemotactic effect for granulocytes and macrophages, and as opsonins they stimulate the phagocytosis of bacteria and foreign material by granulocytes and macrophages (for review, see ref. 4).
2. Thrombin and plasmin are regulators of haemostasis. On the one hand, their effect is the limitation of the local reaction by occlusion of the micro-vessels; on the other hand the lysis of injurious microthrombi.
3. Components of the kinin system regulate dilatation and permeability of microvessels.

There are several interactions between these systems.

The systemic reaction and its induction by inflammatory mediators

The systemic reaction is characterized by fever, leucocytosis, increased secretion cortisol, catabolism with negative nitrogen balance, decrease in serum levels of iron and zinc, and alteration of the cellular and humoral components of the immune systems (Figure 1). In the liver the synthesis and secretion of some proteins is induced. These proteins which circulate in blood plasma are the called 'acute-phase proteins'. The systemic reaction is mediated by signal substances, which are produced at the site of local injury and transported with the blood to their target organs, where they act on specific receptors. These signal substances are also called 'inflammation hormones' or 'mediators'. The presently known signal substances inducing the systemic acute-phase reaction are shown in Table 5.

In contrast to classical hormones, the mediators of the acute-phase response have two peculiar properties: the pleiotropic action and network interaction of different mediators. Pleiotropic action means that each signal substance (mediator) induces a variety of effects and has several target organs (Figure 2). So IL-6 stimulates the synthesis and secretion proteins in the liver, the release of ACTH from the hypophysis, haematopoiesis in the bone marrow, the transformation of B cells to plasma cells, the maturation of T cells to cytotoxic cells, and in the central nervous system the differentiation of neuronal cells (for review see refs 7–9). However, these effects are

Table 5 Signal substances (produced by local acute-phase reaction)

Interleukin 1 (IL-1)
Interleukin 6 (IL-6)
Tumour necrosis factor (TNF)
Interferons (IFN)
Colony-stimulating factor (CSF)

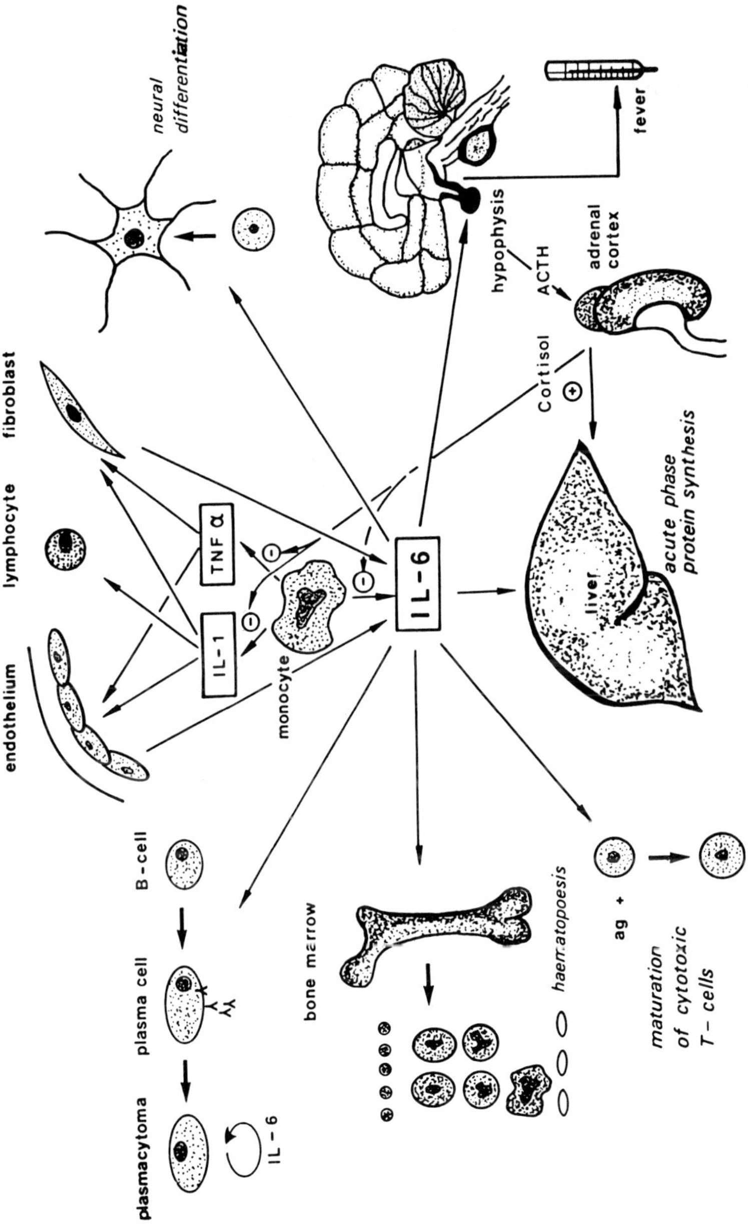

Figure 2 Pleiotropic action and network action of interleukins

predominantly demonstrated *in vitro*. Whether they play a role *in vivo*, given the real concentrations of the mediator at its specific receptor site, remains open. Local concentrations cannot yet be measured directly. Therefore it is unknown whether, and to what degree, the pleiotropic action of a mediator is realized in the organism *in vivo*.

The network action is based on the manifold interactions between different mediators. Such interactions exist with respect to the synthesis and degradation of mediators, but also with respect to their action on specific receptors at the target organ. So the synthesis of IL-6 is stimulated by IL-1 and TNF. On the other hand, there are examples of antagonistic effects of different mediators on cell proliferation and protein metabolism (for review see refs 7–10). However, the suggestion of a network action is again based on *in vitro* experiments. Whether the interactions are realized *in vivo* in the organism must be clarified by further investigations.

IL-6 is the major regulator of the hepatic reaction during the acute-phase response (for review see refs 7–10). The stimulation of synthesis and secretion of acute-phase proteins by the liver may be its most important function.

IL-6 is a phosphoglycoprotein, which is produced at the site of local injury by monocytes and macrophages and, to a smaller extent, also by fibroblasts and endothelial cells. IL-6 synthesis is stimulated by IL-1 and TNF, and is repressed by glucocorticoids. Since IL-1 and TNF, like IL-6, are also synthesized only after previous stimulation, the question arises which substances may act as the initial endogenous starter of the mediator cascade. The 'starter' of IL-6 synthesis could be the platelet-derived growth factor released from platelets. After their contact with injured endothelial cells, synthesis of IL-6 and of other mediators (IL-1, TNF) may take place. Also in the Kupffer cells of the liver, synthesis of IL-6 and of other mediators (IL-

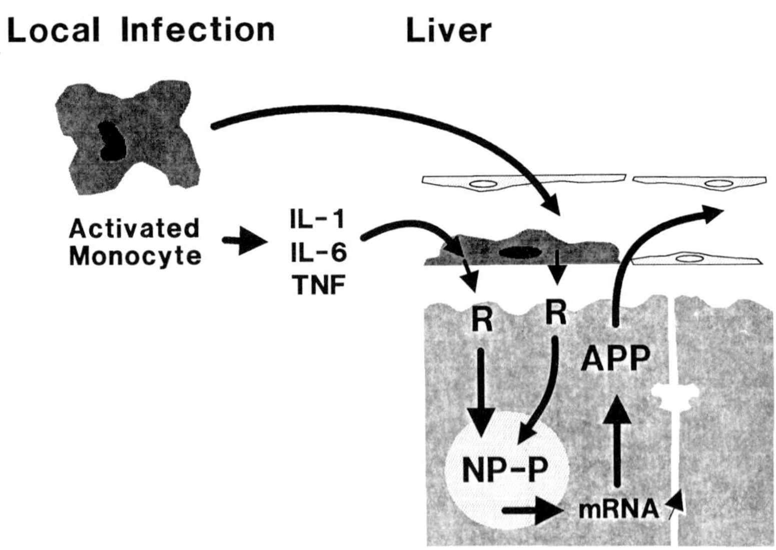

Figure 3 Induced synthesis of acute-phase proteins by IL-6

1, TNF) may take place. Mediators may reach the liver with the blood and stimulate IL-6 synthesis in the Kupffer cells. This could mean an amplification of the IL-6 effect (Figure 3).

If IL-6 is administered exogenously, 80% of this mediator is bound to a specific receptor in the sinusoidal membrane of hepatocytes. The IL-6 receptor is a glycoprotein with a domain of 90 amino acids similar to immunoglobulins. The synthesis of the receptor in the hepatocytes is induced during extrahepatic inflammation[11]. This induction is mediated by IL-6, IL-1 and glucocorticoids. The induction of the receptor is regulated on the pretranslational level (for review see refs 7–10).

The sequence of intracellular reactions following the binding of IL-6 to the receptor protein, with the final result of increased synthesis of acute-phase proteins, is as yet unclear. A second membrane glycoprotein and subsequent activation of a tyrosine kinase are probably involved[12]. It has been shown that the last step leading to increased transcription of acute-phase genes consists of the activation of a nuclear protein, which – upon activation – binds to enhancer elements of acute-phase protein genes. The enhancer elements of several acute-phase genes share common nucleotide sequences[13] (for review see refs 10 and 14). Therefore, induction of the whole set of acute-phase genes may follow a common mechanism.

The physiological functions of acute-phase proteins

The acute-phase proteins in man are listed in Table 6. The most important functions of acute-phase proteins include their antiproteolytic effect, opsonization effect and immunomodulating effect.

An antiproteolytic effect applies to several acute-phase proteins: α_1-antitrypsin and α_1-antichymotrypsin inhibit the leucocyte elastase and cathepsin G[15,16]. C_1-inactivator is an antiprotease, which inhibits components of the complement system, but also plasmin and kallikrein[17–19]. The proteolytic cascades induced during acute inflammation would probably result in shock if not controlled by the antiproteolytic effect of acute-phase proteins[20] (Figure 4).

C-reactive protein (CRP) binds to phosphorylcholine, an integral constituent of the cellular and bacterial membranes (see refs 21 and 22). After coating of a foreign particle by its interaction with CRP the complement component, C_3b, can be attached to it. This allows phagocytosis by macrophages mediated through their C_3-b receptors. The binding of CRP to chromatin and fragments of DNA derived from necrotic cells[23,24] and the lectin-like binding of CRP to the carbohydrate moiety of membrane glycoproteins[25] favours the removal of cells, bacteria and their fragments by macrophages (Figure 5).

Several acute-phase proteins are immunomodulators (Table 7). CRP activates monocytes[26,27]. Serum amyloid A and α_1-antiprotease suppress antigen-dependent reactions of lymphocytes[28,29]. α_1-Acid glycoprotein inhibits

Table 6 Human acute-phase proteins

Increasing	*Decreasing*
C-reactive protein	Albumin
Serum amyloid A	Transferrin
Fibrinogen	Transthyretin
Haptoglobin	α_1-Lipoprotein
α_1-Antitrypsin	Inter α_2-antitrypsin
α_1-Antichymotrypsin	α_2-HS-Glycoprotein
α_1-Acid glycoprotein	
Complement factor C3	
C_1-Inactivator	
Caeruloplasmin	
α_2-Antiplasmin	

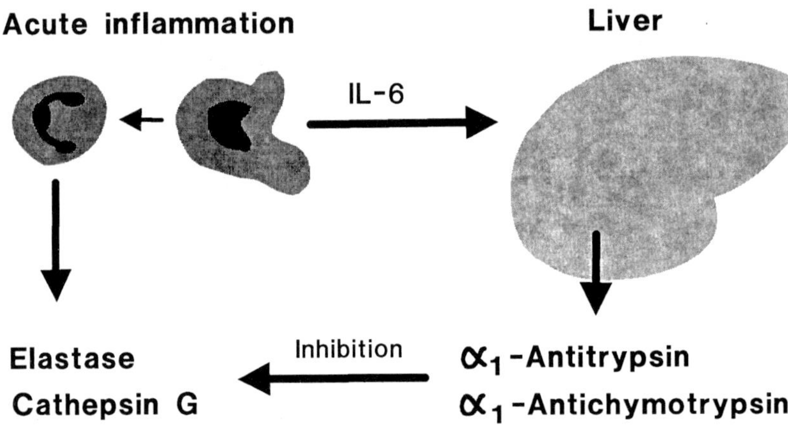

Figure 4 Antiproteolytic effect of acute-phase proteins in extrahepatic inflammation

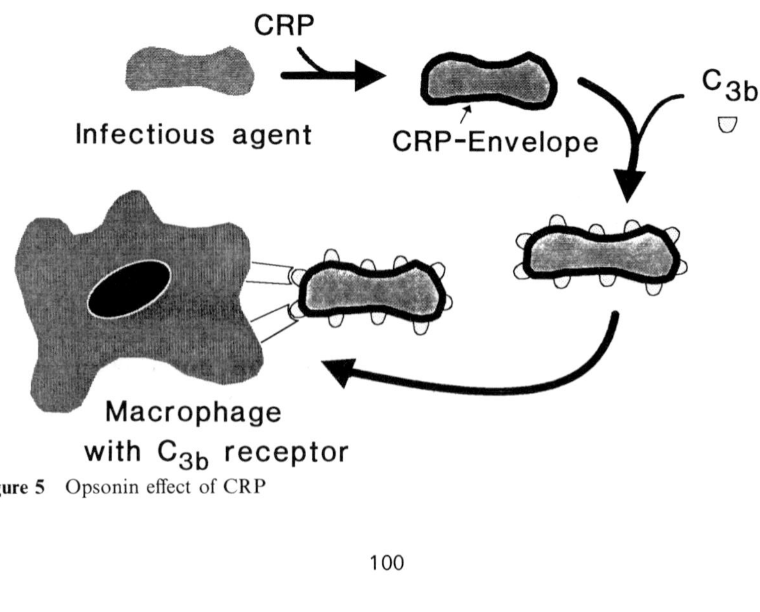

Figure 5 Opsonin effect of CRP

Table 7 Immunomodulation by APP

CRP:	activation of monocytes
SAA; α_1-AP:	suppression of lymphocytes proliferation
α_1-AG:	inhibition of antibody synthesis and cytotoxic T cells

CRP = C-reactive protein α_1-AP : α_1-Antiprotease
SAA = Serumamyloid A α_1-Ag : α_1-Acid glycoprotein

the proliferation of lymphocytes, the production of antibodies and the activity of cytotoxic T cells[30].

Clinical consequences

The experimental results demonstrate that a mutual interaction exists between the site of a local extrahepatic infection and the liver. At the site of local infection proteolytic cascades are induced. Their overshooting would result in tissue destruction and shock. The signal substances, especially IL-6, produced at the site of local inflammation, induce the hepatic synthesis and secretion of acute-phase proteins. These proteins are antagonists (inhibitors) of the proteolytic enzymes (Figure 6). Some of the acute-phase proteins are important for the scavenger function of macrophages by stimulating phagocytosis of cellular and bacterial fragments. Furthermore, the acute-phase proteins can modulate the immune functions. Therefore there is a mutual interaction establishing a feedback regulation between liver and extrahepatic sites of local infection.

For diagnostic purposes the concentrations of mediators, especially those of TNF and IL-6, in the blood are an extremely sensitive parameter for the activity of an inflammation. TNF is instantly released; IL-6 is rapidly (within 1.5–4 h) released and remains detectable in the plasma only for a short time. As a monitor, IL-6 therefore reacts more rapidly than sedimentation rate, CRP, or leucocyte counts to a local inflammation.

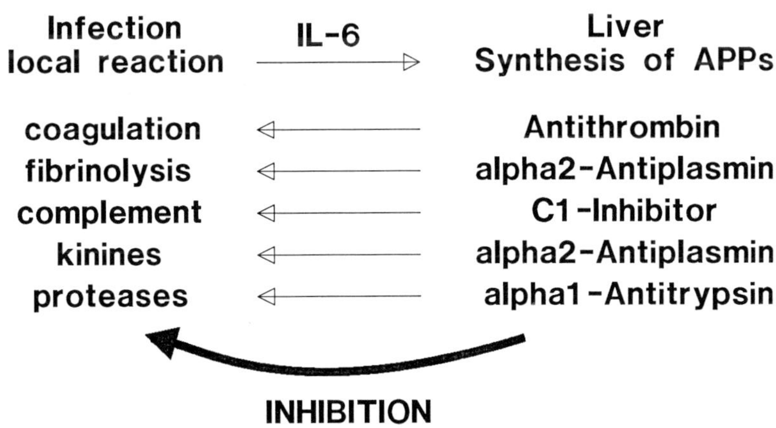

Figure 6 Interaction of infections and the liver

New therapeutic approaches may result from the application of IL-6, IL-6 antagonists, or IL-6 receptor blockers. Furthermore, the process of inflammation may be influenced by the administration of certain acute-phase proteins produced with recombinant DNA technology.

It can be assumed that interleukins and TNF are probably involved in the pathogenesis of liver diseases, e.g. fulminant hepatitis, alcoholic hepatitis and primary biliary cirrhosis.

Summary of section 2

1. Signal substances released by various cell types in the area of local inflammation mediate systemic reactions.
2. Synthesis and secretion of the acute-phase proteins by the liver are stimulated by IL-6 released from monocytes and Kupffer cells.
3. The acute-phase proteins act as antiproteases, immune modulators and/or enhancers of opsonization.
4. Mutual interactions exist between a local extrahepatic infection with inflammation and the liver.

3. INFLUENCE OF LIVER DISEASES ON INFECTIONS

It has been demonstrated that the liver is an important organ for the unspecific immune reaction. Furthermore, a mutual interaction exists between sites of local extrahepatic infection and the liver. Therefore one can expect that liver diseases leading to a reduced hepatic organ function influence the occurrence and the course of extrahepatic infectious diseases.

The incidence of bacterial infections in patients with decompensated cirrhosis is increased. In the most detailed study of Rimola *et al.*[31], 46% of the patients with decompensated cirrhosis were infected at admission to the hospital, or developed bacterial infection during the early hospital stay. This incidence is nearly four times greater than that occurring in the general hospitalized population (12%). Also hospital-acquired infections are significantly more frequent in patients with cirrhosis (38%) than in a control group without liver diseases (2–11%)[31]. The most common infections were urinary tract infections, bacteraemia and spontaneous bacterial peritonitis, followed by respiratory and cutaneous infections (Table 8). Causative microorganisms

Table 8 Bacterial infections in cirrhosis[31]

	No.	Percentage
Patients with proven infection	86	45.9
Urinary tract infection	54	28.9
Bacteraemia	31	16.6
Respiratory infection	12	6.4
Skin infection	11	5.9
Spontaneous bacteraemic peritonitis	9	4.8
Patients with possible infection	14	7.5

are predominantly enteric bacteria such as *E. coli*, *Klebsiella* and *Proteus*. Non-enteric bacteria are infrequently found[31].

The pathogeneses of the high incidence of bacterial infections in chronic liver diseases are not completely understood. Probably the reduced activity of the RES resulting from the destruction of liver parenchyma, dysfunction of Kupffer cells and from haemodynamic bypass of the RES by portacaval anastomoses plays the predominant role. A reduced ability of the Kupffer cells for phagocytosis of bacteria and of bacterial toxins was demonstrated in animal experiments and in patients with liver cirrhosis[32–34]. In addition, the ability of leucocytes for chemotactic migration and phagocytosis is reduced[35–39].

A reduced plasma concentration and activity has been demonstrated for several components of the complement system[39–41]. Alcohol abuses and malnutrition can depress the phagocytosis of bacteria by macrophages and granulocytes, thereby increasing the incidence of infections[42]. An increased permeability of the intestinal mucosal barrier in alcoholic liver diseases is discussed as an additional important factor in the pathogenesis of infections[43]. Finally, invasive procedures may increase the incidence of infections (Table 9).

The clinical symptoms of infections in chronic liver diseases depend on the main localization of the infectious inflammatory process. The clinical picture and the degree of symptoms vary considerably. Only 50% of the patients have fever. Septic shock occurs in only 10% of patients. Leucocytosis is not obligatory, 10% of the patients present with leucopenia. Cases with septic shock are associated with metabolic acidosis caused by an increase of lactate concentration, hypoglycaemia and hypoxaemia. An important and frequent complication is spontaneous bacterial peritonitis. Therefore in any case of unexplained deterioration of hepatic function, the possibility of concomitant bacterial infection must be suspected.

The bacteriological investigation of blood and ascitic fluid is compulsory; however, blood and ascitic fluid cultures are frequently negative in cirrhotics with an otherwise typical clinical picture. These patients must therefore be treated in a similar way to patients with 'proved' infection.

The prognosis in these cases is poor. The mortality rate of patients with decompensated cirrhosis, bacterial infection and spontaneous bacterial peritonitis has been reported[31] to range between 20% and 60%. The prognosis depends on the degree of liver failure, the type of infectious agent and the time interval between the first symptoms and the beginning of antibiotic therapy.

Table 9 Mechanisms of frequent bacterial infections in cirrhosis

Impaired RES phagocytic activity by shunting of portal blood and/or reduced function of Kupffer cells
Reduced serum complement (C4, C5a)
Abnormalities of neutrophil function (phagocytosis, intracellular killing, metabolic activity)
Reduced opsonization, humoral activity
Increased permeability of the intestinal mucosal barrier to enteric bacteria
Alcoholism and malnutrition depress granulocyte function and RES activity
Invasive procedures (oesophageal tamponade, central venous catheterization, peritoneovenous shunt)

Cephalothin or ampicillin, in combination with an aminoglycoside, have been suggested for antibiotic treatment. Careful observation of renal function is necesary because these patients are predisposed to develop aminoglycoside nephrotoxicity. Often a discrepancy between the result of *in vitro* susceptibility tests and *in vivo* efficacy of antibiotics is found.

Summary of part 3

1. The incidence of bacterial infections is high in patients with liver diseases, especially in liver cirrhosis.
2. The main reason is a reduced activity of the unspecific immune system due to a decreased activity of the MPS.
3. In addition, the function of the granulocytes is disturbed and the components of the complement system are reduced.
4. The symptoms of infections are commonly atypical in the presence of chronic liver disease. Fever and leucocytosis are not obligatory.
5. Antibiotic treatment is necessary when clinical symptoms of infection are present in patients with chronic liver disease, even when bacteriological examinations are negative.
6. Extrahepatic infections should be considered as possible reasons for aggravation of chronic liver disease.

References

1. Thomas, H. C., McSween, R. N. M. and White, R. G. (1973). Role of the liver in controlling the immunogenicity of commensal bacterial in the gut. *Lancet*, **1**, 1288–91
2. Croften, R. W., Martina, M. C., Diesselhoff-Den Dulk, M. M. C. and van Furth, R. (1978). The origins, kinetics and characteristics of the Kupffer cells in the normal steady state *J. Exp. Med.*, **148**, 1–17
3. Back, P. and Kluge, P. (1987). Leberschäden bei Infektionskrankheiten. In Gerok, W. (ed.), *Hepatologie*, pp. 441–60. Munich: Urban & Schwarzenberg
4. Roitt, I. M., Brostoff, J. and Male, D. K. (1985). *Immunology* (London: Gower Medical)
5. Kushner, I. (1982). The phenomenon of the acute phase response *Ann. N.Y. Acad. Sci.*, **389**, 38–48
6. Koj, H. (1985). Definition and classification of acute phase proteins. In Gordon, A. H. and Koj, A. (eds), *The Acute Phase Response to Injury and Infections*, pp. 139–232. Amsterdam: Elsevier
7. Andus, T., Heinrich, P. C., Castell, J. C. and Gerok, W. (1989). Interleukin-6: ein Schlüsselhormon der Akutphase-Reaktion *Dtsch. Med. Wochenschr.*, **114**, 1710–16
8. Castell, J. V., Andus, T., Kunz, D. and Heinrich, P. C. (1989). Interleukin-6. The major regulator of acute-phase-protein synthesis in man and rat *Ann. N.Y. Acad. Sci.*, **557**, 87–99
9. Bauer, J. (1989). Interleukin-6 and its receptor during homeostasis, inflammation and tumor growth. *Klin. Wochenschr.*, **67**, 697–706
10. Heinrich, P. C., Castell, J. V. and Andus, T. (1989). Interleukin-6 and the acute phase response. *Biochem. J.* (In press)
11. Bauer, J., Lengyel, G., Bauer, T. M., Acs, G. and Gerok, W. (1989). Regulation of interleukin-6 receptor expression in human monocytes and hepatocytes. *FEBS Lett.*, **249**, 27–30
12. Taga, T., Hibi, M., Hirata, Y., Yamasaki, K., Yasukawa, K., Matsuda, T., Hirano, T. and Kishimoto, T. (1989). Interleukin-6 triggers the association of its receptor with a possible signal transducer pg 130. *Cell*, **58**, 572–81
13. Oliviero, S. and Cortese, R. (1989). The human haptoglobin gene promoter: interleukin-6-

responsive elements interact with a DNA-binding protein induced by interleukin-6. *EMBO J.*, **8**, 1145–51
14. Fey, G. H. and Fuller, G. M. (1987). Regulation of acute phase gene expression by inflammatory mediators. *Mol. Biol. Med.*, **4**, 323–38
15. Travis, J. and Salvesen, G. S. (1983). Human plasma proteinase inhibitors. *Ann. Rev. Biochem.*, **52**, 655–709
16. Harpel, P. C. (1983). Protease inhibitors – a precarious balance. *N. Engl. J. Med.*, **309**, 725–6
17. Sim, R. B., Reboul, A., Arlaud, G. J., Villiers, C. L. and Colomb, M. G. (1979). Interaction of 125 I-labeled complement subcomponents C1r and C1s with proteinase inhibitors in plasma. *FEBS Lett.*, **97**, 111–14
18. Harpel, P. C. and Cooper, N. R. (1975). Studies on human plasma C1 inactivator-enzyme interaction. *J. Clin. Invest.*, **55**, 593–604
19. Harpel, P. C., Lewin, M. F. and Kaplan, A. P. (1985). Distribution of plasma Kallikrein between C1 inaktivator and alpha-2-macroglobulin in plasma. *J. Biol. Chem.*, **260**, 4257–63
20. Colmann, R. W. (1989). The role of plasma proteases in septic shock. *N. Engl. J. Med.*, **320**, 1207–9
21. Andersen, J. K., Stroud, R. M. and Volonakis, J. E. (1978). Studies on the binding specificity of human CRP for phosphorylcholine. *Fed. Proc.* **37**, 1495
22. Volonakis, J. E. and Narkates, A. J. (1981). Interaktions of CRP with artificial phosphatydilcholine bilauers and complement. *J. Immunol.*, **126**, 1820–5
23. Robey, R. A., Jones, K. D., Tanaka, T. and Liu, T. Y. (1984). Binding of CRP to chromatin and nucleosome core particles. *J. Biol. Chem.*, **259**, 7311–16
24. Shepard, E. G., Van Helden, P. D., Strauss, M., Böhm, L. and De Beer, F. G. (1986). Functional effects of CRP binding to nuclei. *Immunology*, **58**, 489–94
25. Soelter, J. and Uhlenbruck, G. (1986). The role of phosphate groups in the interaction of human CRP with galactan polysaccharides. *Immunology*, **58**, 139–44
26. Zahedi, K. and Mortensen, R. F. (1986). Macrophage tumoricidal activity induced by human CRP. *Cancer Res.*, **46**, 5077–83
27. Zeller, J. M., Landay, A. L., Lint, T. F. and Gewurz, H. (1986). Enhancement of human peripheral blood monocyte respiratory burst activity by aggregated CRP. *J. Leuk. Biol.*, **40**, 769–83
28. Benson, M. D. and Aldo-Benson, M. (1979). Effect of purified protein SAA in immune response in vitro: mechanisms of suppression. *J. Biol. Chem.*, **122**, 2077–82
29. Aroba, P. K., Miller, M. C. and Aronson, L. D. (1978). Alpha-1-antitrypsin is an effector of immunological stasis. *Nature*, **274**, 589–90
30. Cheresh, D. A., Haynes, D. H. and Distasio, J. A. (1984). Interaction of an acute phase reactant, alpha-1-acid glycoprotein with the lymphoid cell surface: a model for non-specific immune suppression. *Immunology*, **51**, 541–8
31. Rimola, A., Arroyo, V. and Rodes, J. (1986). Infective complications in acute and chronic liver failure: basis and control. In Williams, R. (ed.), *Liver Failure*, pp. 93–111. (Edinburgh: Churchill Livingstone)
32. Rimola, A., Soto, R., Bory, F., Arroyo, V., Piera, C. and Rodes, J. (1984). Reticuloendothelial system phagocytic activity in cirrhosis and its relation to bacterial infections and prognosis. *Hepatology*, **4**, 53–8
33. Lahnborg, G., Friman, L. and Bergheim, L. (1981). Reticuloendothelial function in patients with alcoholic liver cirrhosis. *Scand. J. Gastroenterol.*, **16**, 481–9
34. Richards, P. S. and Saba, T. M. (1985). The phagocytic activity of the reticuloendothelial system (RES) in the liver is important in host resistance to shock. *Hepatology*, **5**, 32–7
35. De Meo, A. N. and Andersen, B. R. (1972). Defective chemotaxis associated with a seruminhibitor in cirrhotic patients. *N. Engl. J. Med.*, **286**, 735–40
36. Feliu, E. (1977). Blood polymorphonuclear dysfunction in patients with alcoholic cirrhosis. *Eur. J. Clin. Invest.*, **7**, 571–7
37. Yousif-Kadaru, A. G. M., Rajkovic, I. A., Wyke, R. J. and Williams, R. (1984). Defects in serum attractant activity in different types of chronic liver disease. *Gut*, **25**, 79–84
38. Rajkovic, I. A. and Williams, R. (1986). Abnormalities of neutrophil phagocytosis, intracellular cilling and metabolic activity in alcoholic cirrhosis and hepatitis. *Hepatology*, **6**, 252–62

39. Fox, R. A., Dudley, F. J. and Sherlock, S. (1971). The serum concentration of the third component β1c/β1a in liver disease. *Gut*, **12**, 574–8
40. Finlayson, N. D. C., Krohn, K., Fauconnet, M. H. and Anderson, K. E. (1972). Significance of serum complement levels in chronic liver disease. *Gastroenterology*, **63**, 653–9
41. Potter, B. J., Trueman, A. M. and Jones, E. A. (1973). Serum complement in chronic liver disease. *Gut*, **14**, 451–6
42. Bjorneboe, M. and Prytz, H. (1976). The mononuclear phagocytic functions of the liver. In Ferguson, A. and McSween, R. N. M. (eds), *Immunological Aspects of the Liver and Gastrointestinal Tract*, pp. 251–89. (Lancaster: MTP Press)
43. Bode, C., Kugler, V. and Bode, J. C. (1987). Endotoxemia in patients with alcoholic and non-alcoholic cirrhosis and in subjects with no evidence of chronic liver disease following acute alcohol excess. *J. Hepatol.*, **4**, 8–14

Section II: The Liver in Bacterial and Spirochaetal Infections

8
The liver in tuberculosis and sarcoidosis

F.-D. GOEBEL and C. ZIETZ

TUBERCULOSIS

Hepatic tuberculosis – at least in our area – appears to be a rare disease. It occurs in two different forms:

1. involvement of the liver in disseminated miliary tuberculosis which represents the more frequent type and
2. a primary tuberculosis of the liver: tuberculous hepatitis.

In several larger series published primarily from South Africa out of 341 patients with tuberculous liver disease 302 suffered from miliary tuberculosis and only 39 patients had primary liver tuberculosis[1–4]. Of the latter group only adults, and no children, were affected. The mean age of the adult cases in the whole series was 45 years, of the children only 2 years. Clinical signs and symptoms were present in most cases but were rather inconclusive.

Although the majority of the patients described in these papers consisted of black mineworkers in South Africa with a high incidence of tuberculosis, in only 47% of the patients was the disease suspected clinically. Patients with hepatic tuberculosis presented with many different signs and symptoms, none of them being pathognomonic (Table 1). The most important clue to the diagnosis of hepatic tuberculosis appeared to be the presence of tuberculosis elsewhere, particularly in the lungs. Where such evidence was

Table 1 Clinical features in hepatic tuberculosis (n = 341)

Hepatomegaly	91%
Pyrexia	75%
Weight loss	64%
Abdominal pain	52%
Splenomegaly	39%
Bowel changes	33%
Night sweats	25%
Jaundice	12%

lacking a correct diagnosis may be extremely difficult, and sometimes has been made either at autopsy or liver biopsy as an incidental finding. Clinically the liver was enlarged in 90% of the patients, tender on palpatation in many cases. About 50% of the patients described complained of frank abdominal pain, unrelated to meals, in most cases localized to the right upper quadrant.

If generalized abdominal pain is present, the patient usually had disseminated tuberculous peritonitis. Associated splenomegaly (39%) represented invariably mycobacterial infection. The reverse, however, does not hold true: in many cases with tuberculosis of the spleen proven at autopsy the organ was of normal size clinically. About 75% had pyrexia; in many cases the diagnosis of 'fever of unknown origin' had been maintained in the past for longer periods of time. Nightsweats, anorexia and weight loss were also prominent findings in these patients. Changes of bowel habits occurred, diarrhoea being about twice as common as constipation, but this might be related to the fact that most patients were Africans. Jaundice was a relatively rare sign, mostly due to intra- or extrahepatic obstruction, but seldom also of haemolytic origin.

As for clinical signs, the laboratory abnormalities are inconclusive as well (Table 2). Elevation of alkaline phosphatase (91%), transaminases (77%), serum gamma-globulin (78%) and hyperbilirubinaemia (21%) point to liver affection in general. Decreased concentration of serum albumin (88%) and sodium (65%) are common findings; moderate reduction of prothrombin index is found in about 38% of the patients.

Hepatic imaging techniques are frequently misleading. Ultrasonography shows increased echogenicity of the liver in some patients, but without any specific feature. Technetium-99 sulphur colloid scan might reveal a pathological uptake indicating diffuse hepatocellular disease. In few instances decreased uptake of isotope in a multicentric fashion is also observed. Abdominal computer tomography reveals results similar to those using ultrasonography, in many cases merely showing enlargement of the liver. In rare instances intrahepatic calcifications might be noted.

The diagnosis of hepatic tuberculosis can be established only in liver tissue obtained by percutaneous liver biopsy, laparoscopy or laparotomy. The histological features will be dealt with in greater detail in another chapter of this volume. Hepatic granulomata with central areas of caseation are the classical morphological signs of hepatic tuberculosis. In the published series Ziehl–Neelsen and Auramin staining reveal acid-fast bacilli in about two-thirds of cases described. A higher yielding rate will be achieved by

Table 2 Pathological laboratory findings in hepatic tuberculosis ($n = 341$)

Elevated alkaline phosphatase	91%
Serum albumin	88%
Serum gamma-globulin	78%
Serum transaminases	77%
Hyponatraemia	65%
Hypoprothrombinaemia	38%
Hyperbilirubinaemia	21%

microbiological culture of biopsy tissue which also permits typing of the organism and drug testing.

The prognosis of patients with tuberculous liver disease depends on several factors. One factor probably is late diagnosis and initiation of therapy. In the series of 96 patients described by Essop *et al.*[2] the mortality rate was very high (42%). The outcome could be related to coexisting liver disease such as cirrhosis or alcoholic hepatitis. Variables adversely affecting mortality rate were: age below 20 years, and predisposing factors such as corticosteroid therapy, chronic renal failure or diabetes mellitus. Coagulopathy and a high caseation score in liver biopsy had negative predictive value. On the contrary, liver enzymes, serum sodium or icterus did not affect the outcome.

In recent years an increase of mycobacterial liver disease has been noted with the spread of the acquired immunodeficiency syndrome[5]. The HIV-related immunosuppression influences not only the incidence of mycobacterial infections (as well as the frequency of certain mycobacterial strains), but also the morphological appearance of the infection in the liver[6]. The incidence of mycobacterial disease in AIDS patients depends on the prevalence of certain strains in the geographical area. In developing countries among all mycobacterial diseases infections of typical tuberculosis prevail, whereas in western countries atypical mycobacteriosis seems predominant. The type of organ involvement is of particular interest. Compared with persons without HIV infection AIDS patients with *Mycobacterium tuberculosis* tend to have extrapulmonary involvement and more often miliary dissemination including liver involvement. Atypical mycobacteria usually involve the reticulo-endothelial system, i.e. liver, spleen, bone marrow, lymph nodes and frequently also the gastrointestinal tract, but seem almost to spare the lungs[8]. The morphological sequelae of mycobacterial infection of the liver depend on the type of agent and the immunological status of the host. Classical tuberculosis tends to be an early complication of the clinical course in HIV disease, fulfilling the criteria of full-blown AIDS only in cases of extrapulmonary or miliary distribution. In contrast, atypical mycobacteriosis appears to be a late infection due to a severely impaired immune system (Table 3).

The reaction of the liver to mycobacterial organisms is highly mediated by immunological mechanisms[9]. Monocytes from the bloodstream invade the affected area and are transformed to macrophages. By phagocytosis the microorganisms are incorporated into the cell. In immunocompetent individuals T lymphocytes stimulate the macrophage by means of lymphokines into an activated macrophage, enabling the cell to destroy the organism. This in turn causes destruction of the macrophage itself, giving the histological picture of caseation. If stimulation of the lymphocytes is inhibited experimentally by cyclosporin A, abundant replication of mycobacteria takes place in the non-activated macrophage[10]. In AIDS the immunosuppression mainly

Table 3 CD4 positive T lymphocytes of patients with HIV infection at the time of diagnosis of mycobacterial infection

Mycobacterium tuberculosis ($n = 11$)	$286 \pm 98\,\mu l$
Atypical Mycobacteria ($n = 16$)	$117 \pm 34\,\mu l$
Controls ($n = 50$)	$847 \pm 366\,\mu l$

consists of a defective cell-mediated immunity due to the lack of T lymphocytes. The histological features of atypical mycobacterial infection fit that pathophysiological explanation: in the absence of macrophage activation an unrestricted amplification of intracellular organisms can be observed, sometimes leading to greatly enlarged cells appearing as foam cells[6].

The characteristic picture of caseating granulomata with a surrounding wall of epithelioid and giant cells, which arouses the suspicion of tuberculous infection on histological grounds, is completely abated in advanced stages of immunoincompetence. Since mycobacteria-laden macrophages without visible tissue reaction are scattered throughout the organ, the liver might appear normal on regular staining, only special stains for AFB will reveal infection and thereby prove severe immunosuppression. Ziehl-Neelsen staining of lymph nodes in particular shows macrophages packed with mycobacteriae. Hence the clinician has to inform the pathologist of any type of immunoincompetence of the patient. Since AIDS patients are at increased risk for tuberculosis as well as atypical mycobacterial infection, some patients are affected by both strains at the same time. They might exhibit at liver biopsy more or less well-preserved granulomata on one side and macrophages full of bacteria without tissue reaction on the other side. This observation also calls for microbiological evaluation and distinction of different types from every liver biopsy material.

SARCOIDOSIS

Sarcoidosis is a systemic granulomatous disorder of unknown cause involving many organs. Depending on the geographical area it is the leading disease, or second most frequent next to tuberculosis, forming granulomata in the liver. In most cases hepatic involvement has no disease character by itself. The characteristic clinical presentations of sarcoidosis include pulmonary infiltrates, lymphadenopathy, fever, infiltrative skin lesions, uveitis and arthritis. The importance of liver granulomata in sarcoidosis is predominantly related to the relatively easy access for diagnostic purposes by liver biopsy. Approximately 60–75% of all patients with sarcoidosis reveal hepatic involvement[11]. The histological feature of sarcoidosis is a granuloma with epithelioid and giant cells without necrosis, but with an inflammatory cell wall consisting mainly of lymphocytes. In the acute phase, and sometimes also in chronic phases, an elevation of 1,25-dihydroxycholecalciferol (vitamin D_3) can be found (Table 4). It is apparently produced by the epithelioid

Table 4 Signs and symptoms of sarcoidosis of the liver

Pulmonary involvement frequent
Multi-organ involvement
Granuloma formation
Elevated serum levels of 1′-25′-dihydroxycholecalciferol
Hypercalcaemia
Hypercalciuria
Elevated angiotensin-converting enzyme (ACE)
Positive Kveim–Siltzbach test

cell itself[12]. This causes hypercalcaemia and consequently hypercalciuria. Increased activity of the angiotensin-converting enzyme (ACE) is found in up to 75% of cases, depending on disease activity. It is not specific, since it is also found in other disorders. In contrast, the Kveim–Siltzbach test, found positive in about 80% of patients with sarcoidosis, appears to be very specific[13]. Unfortunately this test is not uniformly available and not well standardized.

As already stated, very few patients with sarcoidosis show clinically evident involvement of the liver despite frequent granulomatous findings at liver biopsy or autopsy. In rare cases particularly long-standing activity can cause overt liver disease (Table 5). Sometimes the liver is enlarged and the biochemical tests are mildly to moderately abnormal. In those cases with symptomatic hepatic sarcoidosis various complications have been observed. A chronic disorder resembling chronic active hepatitis has been described[14]. Rare cases of portal hypertension, jaundice and even hepatocellular failure have also been observed[15]. In far-advanced cases with long-standing liver disease clinical and histological features of liver cirrhosis may develop[16]. Splenomegaly with ensuing pancytopenia might be the consequence of portal hypertension, but can also occur by granulomatous infiltration within the spleen[15]. The latter situation can be relieved by corticosteroids, which in turn are of no apparent value in chronic liver involvement.

It is interesting – and sometimes productive – to compare instances of apparently distinct disorders in which overlapping clinical and laboratory features suggest the possibility of kinship. Such is the case with sarcoidosis and primary biliary cirrhosis[17]. The clinical and laboratory findings in classical cases are easily distinguished. Yet the two disorders have several features in common (Table 6). The causes of both diseases are unknown, granulomatous changes are found in the liver and both disorders represent systemic diseases. Finally, they have immunological disturbances in common, in particular depression of delayed-type hypersensitivity with reduced skin energy and reversed ratio of helper and suppressor T lymphocytes[18–20]. Descriptions of approximately 35 patients in the literature who have shown

Table 5 Complications of liver sarcoidosis

Intrahepatic cholestasis
Extrahepatic cholestasis
Jaundice
Cirrhosis
Portal hypertension
Hepatocellular failure
Primary biliary cirrhosis?

Table 6 Common features between primary biliary cirrhosis and sarcoidosis

Unknown cause
Granuloma formation
Systemic involvement
Depressed immunity

signs and symptoms of both disorders, either at the same time or in the clinical course over many years, have led to discussion about the relationship between these conditions. Even in advanced stages of sarcoidosis with features of PBC the antimitochondrial antibody test remains negative; in cases of PBC resembling sarcoidosis the Kveim-Siltzbach test never becomes positive[21]. Without identification of the cause of both disorders the question of kinship between those conditions cannot be resolved[22].

References

1. Hersch, C. (1964). Tuberculosis of the liver. A study of 200 cases. *S. Afr. Med. J.*, **38**, 857–63
2. Essop, A. R., Posen, J. A., Hodkinson, J. H. and Segal, J. (1984). Tuberculosis hepatitis: a clinical review of 96 cases. *Q. J. Med.*, **53**, 465–77
3. Farhi, D. C., Mason, U. G. and Horsburgh, C. R. (1985). Pathologic findings in disseminated *Mycobacterium avium-intracellulare* infection. *Am. J. Clin. Pathol.*, **85**, 67–72
4. Maharaj, B., Leary, W. P. and Pudifin, D. J. (1987). A prospective study of hepatic tuberculosis in 41 black patients. *Q. J. Med.*, **63**, 517–22
5. Kehrein, B., Ruf, B., Thalmann, U., Schürmann, D., Brehmer, W., Pohle, H. D. and Jautzke, G. (1988). Mykobakteriosen bei AIDS. *Pathologe*, **9**, 218–27
6. Thomsen, C., Zietz, C., Zoller, W. G., Gokel, J. M., Hehlmann, R. and Goebel, F.-D. (1988). Mykobakterielle Infektion bei Patienten mit erworbenem Immundefektsyndrom. *AIFO*, **3**, 197–201
7. Centers for Disease Control (1987). Diagnosis and management of mycobacterial infection and disease in persons with human immunodeficiency virus infection. *Ann. Intern. Med.*, **106**, 254–6
8. Hawkins, C. C., Gold, J. W. M., Whimbey, E., Kiehn, T. E., Brannon, P., Cammarata, R., Brown, A. E. and Armstrong, D. (1986). *Mycobacterium avium* complex infections in patients with the acquired immunodeficiency syndrome. *Ann. Intern. Med.*, **105**, 184–8
9. Müller-Hermelink, H. K. and Kaiserling, E. (1980). Epitheloidzellreaktionen im lymphatischen Gewebe. In: *Verh. Dtsch. Ges. Path.*, **64** (ed. G. Dohm), pp. 77–102 (Stuttgart: Gustav-Fischer-Verlag)
10. Wiesinger, D. and Borel, J. F. (1979). Studies on the mechanism of action of cyclosporin A. *Immunobiology*, **156**, 454–72
11. Ferguson, R. H. and Paris, J. (1958). Sarcoidosis. Study of 29 cases with a review of splenic, hepatic, mucus membrane, retinal and joint manifestations. *Arch. Intern. Med.*, **101**, 1065–84
12. Adams, J. S., Diz, M. M. and Sharma, O. P. (1989). Effective reduction in the serum 1,25-dihydroxyvitamin D and calcium concentration in sarcoidosis-associated hypercalcemia with short-course chloroquine therapy. *Ann. Intern. Med.*, **111**, 437–8
13. James, D. G. (1984). Sarcoidosis. *Postgrad. Med. J.*, **60**, 234–41
14. Tekeste, H., Latour, F. and Levitt, R. E. (1984). Portal hypertension complicating liver disease: case report and review of the literature. *Am. J. Gastroenterol.*, **79**, 389–96
15. Valla, D., Pessegueiro-Miranda, H., Degott, C., Lebrec, D., Rueff, B. and Benhamou, J.-P. (1987). Hepatic sarcoidosis with portal hypertension. A report of seven cases with a review of the literature. *Q. J. Med.*, **63**, 531–44
16. Pariente, E. A., Joly, J. P., Capron, J. P., Mancheron, H., Flamant, Y. and Barge, J. (1981). Hypertension portale, cholestase et syndrome pulmonaire chez une femme de 58 ans. *Gastroenterol. Clin. Biol.*, **5**, 340–8
17. Heslinga, J. M., Ruiter, D. J., Goud, T. H. and Lens, J. (1982). Sarcoidosis of the liver, complicated by bleeding oesophageal varices. *Netherlands J. Surg.*, **34–5**, 231–4
18. Maddrey, W. C. (1983). Sarcoidosis and primary biliary cirrhosis. *N. Engl. J. Med.*, **308**, 588–90
19. Fagan, E. A., Morre-Gillon, J. C. and Turner-Warwick, M. (1983). Multiorgan granulomas and mitochondrial antibodies. *N. Engl. J. Med.*, **388**, 572–5

20. Pereira-Lima, J. and Schaffner, F. (1987). Chronic cholestasis in hepatic sarcoidosis with clinical features resembling primary biliary cirrhosis. *Am. J. Med.*, **83**, 144–8
21. Ludwig, J. (1988). Etiology of biliary cirrhosis: diagnostic features and a new classification. *Zentralbl. Allg. Pathol. Pathol. Anat.*, **134**, 132–41
22. Eklund, A., Stjernberg, N., Uddenfeldt, P. and Danielsson, A. (1985). Kveim test and mitochondrial antibodies in the differential diagnosis between primary biliary cirrhosis and sarcoidosis. *Sarcoidosis*, **2**, 38–41

9
The liver in sepsis and pyogenic abscess of the liver

A. J. GREENSTEIN

When abscess of the liver is treated by cautery or incision, if the pus which is discharged be pure and white the patients recover (for in this case it is situated in the coats of the liver) but if it resembles the lees of oil as it flows they die (Hippocrates (460–370 BC))[1]

INTRODUCTION

It is not surprising that the liver, the largest composite organ in the body, and a major player on the metabolic scene, is intimately involved in sepsis. The liver is involved in septic processes in at least four different ways. These include extrahepatic sepsis with secondary hepatic dysfunction, intrahepatic sepsis such as pyogenic or amoebic liver abscess, and cirrhosis with infected ascites and spontaneous bacterial peritonitis. Finally the interrelationships of inflammatory bowel disease (IBD) and liver sepsis are legion, ranging from mild histopathological changes, to sclerosing cholangitis with stasis and sepsis, to frank intrahepatic pyogenic abscess. This presentation will discuss the three former septic processes, and make only limited reference to the pyogenic abscess aspects of IBD.

THE LIVER IN SEPSIS

Severe sepsis leads to bacteraemia and shock, and may be life-threatening. Gram-negative sepsis results classically in primary impairment of cellular oxygen uptake and utilization. There is a compensatory hyperdynamic circulation with increased cardiac output. A decrease in peripheral vascular resistance occurs in an attempt to improve the oxygen supply to the cells. There are few reports on the role of the liver in sepsis and shock compared with heart, lung and kidneys, perhaps because the liver disease itself is rarely the direct cause of death[2]. Nevertheless, patients who develop jaundice in association with systemic bacterial infections, with or without concomitant shock, are at increased risk, and have a significant mortality.

We will examine the effects of extrahepatic sepsis on the liver in three groups of patients: the neonate, the infant and the adult. In all three groups there are certain common features, but they differ in many respects including the type of underlying sepsis, the type of underlying bacterial infection, the degree of liver damage, and the mortality rate (see Table 1). Common features include a considerable and disproportionate conjugated hyperbilirubinaemia in most patients, elevated alkaline phosphatase in some, and impairment of renal function with frank pyelonephritis especially in the younger groups. I will now consider each of the groups in turn.

Neonatal sepsis with liver involvement

The neonatal period includes the first week of life. Hamilton and Sass-Kortsak reported on eight such patients[3]. The onset of jaundice was sudden in six, occurring between 4 and 7 days of birth, and gradual in two, occurring within the first 2 days of life. Seven of the eight patients died, six within 24 h. Seven had enteric organism, five *E. coli*, one *Aerobacter aerogenes*, one *Pneumococcus* and one *Pseudomonas* plus *S. sonnei*. Umbilical infection was suspected in some, and positive blood culture was present in the seven who died. Histological liver damage was conspicuous by its absence in these patients.

Table 1 Clinicopathological patterns of disease in patients with extrahepatic sepsis and liver involvement

	Neonate	*Infant*	*Adult*
Mortality	88%[3]	25%[3]	12.5% with abscesses[7] 43% with pneumonia etc.[5]
Urinary dysfunction	Yes	>90%	>66%
Urosepsis	Common	66%	20%
Haemolysis	Yes+++	Yes+	No
Bacterial cultures	*E. coli* 60% Enteric in 88%	*E. coli* in almost all	*Staph. aureus, E. coli* *Pseudomonas, Enterococci* *Paracolon, Proteus,* *Serratia, D. pneumoniae,* etc.
Histological liver damage	None	Bile stasis Pericholangitis Centrilobular Necrosis (15%)	Fatty change Focal hepatitis Centrilobular Lipofuscin
Mean max. lab. values			
Total bilirubin (mg/100 ml)	±20	±14	±9
Conjugated (mg/100 ml)/%	±2/87%	±5/<100%	±7/<100%
White cell count (mm^3)	±20,000	±28,000	±16,000
Alkaline phosphatase (KA units)	±24	±22	≠Unusual*

* Occasional cases with raised AP only reported by Fang *et al.*[8]

The liver in infant sepsis

There are several reports of infants with jaundice in both autopsy[4] and clinical series[3]. These patients differ from the neonatal group in several respects. The prognosis is clearly better, 12 of 16 patients reported by Hamilton surviving[3]. In addition there were marked histological changes in the liver in all patients who died. These included toxic cellular changes, with marked centrilobular necrosis in four of the 10 mortalities in the two series. In addition there was both intracellular and intracanalicular bile stasis, Urosepsepsis, and bacteraemia were features of these cases, especially those who died.

Jaundice in severe bacterial infection in the adult

Jaundice can occur in adult patients in association with severe systemic infection such as pneumonia, pyelonephritis or soft tissue infection[5]. The postoperative period is particularly vulnerable[6,7]. Fahrlander *et al.*[7] described eight patients, with seven survivors; five following surgery on the biliary tract, intestinal tract or ureter, and three infection or pneumonia. Miller *et al.*[5] described the findings on 30 patients, nine with pneumonia, six with pyelonephritis, eight with pelvic infection or peritonitis and six with soft tissue infection and various other miscellaneous causes. The mortality was 43%. The characteristic finding was elevation of bilirubin (mean 8.79 mg/100 ml), mainly direct reacting (6.78 mg/100 ml) (see Table 1). There was a small increase only in alkaline phosphatase, to approximately normal values. Histological findings in 13 were non-specific, ranging from mild to moderate cholestasis, with fatty change and periportal inflammation. Most articles report similar biochemical abnormalities with predominant hyperbilirubinema; but Fang *et al.*[8] described four other cases between 50 and 68 years of age, with abscesses of colon, appendix, lung, or bone, in whom there was a marked elevation in alkaline phosphatase and a minimal increase in bilirubin. All four patients survived, suggesting a better prognosis for this group.

Spontaneous bacterial peritonitis

This lethal development is a terminal event occurring in 10% of patients with advanced cirrhosis and ascites. Most patients are infected by enteric bacteria, especially *E. coli.* Anatomically the portal system lies in close proximity to the lymphatics. Weeping of the lymphatics from the surface of the liver, a characteristic feature of cirrhosis, could transfer bacteria to the ascitic fluid. The source of the enteric bacteria is a dilated sinusoidal system resulting from the post-sinusoidal obstruction of cirrhosis. Although Conn and Fessel[9] report a 97% hospital mortality, Nance[10] suggested a more accurate figure of 85–90%.

THE LIVER IN INFLAMMATORY BOWEL DISEASE

Most changes in inflammatory bowel disease involve histopathological cellular infiltrates or granulomas without sepsis or liver dysfunction, of little clinical significance. The sclerosing cholangitis of ulcerative colitis, and more rarely Crohn's disease, is complicated by multiple strictures, proximal dilatation of the intrahepatic ducts, and in some patients intrahepatic abscess formation. Liver transplantation for advanced cases of sclerosing cholangitis with severe hepatic dysfunction is now being carried out with increasing frequency.

Liver abscess is a rare complication of Crohn's disease[11] and almost unknown in ulcerative colitis. We described six patients, and reviewed another seven case reports from the medical literature[11]. Transperitoneal surgical drainage is advisable for these patients because of concomitant underlying intra-abdominal abscess. Five of the 13 patients died. All mortalities had multiple abscesses; their mean age was 56, 19 years older than the eight survivors, and three received antibiotics alone without drainage. The diagnosis was frequently difficult to make, and obscured by the symptoms of the underlying inflammatory bowel disease, or concomitant intra-abdominal abscess.

PYOGENIC LIVER ABSCESS

The incidence and types of liver infections of gastrointestinal origin vary markedly from one part of the world to the other, and in the United States from one demographic area to another. These infections may be due to bacteria, parasites, or fungi. Schistosomiasis, amoebiasis, echinococcal disease, and clonorchis sinensis are endemic in many areas of the Far East, South America, Africa and the United States. While these parasitic diseases are the major cause of liver infections in selected areas of the world, pyogenic liver abscess is probably the most commonly encountered infection of gastrointestinal origin in the United States. This presentation will discuss pyogenic liver abscess and allude to hepatic amoebiasis, the most commonly encountered liver infections of gastrointestinal origin in the United States.

Pyogenic liver abscess and its grave prognosis were recognized before the Christian era by Hippocrates (460–370 BC)[1], who was able to distinguish between liver abscesses, which were lethal, and cystic disease of the liver, which is seldom of real clinical significance. Celsus (53 BC–AD 7)[12] appreciated that the development of jaundice in association with infections of the liver indicated an extremely grave prognosis; a relationship supported by the high mortality of both intrahepatic and extrahepatic infections with hyperbilirubinaemia. In 1836 Bright[13] gave the first clear description of suppuration of the liver with true abscess formation. The relationship to appendicitis was described by Matterstock[14] and Fitz[15], who each reported 11 cases with this association. Fitz appreciated that liver abscess developed as a consequence of mesenteric thrombophlebitis, which originated in the region of the appendix. In 1938 a detailed description of 47 cases of liver abscess was given by Ochsner and his associates[16], but 75% of their patients suffered from amoebic liver abscess and a much smaller proportion from pyogenic liver abscess.

Over the past 50 years the source of liver abscess has changed considerably. There has been a steep reduction in amoebic liver abscess[17], a marked reduction of appendicitis-related abscess following use of newer antibiotics[18], and an increase in biliary tract-related pyogenic liver abscess. With computerized tomography (CT) or magnetic resonance imaging (MRI) preoperative diagnosis has increased, and autopsy cases have decreased due to earlier and more definitive therapy[18].

Pyogenic liver abscess is a distinct clinical entity in which the absolute distinction from other cystic liver masses requires the aspiration and culture of pyogenic bacteria from the purulent fluid obtained from the abscess cavity. Despite the major changes in aetiology, and the improved prognosis of pyogenic liver abscesses, the incidence of true pyogenic liver abscess has changed little over the past century. Prevalence rates during this century have remained fairly constant, ranging from 0.29% to 1.47% for necropsy series[18–22], and from 0.008% to 0.016% for hospital populations[17,21–23].

Pyogenic liver abscesses may be divided into those of gastrointestinal origin and a separate group of systemic origin. The latter include those caused by bacteraemia, spreading via the hepatic artery, those secondary to penetrating and blunt trauma, and those of unexplained origin, known as cryptogenic. The proportion of cryptogenic abscesses has fallen, with the utilization of more modern diagnostic techniques from 60% to approximately 20%[16,24]. Abscesses of gastrointestinal origin may originate from (1) gallbladder or bile ducts; (2) abdominal viscera, via the portal vein (pylephlebitis suppurativa); and (3) may spread by direct contiguity from adjacent organs such as stomach, duodenum, kidney, or subphrenic spaces. Biliary tract disease is now the most frequent cause of pyogenic liver abscess of gastrointestinal origin, largely because of a rising proportion of elderly patients with gallbladder disease[25,26]. The most common source of pylephlebitis suppurativa used to be appendicitis. Today this is a rare entity, and when present originates from other sources such as pericolonic or peritoneal abscesses due to diverticulitis, inflammatory bowel disease or perforated cancer. Diverticulitis may be overt and easily detected, or occult in nature eluding the most careful diagnostic workups[27]. Inflammatory bowel disease is another important source, particularly Crohn's disease, in which abscess[28] and fistula[29] formation are common. We found a total of six patients with liver abscesses among 1277 patients with Crohn's disease[11]. The development of liver abscess is less common in ulcerative colitis, despite the fact that bacteria have been found within the portal system[30,31]. Other sources include inflammation of the pancreas with either pancreatic necrosis or abscess, colonic carcinoma with perforation and pericolonic abscess, infected haemorrhoids, or Meckel's diverticulum.

The relationship of liver abscess to the anatomical origin of flow in the portal vein has intrigued investigators since the beginning of this century. In 1948 Kinney and Ferrebee[26] likened the portal vein to the Mississippi River. In this river the two tributaries continue to maintain their individual character of two separate channels, even after joining one another to create a single stream. Credence has been lent to their hypothesis by the demonstration that India ink injected into the superior mesenteric vein of a rabbit goes to the right lobe of the liver, while ink injected into the splenic vein goes to the left lobe[32]. In fact, abscesses of the right lobe originate more frequently on the right side, usually from the caecum or other organs in this region, while those of the left lobe usually originate on the left side from sigmoid colon or rectum[26]. Although this theory is intriguing, there are often exceptions, since many abscesses of portal origin are bilateral or contralateral.

Abscesses often extend to the liver directly from contiguous organs, such as stomach, pylorus, gallbladder, kidney, colon or duodenum (Figure 1). Most abscesses occur in the right lobe of the liver, which is by far the larger, and to which gallbladder bile ducts and right colon drain.

Diagnosis

In earlier years the diagnosis of pyogenic liver abscess was usually missed on presentation and was made, if at all, only late in the course of the disease, after long-standing suppuration[33]. The ability to make the diagnosis preoperatively depended upon such advanced signs and symptoms as well-defined right upper quadrant pain or discomfort, a large palpable liver, an

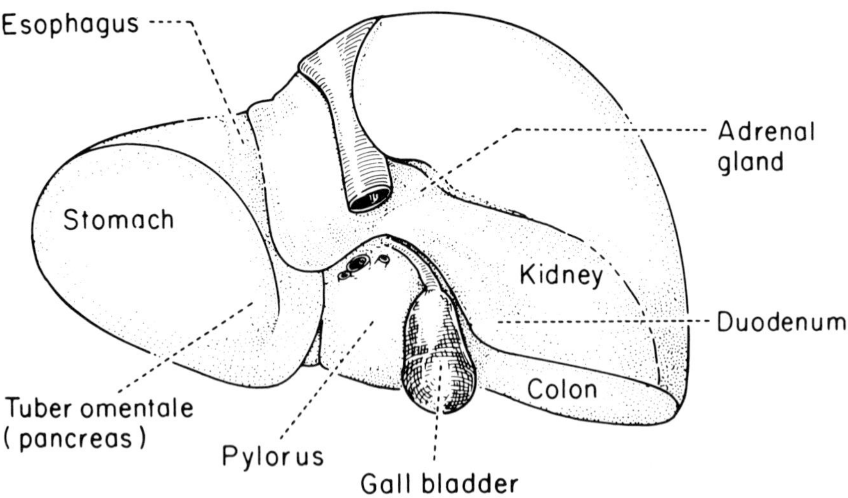

Figure 1 Diagrammatic representation of the posteroinferior surface of the liver showing organs in contact with the liver from which pyogenic liver abscess may originate (reproduced from *Bockus Gastroenterology 4th Edition*, Volume 5 (Liver) (W. B. Saunders) with permission)

acute septic clinical picture, weight loss, and jaundice[21,34]. More recently CT scanning, magnetic resonance imaging, and sonography have allowed earlier diagnosis before the florid clinical picture develops. As a consequence of this earlier recognition, the clinical presentation now tends to be more insidious and the signs more subtle. The clinical manifestations of pyogenic liver abscess are listed in Table 2. Subdivision into earlier and late eras shows a clear distinction with regard to the various clinical signs, with a definite trend to a reduced frequency of pain, rigors, and hepatomegaly in more recent years.

Liver abscess may present in many guises: unexplained fever and leukocytosis[34] with shaking chills[35,36]; insidious malaise, weakness, anorexia, and weight loss, especially in the elderly[34]; and even on occasion the picture of intrathoracic disease with cough, dyspnoea, and pleuritic pain[21].

Laboratory abnormalities are common but are not sufficiently specific to point to the precise diagnosis. They include leucocytosis with a left shift, anaemia, and abnormalities of liver function tests such as increase in bilirubin or alkaline phosphatase[21,27,34]. An elevated bilirubin is almost always a feature of biliary tract infection[21].

Bacteriological cultures were frequently negative or 'sterile' both before[16,37], and in the earlier years after[38–40], the introduction of antibiotics. This frequency of negative cultures in earlier years was due to a high incidence of amoebiasis[16,20] as well as inadequacy of anaerobic culture techniques[41]. The proportion of positive cultures subsequently increased, first between 1934 and 1958 with the recognition of antibiotic-resistant Gram-negative *Proteus Vulgaris*, *Aerobacter aerogenes*, and *Pseudomonas aeruginosa*[19], and later on account of a steadily increasing recovery of anaerobic organisms, including microaerophilic streptococci, bacteroides, fusobacterium, and actinomyces[23,31,42].

Radiological methods are critical to the diagnosis of all forms of localized liver infection. Radiological features on plain X-ray are usually non-specific; they include right-sided pulmonary changes such as elevated or fixed right diaphragm, pleural effusion, basilar atelectasis, and empyema or lung abscess in 20–80% of patients[16,17,21,24,38]. Similar findings are found on the left side in a smaller proportion of cases[17]. A subdiaphragmatic gas or fluid level[38,43,44] may also be seen on occasion. Upper gastrointestinal series may show displacement of the stomach by an enlarged left lobe of the liver in 19% of patients[21].

Angiography is still of value, particularly for small or multiple abscesses or for those in remote areas of the liver; angiographic techniques include selective hepatic arteriography, splenoportography, inferior venacavography, and transumbilical hepatography[17]. Angiography is especially valuable in delineating the liver anatomy if resection is contemplated, since it allows precise localization of the lesion; it is also particularly useful for multiple abscesses and for those associated with malignant tumors[17]. The classic arteriographic features are displacement, elongation, and distortion of intrahepatic arteries with an avascular central area and hypervascular margins at the periphery of the abscess[45–47]. The hepatogram phase shows a differential translucency in amoebic abscess[45]. Splenoportography will

Table 2 Clinical manifestations in pyogenic liver abscess

	Ochsner et al.[16] *(1928)*	*Ochsner et al.*[16] *(1928–37)*	*Pitt and Zuidema*[23] *(1936–65)*	*Lee and Block*[39] *(1965–70)*	*Altemeier et al.*[49] *(1955–70)*	*Rubin et al.*[21] *(1961–73)*	*Balasegaram*[17] *(1965–80)*	*McDonald and Howard*[24] *(1954–80)*	*Greenstein et al.*[18] *(1967–82)*
No. patients	518*	47	12	11	65	50	125	490*	38
Symptoms (%)									
Fever	96	94	96	92	95	87	98	79	95
Pain	90	88	75	54	62	47	97	51	84
Rigors	59	36	92	77	18	38	30	35	71
Nausea/vomiting	33	33	70	31	15	28	68	33	47
Weight loss	†	†	75	69		25	74	31	37
Anorexia	†	†			54	38	65	26	47
Malaise	†	†				30	33	20	34
Signs (%)									
Hepatomegaly	89	61	80	54	49	51	89	50	39
Tenderness right upper quadrant	92	91	76	69	49	47	89	50	42
Jaundice	36	24	52	8	31	20	22	27	24
Pulmonary signs					21	24	36		37

* Collected series
† Prominent and early.

liver$land
03-04-90 15:44:52

demonstrate splenic vein thrombosis or an avascular area. Venacavography will show large posterior segment abscesses as venacaval displacement and narrowing.

Radionuclide scanning, ultrasonography, CT, and MRI are the most valuable diagnostic methods. CT and MRI are today the 'gold standard' among diagnostic modalities, and indeed may make most other techniques obsolete. The use of these techniques heralds a new era in the management of hepatic abscess, allowing earlier diagnosis, more precise localization and accurate percutaneous or surgical drainage.

Scintigraphy, originally using ^{131}I-rose bengal taken up by hepatocytes and ^{131}I-labelled serum taken up by the Kupffer cells, and more recently using technetium-99 sulphur colloid, began to be associated with reduced mortality in the 1960s, providing a diagnostic accuracy up to 98%[48–53]. Ultrasonography remains a valuable diagnostic tool, since it is rapid, relatively inexpensive, non-invasive, does not require use of ionizing radiation, and differentiates solid from fluid masses. While the anterior superior aspect of the dome of the liver is best demonstrated by radionuclide scanning, the area around the gallbladder fossa is better seen by sonography, making these techniques complementary[54]. Resolution by these measures has improved from 4 cm to about 2 cm today[17,54,55]. Differentiation of abscesses from solid tumors can be made except in cases with central necrosis and liquefaction.

Single or multiple abscesses as small as 0.5 cm can be clearly delineated[56] in a high proportion of cases. Although CT is not infallible[57], it is becoming clearer and more reliable year by year. CT is not only valuable in diagnosis but may also be critical in guiding surgical management in at least one-third of cases[58].

Laparoscopy is seldom required today but may occasionally be useful for locating the site of bulging at the surface of the liver[17]; and to rule out or confirm by biopsy the presence of metastatic disease. Endoscopic retrograde cholangiography should be used with circumspection in biliary tract-related liver abscess, since it may aggravate ascending cholangitis[17].

Treatment

Prophylaxis or prevention is the most effective way to reduce mortality from pyogenic liver abscess. Methods of prevention include early decompression of malignant or calculous obstruction of the biliary tree; complete excision of devitalized tissue; and ligation of all transected arteries, veins, and bile ducts in blunt liver trauma, with prophylactic antibiotic administration prior to hepatic artery ligation. Early treatment of intra-abdominal sepsis will also reduce the incidence of pyogenic liver abscess.

Definitive therapy is essential to avoid the potentially 100% mortality of pyogenic liver abscess[16,17,19,23,49,50]. This therapy includes antibiotics, adequate drainage of the liver abscess, and simultaneous eradication of underlying causative factors, especially if the sepsis originates in the gastrointestinal tract.

Antibiotic treatment alone was recommended in some earlier publications that reported a success rate of 80–90%[59–61]. However, it was subsequently recognized that the key to successful treatment, besides antibiotic therapy, was aspiration or surgical drainage of the abscess. Antibiotic therapy includes penicillin or a cephalosporin for Gram-positive cocci and sensitive Gram-negative organisms; metronidazole, clindamycin, or chloramphenicol for anaerobes, especially *B. fragilis*; and an aminoglycoside for resistant Gram-negative organisms. Ranson *et al.*[48] in 1975 found a 78% sensitivity to gentamicin and an 80% sensitivity to chloramphenicol.

Today a large number of newer antibiotics are available. One would recommend cefoxitin alone as the primary mode of therapy. Although some advise unasyn (ampicillin + sulbactam), there is some question as to whether this combination is as effective as the combination of clindamycin and gentamicin[62]. Imipenem alone (thienamycin) is effective against all organisms likely to be found in liver abscesses. These include anaerobes such as *Bacteroides fragilis*, *Enterobacter*, *Serratia*, and coliforms, *Klebsiella*, *Staphylococcus aureus*, and *Streptococcus fecalis*, as well as *Pseudomonas aeruginosa*. It is such a valuable drug that it should be reserved for treatment failures, or patients in whom an organism resistant to cefoxitin, unasyn (ampicillin + sulbactam), or the clindamycin/metronidazole aminoglycoside combination.

As early as 1953, McFadzean *et al.*[63] described successful percutaneous drainage in 14 patients with solitary pyogenic liver abscess, all of whom survived. The initial drainage was carried out blindly, with subsequent radiological guidance provided by replacing the aspirated purulent fluid with air and lipiodol. It was not until the 1970s, however, when Smith *et al.*[64] described ultrasonically guided aspiration of abscesses, and Novy *et al.* described angiographic diagnosis by closed aspiration[37], that percutaneous drainage was again tried. Later in the decade, Gerzof and co-workers described percutaneous drainage using CT and ultrasonographic guidance for detection, localization, and aspiration of liver abscesses[65,66]. Since the early 1980s, successful treatment by percutaneous drainage has become increasingly popular[17,67–70].

The most widely used and successful therapy for pyogenic liver abscess, however, remains open surgical drainage. Surgical exploration should be carried out in all treatment failures, especially when there is concomitant recognized intra-abdominal disease, and after CT localization of loculated or multiple abscesses. The major issue has been and remains whether the serous-lined peritoneal or pleural cavities should be transgressed during the operative procedure (trans-serous route), or whether the surgical approach can avoid or bypass these cavities (extraserous approach), thus limiting the likelihood of peritonitis or pyothorax. In the early years, Ochsner *et al.*[16] found a much higher mortality with the trans-serous (transpleural or transperitoneal) route of drainage than with the extraserous (posterior and anterior extraperitoneal) approach as described by Nather *et al.*[71] and Clairmont *et al.*[72]. As a result extraserous drainage was recommended for several decades.

In 1968, however, a gratifyingly low mortality, two of 21 patients, was reported by Joseph *et al.*[38] utilizing the transabdominal trans-serous approach, while there were two deaths among five patients drained extraperitoneally. Thereafter most authors[23,39,49,50] have recommended the most direct route, generally advising the transabdominal approach. Ranson *et al.*[48] noted that better access to multiple abscesses and wider exploration of the abdomen to locate the source of the abscess were the major advantages of the trans-serous route. Furthermore this route is particularly valuable for access to the left lobe and to the anterior portion of the right lobe of the liver. With simultaneous administration of antibiotics the risk entailed by transgressing the peritoneal or pleural cavity is minimized.

Nevertheless, if an abscess is proved by high-resolution scanning to be solitary and easily accessible to direct extraperitoneal drainage, this route may still be considered, particularly in patients who are critically ill. This extraserous approach was first described by Trendelenberg in 1883[73] for access to the posterior superior aspect of the right lobe, which is the most difficult to reach through the abdomen. It is still valuable for this purpose today, as well as for draining high subhepatic and high intrahepatic abscesses[37,48,74,75].

Whatever route of surgical drainage is utilized, the abscess must be aspirated completely and the roof partially excised. Drains should be left in position for irrigation with antibiotics. Drainage should be continued for as long as 2 months, with concomitant antibiotics up to 4 months following surgery. Steady reduction in size of the abscess cavity should be documented by sonography or by CT scanning.

Liver debridement or liver resection may be necessary in some cases with multiple abscesses or with perforation into adjacent pleura, peritoneum, or pericardium[17]. Chronic fibrotic abscesses with well-defined thick walls, first described by Beaver[76], require hepatic resection[17,74]. Occasionally, hepatic resection or lobectomy is also required for post-traumatic pyogenic abscesses, for major laceration of a lobe of the liver, for haemobilia[17], or for abscesses of the left lateral segment[21,24,77].

Prognosis

Prognosis of pyogenic abscess has steadily improved over the past half-century (Table 3), with case fatality rates falling from a range of 60–80%[21,24,77,78] to 16–38% or lower[18]. Factors contributing to this decreasing mortality include earlier diagnosis and more accurate localization by imaging

Table 3 Mortality in pyogenic liver abscess – the influence of multiplicity

	Era	*No. of patients*	*Solitary (%)*	*Multiple (%)*	*Overall (%)*
Pitt *et al.*[23]	1952–72	80	31	88	65
Warren *et al.*[77]	1923–66	20	33	81	60
McDonald and Howard[24]	1954–80	586*	24	76	57
Heymann[78]	1938–76	29	21	77	48
Lazarchik *et al.*[50]	1960–70	75	25	61	40
Greenstein *et al.*[18]	1967–82	38	16	32	24

* Collected series.

techniques, improved bacteriology, particularly with anaerobic cultures, more effective perioperative antibiotic therapy, and planned percutaneous aspiration or transabdominal surgical drainage.

The major factors affecting mortality include the age of the patient, the number of abscesses (Table 4), the development of complications, and the presence of associated diseases such as cancer. Polymicrobial bacteraemia and impaired liver function, manifested by jaundice and hypoalbuminaemia, are also important risk factors. Mortality is highest in the very young and in the elderly, with reports of case fatality rates as high as 80% in these two groups[21,23,79].

The number of abscesses is a particularly crucial prognostic factor; mortality is highest with multiple abscesses[35], usually due to ascending cholangitis, and lower with solitary abscesses spreading to the liver via the vascular system (Table 4). Indeed in our series[18], multiplicity was the most important single determinant of mortality, carrying a case fatality rate twice as high as for solitary abscess (Table 4).

Complications associated with a higher mortality include septicaemia or bacteraemia[18,23], subphrenic or subhepatic abscess[17,49], and rupture of the abscess into the peritoneal cavity, the pleural cavity, or the lung[17,23]. Additional complications are liver failure, haemobilia, haemorrhage into the liver abscess, empyema, haemoptysis, and meningitis[17,21,49]. Commonly associated diseases that contribute to mortality risk include diabetes mellitus[49,78], polycystic disease[49], lymphoblastic leukaemia[49], and cirrhosis. Pylephlebitis suppurativa, associated with a prohibitive mortality[16,19], is rare today.

Table 4 Major factors influencing mortality among 38 patients with pyogenic liver abscess[18]

	Survivors	*Deaths*	*Total*	*Mortality (%)*	*Significance (d.f. = 1)*	
	(n = 29)	*(n = 9)*	*(n = 38)*	*(24%)*	χ^2	*p*
Solitary abscess	16	3	19	16		n.s.
Multiple abscess	13	6	19	32		
>60 years old	12	7	19	37	3.6	<0.06
<60 years old	17	2	19	11		
With cancer	2	4	6	67	7.3	<0.01
Without cancer	27	5	32	16		
With hypoalbuminaemia	23	8	32	26		n.s.
Without hypoalbuminaemia	6	1	7	14		
With clinical jaundice	5	4	9	44	2.8	<0.10
Without jaundice	24	5	29	17		
Elevated bilirubin	18	7	25	28		n.s.
Normal bilirubin	11	2	13	15		
Biliary origin	12	5	17	29		n.s.
Non-biliary origin	17	4	21	19		
Bacteriology of abscess						
Polymicrobial	9	4	13	31		n.s.
Monomicrobial	15	4	19	21		
Sterile	4	0	4	0		
No culture available	1	1	3	50		
Bacteriology of blood						
Positive blood culture	4	6	10	60	9.5	<0.005
Negative blood culture	25	3	28	11		

Differential diagnosis

The most important differential diagnosis to make is that of amoebic liver abscess, especially in visitors from South America or patients returning from areas where amoebiasis is endemic. This can be made by stool examination, or serology (amoebic complement fixation, immunoelectrophoresis or haem agglutination)[80]. It is important to bear in mind that secondary bacterial infection may complicate amoebic abscess. Nevertheless, specific antibiotic therapy such as metronidazole, chloroquine or emetine may result in rapid cure of amoebic abscess with or without concomitant drainage.

In patients from the Far East multiple liver abscesses can result from infestation with *Fasciola hepaticum* or *Clonorchis sinensis*, which will cause recurrent abscesses and ultimately perhaps cholangiocarcinoma.

In our study of patients with pyogenic liver abscess[18], we have noted changes in the population at risk. In the earlier years of our series extrahepatic intra-abdominal infection caused all the deaths, while in more recent years obstructive or metastatic cancer was noted with increasing frequency[18]. Miedema *et al.* have also noted a high cancer incidence with 20 of 106 deaths due to advanced carcinoma[81]. Abscesses now occur chiefly in patients who in previous years would have died sooner, especially terminal cancer patients with impaired immune response. In our series[18] bacteraemia occurred in six of the nine patients who died, and was of biliary origin in five. Thus the highest mortality still occurs in elderly patients with multiple abscesses and bacteraemia associated with biliary obstructive disease; and in those with underlying malignancy. The former should be preventable by early surgical exploration prior to abscess formation. The prognosis of the latter will always be determined by that of the underlying malignancy.

Addendum

At the time of writing, June 1989, an important contribution was made to the question of liver injury in severe extrahepatic sepsis[82]. Pirovino *et al.* of Bern, Switzerland, compared nine jaundiced patients with extrahepatic sepsis, with a control group of five without jaundice by quantitative liver function tests. They found a severely deranged organic anion transport system (abnormal BSP clearance and retention; elevated serum bile acids), both in jaundiced and non-jaundiced septic patients. By contrast they found normal synthetic (clotting factors), cytosolic (galactose elimination capacity) and microsomal (caffeine clearance) functions. This indicates that the syndrome of jaundice is a functional disorder reversible upon control of infection.

References

1. Hippocrates. In: *The Genuine Works of Hippocrates*, translated from the Greek with a preliminary discourse and annotations by Francis Adams, LL.D., Vols I and II, 1886, William Wood & Co., New York, pp. 57–8, 266–7
2. Shearman, D. J. C. and Finlayson, N. D. C. (eds) (1982) *Diseases of the Gastrointestinal Tract and Liver*, (Edinburgh: Churchill Livingstone).

3. Hamilton, J. R. and Sass-Kortsak, A. (1963). Jaundice associated with severe bacterial infection in young infants. *J. Pediatr.*, **63**, 121–32
4. Bernstein, J. and Brown, A. K. (1962). Sepsis and jaundice in early infancy. *Pediatrics*, **29**, 873–82
5. Miller, D. J., Keeton, G. R., Webber, B. L., Pathol, F. F. and Saunders, S. J. (1976). Jaundice in severe bacterial infection. *Gastroenterology*, **71**, 94–7
6. Miller, D. F. and Irvine, R. W. (1969). Jaundice in acute appendicitis. *Lancet*, **1**, 321–3
7. Fahrlander, H., Huber, F. and Gloor, F. (1964). Intrahepatic retention of bile in severe bacterial infections. *Gastroenterology*, **47**, 590–9
8. Fang, M. H., Ginsberg, A. L. and Dobbins III, W. O. (1980). Marked elevation in serum alkaline phosphatase activity as a manifestation of systemic infection. *Gastroenterology*, **78**, 592–7
9. Conn, H. O. and Fessel, J. M. (1971). Spontaneous bacterial peritonitis in cirrhosis: Variations on a theme. *Medicine*, **50**, 161–97
10. Nance, F. C. (1985). Disease of the peritoneum, mesentery and omentum. In Berk, J. E. (ed.) *Bokus, Gastroenterology*, Vol. 7, Chapter 228, (London: W. B. Saunders)
11. Greenstein, A. J., Sachar, D. B., Lowenthal, D., Goldofsky, E. and Aufses, A. H. Jr. (1985). Pyogenic liver abscess in Crohn's disease. *Q. J. Med.* (new series), **56**, **220**, 505–18
12. Celsus, A. C. In: *A. Cornelius Celsus of Medicine. In Eight Books*, translated with notes critical and explanatory by James Greive, MD, London, 1756, Printed for D. Wilson and T. Durham, at Plato's Head in the Strand, Chapter VIII, pp. 69–71.
13. Bright, J. (1836). Observations on jaundice. *Guys Hospital Reports*, **1**, 638–48
14. Matterstock, G. K. (1938). Quoted by Ochsner, A., DeBakey, M. and Murray, S. In *Pyogenic abscess of the liver. Am. J. Surg.*, **40**, 292–329
15. Fitz, R. H. (1886). Perforating inflammation of the vermiform appendix; with special reference to its early diagnosis and treatment. *Am. J. Med. Sci.*, **91/92**, 321–45
16. Ochsner, A., DeBakey, M. and Murray, S. (1938). Pyogenic abscess of the liver. II. An analysis of forty-seven cases with review of the literature. *Am. J. Surg.*, **40**, 292–319
17. Balasegaram, M. (1981). Management of hepatic abscess. In Ravitch, M. M. (ed.), *Current Problems in Surgery*, Vol. XVIII, No. 5, May 1981. (Chicago: Year Book Medical Publishers)
18. Greenstein, A. J., Lowenthal, D., Hammer, G., Schaffner, F. and Aufses, A. H., Jr (1984). Continuing changing patterns of disease in pyogenic liver abscess: a study of 38 patients. *Am. J. Gastroenterol.*, **79**, 217–26
19. Sherman, J. D. and Robbins, S. L. (1960). Changing trends in the casuistics of hepatic abscess. *Am. J. Med.*, **28**, 943–80
20. Keefer, C. S. (1934). Liver abscess: A review of eighty-five cases. *N. Engl. J. Med.*, **211**, 21–4
21. Rubin, R. H., Swartz, M. N. and Malt, R. (1974). Hepatic abscess: changes in clinical, bacteriologic and therapeutic aspects. *Am. J. Med.*, **57**, 601–10
22. DeBakey, M. E. and Creech, O. Jr. (1963). Hepatic abscess. In Schiff, L. (ed.), *Diseases of the Liver*, 2nd edn, pp. 728–64.
23. Pitt, H. A. and Zuidema, G. D. (1975). Factors influencing mortality in the treatment of pyogenic hepatic abscesses. *Surg. Gynecol. Obstet.*, **140**, 228–34
24. McDonald, A. P. and Howard, R. J. (1980). Pyogenic liver abscess. *World J. Surg.*, **4**, 369–80
25. Schwartz, S. I. (1964). *Surgical Diseases of the Liver* (New York: McGraw-Hill), pp. 143–66
26. Kinney, T. and Ferrebee, J. W. (1948). Hepatic abscess. Factors determining its localization. *Arch. Pathol.*, **45**, 41–6
27. Wallack, M. K., Brown, A. S., Austrian, R. and Fitts, W. T. Jr (1976). Pyogenic liver abscess secondary to asymptomatic sigmoid diverticulitis. *Ann. Surg.*, **184**, 241–3
28. Greenstein, A. J., Sachar, D. B., Greenstein, R. J., Janowitz, H. D. and Aufses, A. H. Jr (1982). Intraabdominal abscess in Crohn's (ileo) colitis. *Am. J. Surg.*, **143**, 727–30
29. Steinberg, D. M., Cooke, W. T. and Alexander-Williams, J. (1973). Abscess and fistulae in Crohn's disease. *Gut*, **14**, 865–9
30. Brooke, B. N. and Slaney, G. (1958). Portal bacteraemia in ulcerative colitis. *Lancet*, **1**, 1206–7
31. Bargen, J. A. and Lansbury, J. (1933). The association of multiple hepatic abscesses and

chronic ulcerative colitis. *Med. Clin. N. Am.*, **16**, 1427–31
32. Serege, H. (1901). Contribution a l'etude de la circulation du sang fort dans le foie, et des localisations lobaires hepatiques. *J. Med. Bordeaux*, **31**, 271–5
33. Palmer, E. D. (1935). The changing manifestations of pyogenic liver abscess. *J. Am. Med. Assoc.*, **231**, 192
34. Butler, T. J. and McCarthy, C. F. (1969). Pyogenic liver abscess. *Gut*, **10**, 389–99
35. Pyrtek, L. J. and Bartus, S. A. (1965). Hepatic pyemia. *N. Engl. J. Med.*, **272**, 551–4
36. Young, A. E. (1976). The clinical presentation of pyogenic liver abscess. *Br. J. Surg.*, **63**, 216–19
37. Rothenberg, R. E. and Lindner, W. (1934). The single pyogenic liver abscess. *Surg. Gynecol. Obstet.*, **59**, 31–40
38. Joseph, W. L., Kahn, A. M. and Longmire, W. P., Jr (1968). Pyogenic liver abscess. Changing patterns in approach. *Am. J. Surg.*, **115**, 63–8
39. Lee, J. F. and Block, G. E. (1971). The changing clinical pattern of hepatic abscesses. *Arch. Surg.*, **104**, 465–70
40. Ostermiller, W. and Carter, R. (1967). Hepatic abscess. *Arch. Surg.*, **94**, 353–6
41. Sabbaj, J., Sutter, V. L. and Finegold, S. M. (1972). Anaerobic pyogenic liver abscess. *Ann. Intern. Med.*, **77**, 629–38
42. Satiani, B. and Davidson, E. D. (1978). Hepatic abscesses. Improvement in mortality with early diagnosis and treatment. *Am. J. Surg.*, **135**, 647–50
43. Harley, H. R. S. (1970). Radiology in diagnosis and control of surgical treatment of subphrenic and liver abscesses. *Proc. R. Soc. Med.*, **63**, 319–22
44. Foster, S. C., Schneider, B. and Seaman, W. B. (1970). Gas-containing pyogenic intrahepatic abscesses. *Radiology*, **94**, 613–18
45. Viana, R. L. (1975). Selective arteriography in the diagnosis and evaluation of amebic abscess of the liver. *Dig. Dis.*, **20**, 632–7
46. Bosniak, M. A. and Phanthumachinda, P. (1966). Value of arteriography in the study of hepatic disease. *Am. J. Surg.*, **112**, 348–55
47. Novy, S. B., Wallace, S., Goldman, A. M. and Ben-Menachem, Y. (1974). Pyogenic liver abscess. Angiographic diagnosis and treatment by closed aspiration. *Am. J. Roentgen Rad. Nucl. Med.*, **121**, 388–95
48. Ranson, J. H. C., Madayag, M. A., Localio, S. A. and Spencer, F. C. (1975). New diagnostic and therapeutic techniques in the management of pyogenic liver abscesses. *Ann. Surg.* **181**, 508–18
49. Altemeier, W. A., Schowengerdt, C. G. and Whiteley, D. H. (1970). Abscesses of the liver: surgical considerations. *Arch. Surg.* **101**, 258–66
50. Lazarchick, J., Nichols, D. R. and Washington, J. A. (1973). Pyogenic liver abscess. *Mayo Clin. Proc.*, **48**, 349–55
51. McAfee, J. G., Ause, R. G. and Wagner, H. N., Jr (1965). Diagnostic value of scintillation scanning of the liver. *Arch. Intern. Med.*, **116**, 95–110
52. Cuaron, A. and Gordon, F. (1970). Liver scanning: analysis of 2,500 cases of amebic hepatic abscesses. *J. Nucl. Med.*, **11**, 435–9
53. Covington, E. E. (1970). The accuracy of liver photoscans. *Am. J. Roentgenol.*, **109**, 742–4
54. Lawson, T. L. (1977). Hepatic abscess-ultrasound as an aid to diagnosis. *Am. J. Dig. Dis.*, **22**, 33–7
55. Richardson, R., Norton, L. W., Eule, J. and Eiseman, B. (1975). Accuracy of ultrasound in the diagnosing of abdominal masses. *Arch. Surg.*, **110**, 933–9
56. Alfidi, R. J., Haaga, J. R., Havrilla, T. R., Pepe, R. G. and Cook, S. A. (1976). Computed tomography of the liver. *Am. J. Roentgenol.*, **127**, 69–74
57. Stephens, D. H., Sheedy, P. F., II, Hattery, R. R. and MacCarty (1977). Computed tomography of the liver. *Am. J. Roentgenol.*, **128**, 579–90
58. Buchman, T. G. and Zuidema, G. D. (1981). The role of computerized tomographic scanning in the surgical management of pyogenic hepatic abscess. *Surg. Gynecol. Obstet.*, **153**, 1–9
59. Cronin, K. (1961). Pyogenic abscess of the liver. *Gut*, **2**, 53–9
60. Maher, J. A. Jr, Reynolds, T. B. and Yellin, A. E. (1979). Successful medical treatment of pyogenic liver abscess. *Gastroenterology*, **77**, 618–22
61. Herbert, D. A., Rothman, J., Simmons, F., Fogel, D. A., Wilson, S. and Ruskin, J. (1982). Pyogenic liver abscesses: successful non-surgical therapy. *Lancet*, **1**, 134–6

62. Yellin, A. E. *et al.* (1985). The role of *Pseudomonas* species in patients treated with ampicillin and sulbactam for gangrenous and perforated appendicitis. *Surg. Gynecol. Obstet.*, **161**, 303–6
63. McFadzean, A. J. S., Chang, K. P. S. and Wong, C. C. (1953). Solitary pyogenic abscess of the liver aspiration of antibiotics. *Br. J. Surg.*, **41**, 141–52
64. Smith, E. H. and Bartrum, R. J. (1974). Ultrasonically guided percutaneous aspiration of abscesses. *Am. J. Roentgenol.*, **122**, 308–12
65. Gerzof, S. G., Robbins, A. H., Johnson, W. C., Birkett, D. H. and Nabseth, D. C. (1981). Percutaneous catheter drainage of abdominal abscesses. A five-year experience. *N. Engl. J. Med.*, **305**, 654–7
66. Gerzof, S. G., Robbins, A. H., Birkett, D. H., Johnson, W. C., Pugatch, R. D. and Vincent, M. E. (1979). Percutaneous catheter drainage of abdominal abscesses guided by ultrasound and computed tomography. *Am. J. Roentgenol.*, **133**, 1–8
67. Kimura, M., Tsuchiya, Y., Ohto, M. *et al.* (1981). Ultrasonically guided percutaneous drainage of solitary liver abscess: successful treatment in four cases. *J. Clin. Gastroenterol.*, **3**, 61–5
68. Berger, L. A. and Osborne, D. R. (1982). Treatment of pyogenic liver abscesses by percutaneous needle aspiration. *Lancet*, **1**, 132–4
69. Martin, E. C., Karlsen, K. B. and Frankuchere, E. (1981). Percutaneous drainage in the management of hepatic abscess. *Surg. Clin N. Am.*, **61**, 157–67
70. Crass, J. R. (1983). Liver abscess as a complication of regional enteritis: Interventional considerations. *Am. J. Gastroenterol.*, **78**, 747–9
71. Nather, C. and Ochsner, A. (1923). Retroperitoneal operation for subphrenic abscess. *Surg. Gynecol. Obstet.*, **37**, 66–71
72. Clairmont, P. and Meyer, M. (1926). Erfahrungen ueber die behandlung der appendicitis (treatment of appendicitis). *Acta Chir. Scand.*, **60**, 55–134
73. Trendelenberg, F. (1885). Echinococcus der pleura. In Madelung, O. W. (ed.), *Beitrage Mecklen-burgischer Arttze zur lehre von der Echinococcen-Krankheit*, pp. 87–90. (Stuttgart: Enke)
74. Ariel, I. M. and Kazarian, K. K. (1971). Intrahepatic abscesses – clinical features and treatment. In Ariel, I. M. and Kazarian, K. K. (eds.) *Diagnosis and Treatment of Abdominal Abscesses*, pp. 207–25. (Baltimore: Williams & Wilkins)
75. Boyd, D. P. (1958). The anatomy and pathology of the subphrenic spaces. *Surg. Clin. N. Am.*, **38**, 619–26
76. Beaver, D. C. (1931). Granulomatous abscess of the liver of pyogenic origin. *Am. J. Pathol.*, **7**, 259–76
77. Warren, K. W. and Hardy, K. J. (1968). Pyogenic liver abscess. *Arch. Surg.*, **97**, 40–4
78. Heymann, A. D. (1979). Clinical aspects of grave pyogenic abscesses of the liver. *Surg. Gynecol. Obstet.*, **149**, 209–13
79. Dehner, L. P. and Kissane, J. M. (1969). Pyogenic hepatic abscesses in infancy and childhood. *J. Pediatr.*, **74**, 763–73
80. Greenstein, A. J. *et al.* (1985). Amebic liver abscess: A study of 11 cases compared with a series of 38 patients with pyogenic liver abscess. *Am. J. Gastroenterol.*, **80**, 472–8
81. Miedema, B. W. and Dineen, P. (1984). The diagnosis and treatment of pyogenic liver abscesses. *Ann. Surg.*, **200**, 328–35
82. Pirovino, M., Meister, F., Rubil, E. and Karlaganis, G. (1989). Preserved cytosolic and synthetic liver infection. *Gastroenterology*, **96**, 1589–95

10
The liver in leptospirosis

R. C. JOHNSON

Leptospirosis, a zoonosis of worldwide dimensions, is responsible for an acute febrile illness of humans. The causal organism can be any one of a large number of serovars (antigenic types) of *Leptospira interrogans* that infect a variety of wild and domestic animals. Infected animals shed the spirochaetes in their urine and contaminate soil and water. Humans become infected by direct contact with infected urine or indirectly by exposure to moist soil and water contaminated with infected urine. The disease varies from a mild influenza-like illness to severe renal and hepatic impairment and death in a small proportion of cases[1].

AETIOLOGY

Leptospires are very thin (0.1 μm × 6–20 μm) tightly, coiled spirochaetes with hooked ends and display a unique flexuous type of motility. Translational movement of leptospires is enhanced as the viscosity of the milieu increases. The ultrastructural features of *Leptospira* are responsible for unique motility which probably plays a critical role in the highly invasive nature of these spirochaetes. The peripheral structure of spirochaetes is a multi-layered outer membrane. Enclosed by the outer membrane is the helical protoplasmic cylinder which consists of the peptidoglycan layer, cytoplasmic membrane, and the cytoplasmic contents of the cell. The two endoflagella lie between the outer membrane and the protoplasmic cylinder and are attached to the latter at subterminal positions. The free ends of the endoflagella extend toward the cell centre. Because of their narrow diameter, unstained leptospires cannot be seen with the bright-field microscope but are readily visualized with dark-field microscopy[2].

Although a number of distinct genetic groups exist in the genus *Leptospira* only two species are recognized, the free-living *L. biflexa* and the pathogenic *L. interrogans*[2]. More than 200 serovars of *L. interrogans* have been isolated from over 160 different mammalian species[3]. Rodents, small marsupials, cattle, pigs and dogs are often renal shedders of leptospires. Some serovars appear to be adapted to specific mammalian hosts. The more common associations recognized are *hardjo* with cattle; *pomona* with pigs and cattle; *canicola* with dogs and *icterohaemorrhagiae* and *copenhageni* with rats. However, these serovars may also infect many different animals. The number of serovars present vary with the geographical area. Leptospirosis in the temperate zone is usually due to a relatively small number of serovars. Leptospires multiply in the renal tubules of mammalian hosts and are shed in the urine for varying periods of time. Maintenance hosts such as rodents may be leptospiruric throughout their lifetimes, whereas domestic animals may be heavy shedders of leptospires for several months[4]. Humans may excrete organisms for several weeks. Pathogenic leptospires may remain infectious for several weeks in moist soil and for several months in water. Person-to-person transmission has been reported but is a rare occurrence. Human leptospirosis is most commonly acquired by direct contact with infected urine or indirectly by exposure to moist soil and water contaminated with infected urine. Leptospires enter through broken skin or mucosal membranes and are rapidly disseminated haematogenously from the site of entry. Initial multiplication is believed to occur in the blood and the liver.

CLINICAL MANIFESTATIONS

The clinical manifestations of leptospirosis range from mild and self-limiting to severe and possibly fatal. The severity of the disease is largely determined by the virulence of the infecting strain. The severe icteric form, often referred to as Weil's disease, is frequently associated with *icterohaemorrhagiae* but may be caused by a variety of serovars. Typically, leptospirosis is a biphasic disease consisting of the leptospiraemic or acute phase followed by the leptospiruric or immune phase. After an incubation period of 1–2 weeks the leptospiraemic phase commences abruptly with signs and symptoms that frequently consist of severe headache, fever, chills, malaise, myalgia, and conjunctival suffusion. Headache is intense, the calf, back and abdominal muscles are often tender, and anorexia, nausea and vomiting are frequently experienced. The conjunctival suffusion of leptospirosis is without inflammatory exudates. In severe cases of leptospirosis, jaundice appears during the first week of illness and reaches maximal intensity 4–7 days later. Leptospires may be isolated from the blood and cerebrospinal fluid during this stage[1,5–7].

Increasing titres of antibodies during the second week usher in the leptospiruric or immune phase of the disease. With the exception of the kidney, eye, and possibly the brain, antibodies bring about the elimination of leptospires from the host. Short febrile relapses and signs of meningeal irritation are often observed, but the symptoms may be quite variable. The presence of leptospires in the urine is not associated with impairment of renal function. Ten per cent of cases may experience uveitis which is usually transient and self-limited. The biphasic nature of leptospirosis is not always manifested. It is absent in mild cases where the appearance of antibodies results in the alleviation of signs and symptoms. The phases are indistinguishable in patients with severe icteric illness.

The intensity of jaundice is directly related to the degree of hepatic dysfunction. Renal failure, haemorrhagic manifestations and cardiovascular collapse frequently occur in severely jaundiced patients. Central nervous system involvement occurs but may be unnoticed because of the marked malfunction of the kidney and the liver. Mortality rates of untreated cases vary from 5% to 30% and are most frequently associated with renal failure during the second and third week of the disease[1,5–7].

PATHOLOGY

Although the pathology associated with human leptospirosis has been well described, little information concerning the mechanisms responsible for tissue damage is available. Once the leptospires penetrate the skin or mucous membranes they are rapidly disseminated throughout the body. They invade essentially all tissues, including the eye and the cerebrospinal fluid where they elicit little or no inflammatory response. Leptospiral toxins have been postulated to be responsible for the resulting pathology but no toxins have been conclusively identified[1].

Progressive hepatic and renal dysfunction account for the majority of the fatal cases of leptospirosis. Haemorrhages and bile staining of tissues are observed in these cases. The haemorrhages are widespread but are more pronounced in the skeletal muscles, kidneys, adrenals, liver, stomach, spleen and lungs.

Jaundice is the most notable clinical manifestation of liver dysfunction[1]. Microscopic alterations in the liver are minimal and correlate poorly with the degree of functional impairment. It is generally believed that hepatocellular injury occurs at the subcellular level, since hepatocellular necrosis is minimal and no residual hepatic dysfunction remains following recovery. Serum glutamic oxaloacetic transaminase and serum glutamic transaminase activities are only slightly elevated regardless of the degree of hyperbilirubinaemia, reflecting the absence of significant liver cell necrosis. An intracellular block to bilirubin excretion appears to be the primary mechanism involved. A marked increase in serum creatine phosphokinase in combination with minimal elevation in transaminases in jaundiced patients may facilitate differentiating leptospirosis from other forms of acute hepatitis. Hepatic enlargement is common when jaundice is present. Histopathological changes include proliferation and enlargement of Kupffer cells, cloudy swelling of parenchymal cells, disruption of liver cords and bile stasis in biliary canaliculi. Leptospires are rarely demonstrated in the liver when major hepatic dysfunction is present[1].

Renal manifestations are common in all forms of leptospirosis, but renal failure is most likely to occur in patients with severe hepatic dysfunction. Proteinuria, pyuria, haematuria and azotaemia are the primary manifestations of renal dysfunction. Renal failure in leptospirosis is primarily the result of acute tubular necrosis associated with oliguria. Azotaemia, which usually peaks during the first week, is due to tubular necrosis and reduced renal blood flow. Leptospires have been demonstrated in the lumina of the renal tubules. Severely jaundiced patients are most likely to experience haemorrhagic manifestations, probably due to diffuse vasculitis with capillary injury. These manifestations include epistaxis, haemoptysis, gastrointestinal bleeding, haemorrhagic pneumonitis and subarachnoid haemorrhage. Hypoprothrombinaemia and thrombocytopenia have been observed in some patients[1,10].

LABORATORY FEATURES

Leucocyte counts may be low to slightly elevated in anicteric cases. In contrast, jaundiced patients may have counts as high as 70,000 cells per cubic millilitre. During early leptospirosis it is not uncommon to encounter neutrophilia of greater than 70%. Thrombocytopenia and an elevated erythrocyte sedimentation rate may also be present.

Abnormal urinalyses are common during the leptospiraemic stage. The most frequent abnormality is a mild proteinuria. An increase in the cellular elements in both phases of the disease necessarily reflects the degree of renal involvement. These abnormalities are transient in anicteric leptospiroses. Azotaemia and oliguria are associated with jaundice. Serum creatine phosphokinase are elevated early in the disease and this, in combination with only slight increases in transaminases, helps to differentiate leptospirosis from viral hepatitis[1].

DIAGNOSIS

A definitive diagnosis of leptospirosis is based on culture of the organism, seroconversion, or a four-fold or greater elevation in titre of agglutinating antibodies. Leptospires may be isolated from the blood and spinal fluid during the first week of illness and from the urine during the following 2 weeks. In fatal cases of leptospirosis the organisms may be present in the kidneys and to a lesser extent in the liver.

Leptospires are readily cultivated in the laboratory. Media enriched with rabbit serum or bovine serum albumin (BSA)–Tween 80 are commonly used. Semisolid (0.2% agar) BSA–Tween 80 medium is recommended for the isolation of leptospires and 100–200 μg/ml of 5′-fluorouracil should be incorporated into the medium if potentially contaminated specimens such as urine are to be cultured. Whole blood and spinal fluid should be inoculated immediately into media, whereas urine should be diluted 1:10 and 1:100 before inoculation. Direct examination of specimens by dark-field microscopy is not recommended[8].

The microscopic agglutination test is used as the standard serological procedure. Antibodies usually appear after the sixth day of illness. Because of cross-agglutination reactions between some serovars, the infecting serovar must be isolated for a correct identification[8].

PROGNOSIS

The prognosis is dependent upon the combination of the virulence of the infecting serovar and the general condition of the patient. There is a good correlation between virulence and the development of jaundice. Mortality is rare in anicteric cases and ranges from 5% to 30% in untreated jaundiced patients[1,6,9].

TREATMENT

In vitro susceptibility studies suggest that leptospires are sensitive to the commonly used antibiotics except chloramphenicol. Information concerning the efficacy of antibiotic therapy in human leptospirosis has been conflicting. Antibiotics commonly used are penicillins and tetracyclines. However, because leptospirosis is usually a non-fatal disease with a highly variable clinical course, the effectiveness of antimicrobial therapy has been difficult to evaluate. Recent double-blind studies have demonstrated that doxycycline (200 mg per week) is a highly effective prophylaxis[11]. In addition, doxycycline (100 mg twice daily for 7 days) shortened the duration of fever and most other symptoms when started within 4 days of disease onset[12]. It is generally believed that antimicrobial drugs must be administered within 4 days of the onset of illness to be beneficial. However, the results of another randomized, placebo-controlled, double-blind study of intravenous penicillin treatment of severe, advanced leptospirosis demonstrated that every measurable aspect of the disease was favourably affected[13]. These authors recommended that intravenous penicillin should be given to patients with severe leptospirosis, even if therapy can be initiated only late in the course of the disease. Azotaemia and jaundice require careful monitoring of fluids and electrolytes. Peritoneal dialysis or haemodialysis should be considered for patients with azotaemia.

PREVENTION

Vaccination of livestock and pets decreases or prevents renal shedding of leptospires and is the major control measure for leptospirosis. The vaccine must contain the serovars present in the area since the immunity induced by vaccination is serovar-specific. Rodent control may be another important preventive measure. Little information is available on vaccination of humans[14].

References

1. Feigen, R. D. and Anderson, D. C. (1975). Human leptospirosis. *CRC Clin Sci.*, **5**, 413–67
2. Johnson, R. C. and Faine, S. (1984). Leptospira. In Krieg, N. R. and Holt, J. G. (eds), *Bergey's Manual of Systematic Bacteriology*, Vol. 1, pp. 62–7. (Baltimore: Williams & Wilkins)
3. Leptospiral serotype distribution lists according to host and geographic area. Centers for Disease Control, Atlanta, US Dept. Health Education and Welfare, 1966 (Supplement 1975)
4. Kaufmann, A. F. (1976). Epidemiological trends of leptospirosis in the United States, 1965–

1974. In Johnson, R. C. (ed.), *The Biology of Parasitic Spirochetes*, pp. 177–89. (New York: Academic Press)

5. Diaz-Rivera, R. S., Hall, H., Ramos-Mirales, K. Y. *et al.* (1963). Leptospirosis in Puerto Rico. Clinical aspects of human infection. *Zoonosis Res.*, **2**, 159–77
6. Berman, S. J., Tsar, C. C., Homes, K. *et al.* (1973). Sporadic anicteric leptospirosis in South Vietnam. A study in 150 patients. *Ann. Intern. Med.*, **79**, 167–73
7. Heath, C. W., Jr, Alexander, A. D. and Galton, M. M. (1965). Leptospirosis in the United States, analysis of 483 cases in man, 1949–1961. *N. Engl. J. Med.*, **273**, 857–64; 915–22
8. Alexander, A. D. Leptospira. In Lennette, E. H., Balows, A., Hausler, W. H. Jr and Shadomy, H. J. (eds), *Manual of Clinical Microbiology*, 4th edn, pp. 473–8. (Washington, DC: American Society for Microbiology)
9. Edwards, G. A. and Domm, B. M. (1960). Human leptospirosis. *Medicine*, **39**, 117–56
10. Barrett-Connor, E., Child, C. M. and Carter, M. J. (1970). Renal failure in leptospirosis. *Southern Med. J.*, **63**, 580–3
11. Takafuji, E. T., Kirkpatrick, J. W., Miller, R. N. *et al.* (1984). An efficacy trial of doxycycline chemophylaxis against leptospirosis. *N. Engl. J. Med.*, **30**, 497–500
12. Mclain, J. B. L., Ballou, W. R., Harrison, S. M. *et al.* (1984). Doxycycline therapy for leptospirosis. *Ann. Intern. Med.*, **100**, 696–8
13. Watt, G., Padre, M. A., Tuazon, L., Calubaquib, E., Santiago, E., Ranoa, C. P. and Laughlin, L. W. (1988). Placebo-controlled trial of intravenous penicillin for severe and late leptospirosis. *Lancet*, **1**, 433–5
14. Faine, S. (1982). Guidelines for the control of leptospirosis. Offset publication no. 67. (Geneva: World Health Organization)

11
The liver in infectious and chronic inflammatory bowel disease: morphological findings

R. N. M. MacSWEEN

INTRODUCTION

The liver is strategically placed between the portal venous circulation and the systemic circulation. In this position it may have an important role in modulating the potentially harmful effects of gut-derived microorganisms, toxins and antigens. The concept of the liver acting as a 'filter' on the portal venous blood is not a new one, but it has been modified in the light of recent studies. In particular the contributory role of the spleen has been recognized[1-3]. As an integral part of the immune system whose humoral products are secreted into the portal vein, the spleen is ideally situated to provide opsonins necessary to enhance the clearance of gut-derived organisms by Kupffer cells, antibodies which will complex with gut-derived antigens thus facilitating their sequestration in the liver, and cytokines which will directly modulate immunological and defence mechanisms, in some of which hepatocytes have a central role. We should consider the liver as a filter acting in series with the spleen (Figure 1a). In addition, however, it may act as a filter in parallel with the spleen, gut-derived antigens passing into the systemic circulation via the lymphatic channels and being simultaneously delivered to the spleen and liver via the systemic circulation (Figure 1b).

The importance of these mechanisms should be borne in mind in considering the changes which may occur in the liver in the presence of infectious and inflammatory disease in the gastrointestinal tract. The interactions may be complex. Changes in the gut flora and/or changes in gut mucosal permeability may increase portal venous levels of several factors which may alter liver macrophage function with resultant injurious effects both within the liver and at extrahepatic sites[4,5]. Furthermore, chronic liver injury accompanied by intrahepatic or extrahepatic portal venous shunting (as in primary sclerosing cholangitis) may also lead to extrahepatic systemic effects. These may include inappropriate immune responses with resulting

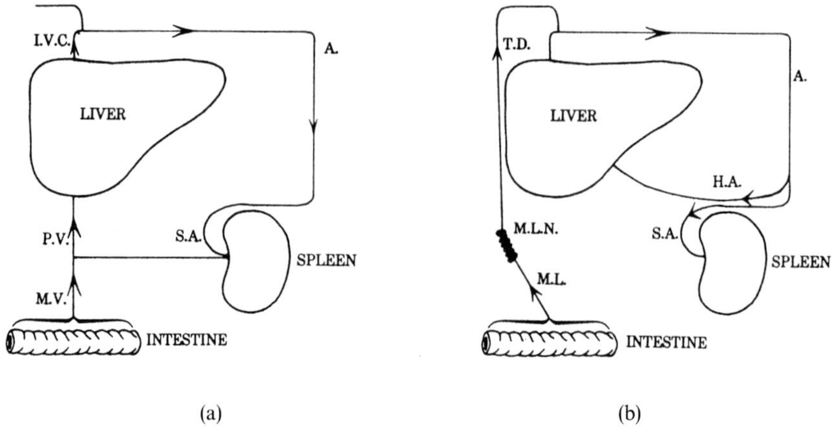

Figure 1 Concept of the liver acting as a 'filter' on the portal venous blood. In (**a**) the liver acts 'in series' with the spleen; opsonins, antibodies and cytokines in the splenic venous blood may modulate the handling by the liver of gut-derived microorganisms and antigens and may affect the release of acute-phase proteins by hepatocytes. In (**b**) the liver acts 'in parallel' with the spleen in dealing with gut-derived microorganisms and antigens which pass via the mesenteric lymphatics. M.V. = mesenteric vein; P.V. = portal vein; S.V. = splenic vein; I.V.C. = inferior vena cava; A. = aorta; S.A. = splenic artery; H.A. = hepatic artery; M.L. = mesenteric lymphatics; M.L.N. = mesenteric lymph nodes; T.D. = thoracic duct

immunological abnormalities which are secondary to the liver injury rather than being primary phenomena.

NON-SPECIFIC MORPHOLOGICAL CHANGES

In both acute and chronic inflammatory bowel disease the morphological changes in the liver may simply comprise non-specific reactive hepatitis. Fatty change may also occur. The features of non-specific reactive hepatitis[6,7] have already been discussed in this symposium (Desmet, chapter 3). The essential feature in making the histological diagnosis is that the changes are always focal even when they are intense and widespread. Thus, some portal tracts may appear normal while others contain a marked mononuclear cell infiltrate (neutrophil polymorphs are present only in small numbers). Similarly, the reactive Kupffer cell hyperplasia, the intrasinusoidal accumulation of mononuclear cells, the focal macrophage aggregates (sometimes producing a granulomatoid or granuloma-like appearance) and the occasional acidophil bodies are irregularly and unevenly distributed within the acini.

INFECTIOUS AND ACUTE INFLAMMATORY BOWEL DISEASES

The hepatic changes which may accompany some of these are summarized in Table 1; a number of them are dealt with elsewhere in this monograph

Table 1 Morphological changes in the liver in acute and infectious inflammatory bowel disease

A.	Bacterial infections	
	Various Gram-positive and Gram-negative organisms	Septicaemic changes; cholangitis, hepatic abscess
	Gram-negative organisms and anaerobic bacilli – septic/endotoxic shock	'Cholangitis lenta'
	Yersinia enterocolitica	Hepatic abscess
	Shigella	Cholestatic hepatitis
	Salmonella	Cholestatic hepatitis; 'typhoid nodule'
B.	Mycotic infections	'Mycetomas' secondary to gut involvement
	Actinomycosis israelii	Actinomycotic abscess
C.	Parasitic infections	
	Entaemoeba histolytica	Amoebic abscess
	Giardia lamblia[21]	Granulomas, cholangitis
	Ascaris lumbricoides	Granulomas, cholangitis, primary recurrent pyogenic (oriental) cholangitis
	Enterobius vermicularis[22]	Granulomas
D.	Miscellaneous	
	Coeliac disease	Non-specific reactive hepatitis, chronic hepatitis[24]. Coexistence with primary biliary cirrhosis[25] and primary sclerosing cholangitis[26]
	Whipple's disease	Granulomas, PAS-positive macrophage aggregates
	Eosinophilic gastroenteritis[23]	Granulomas
	Opportunistic infections	
	Cryptosporidium / *Helicobacter* (campylobacter)	AIDS-related sclerosing cholangitis

The majority of these are discussed in this chapter or elsewhere in the monograph, and the appropriate references will be found there. The superscripts indicate other cited references

and are not discussed further.

The cholestatic syndrome complicating septic/endotoxic shock may sometimes occur when the primary infection is in the bowel, but it may also occur with primary infections in the urinary tract, the lungs and elsewhere. Morphologically, the liver shows perivenular cholestasis accompanied by prominent bilirubinostasis in dilated cholangioles and with an accompanying acute cholangiolitis – so-called cholangitis lenta[8–10] (Figure 2). There is little or no inflammation within the portal tracts. The mechanisms responsible for this cholestatic syndrome are not clear, but there may be direct endotoxic injury at the cholangiolar level[11].

Liver abscesses may sometimes complicate intestinal infection due to *Yersinia enterocolitica*[12]. This is most often seen in patients with haemochromatosis (either primary or secondary). *Y. enterocolitica* is an iron-dependent Gram-negative bacillus which is entirely dependent on exogenous iron for growth. This may afford an explanation why hepatic abscesses are most often seen in association with iron overload.

The cholestatic hepatitis which may occur in shigellosis and in salmonella infection has been attributed to gut-derived toxins[13]. The intrahepatic typhoid nodule is similar to that seen in the gut mucosa[13].

Ascaris lumbricoides, an intestinal roundworm, may affect the liver both

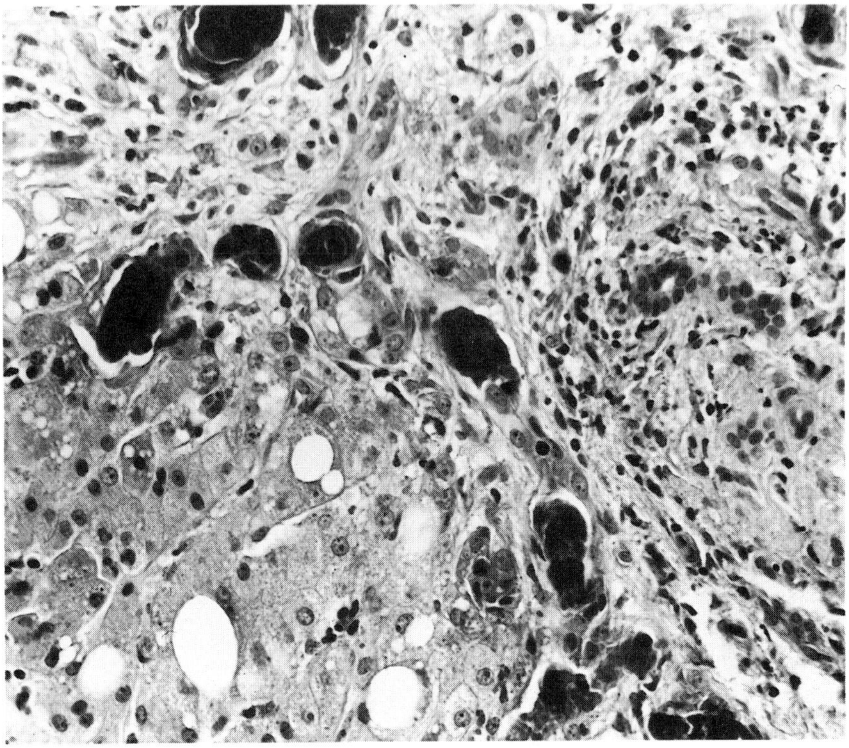

Figure 2 The liver in sepsis/endotoxic shock: note the numerous bile concretions in dilated cholangioles, accompanied by a cholangiolitis (H&E ×400)

in the migratory larval and intestinal adult stages[13]. It has also been implicated in primary recurrent pyogenic (oriental) cholangitis, along with other parasitic infections, however. This prompted Seel and Park[4] to suggest the term 'oriental infestational cholangitis' for this syndrome. It is still not clear, however, why this condition is peculiar to the Far East and is seldom seen in other areas where similar parasitic infections are common.

In Whipple's disease non-specific hepatic granulomas occur[15]. In addition PAS-positive macrophage aggregates (Figure 3) and Kupffer cells have been shown to contain the causal 'sickle-form' bacillus[16,17].

Hepatobiliary complications may accompany opportunistic infections of the gastrointestinal tract. There are a number of case reports of an acquired AIDS-related sclerosing cholangitis[18,19], demonstrable on ERCP and sometimes accompanied by suprapapillary bile duct dilatation. In many cases there has been simultaneous infection with cryptosporidia, cytomegalovirus and campylobacter-like organisms. Histologically there is a severe acute or chronic cholangitis, and cryptosporidia may be present on the luminal surface of the biliary epithelium. The mechanism of the bile duct injury is probably multifactorial and the result of infection by more than one microbial agent[19]. It is of interest, however, that a similar acquired sclerosing cholangitis has

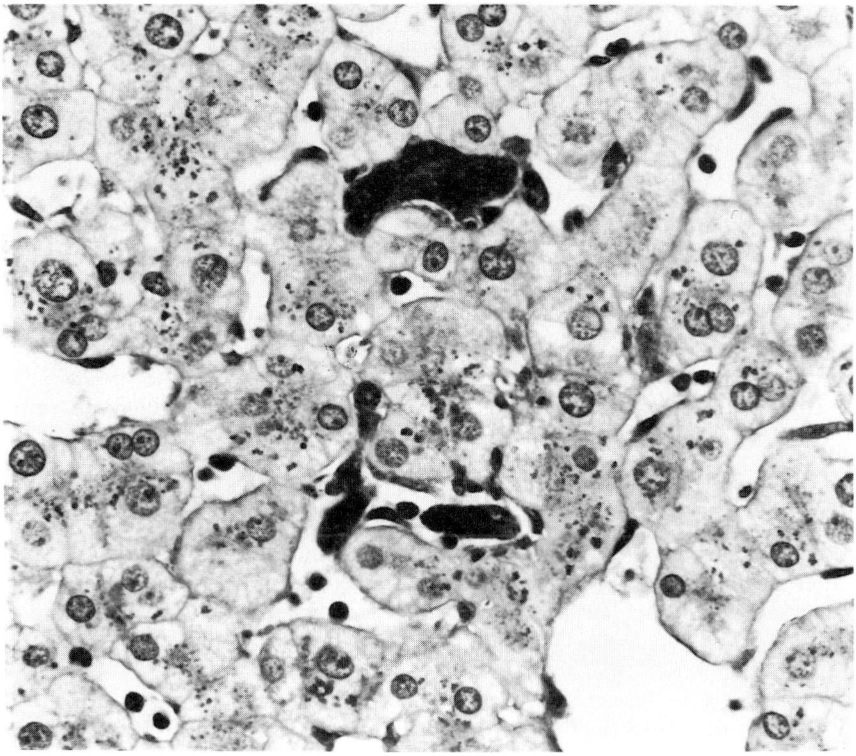

Figure 3 Liver involvement in Whipple's disease; prominent PAS-positive macrophages are present in perivenular sinusoids (PAS × 500). (Section kindly provided by Dr C. Kooijman, Utrecht)

been reported in congenital and familial immunodeficiency states[20]; further understanding of these syndromes may shed light on the pathogenetic mechanisms in primary sclerosing cholangitis.

CHRONIC INFLAMMATORY BOWEL DISEASE

The hepatic lesions which may complicate chronic inflammatory bowel diseases are summarized in Table 2, together with their approximate frequency. To this should be added occasional cases of pyogenic abscess complicating Crohn's disease (Greenstein, chapter 9). In addition, non-specific reactive hepatitis will be present in the majority of cases.

The true prevalence of chronic active hepatitis (CAH) is uncertain. Wee and Ludwig (1985)[27] suggested that some cases of CAH may probably be due to transfusion-related non-A, non-B (HCV) hepatitis. Earlier reports may have been an overestimate due to the difficulty in distinguishing CAH from primary sclerosing cholangitis (PSC). The morphological features in CAH which help distinguish it from sclerosing cholangitis are: a predomi-

Table 2 Liver involvement in chronic inflammatory bowel disease

	Approximate frequency
Fatty liver	30%
Primary sclerosing cholangitis	5–?10%
Chronic active hepatitis	1–2%
Cirrhosis	2–5%
Granulomas	5%
Amyloidosis	Rare
Bile duct carcinoma	×15– ×30 Increased risk*

*As compared with a normal population

nantly lymphocytic infiltrate in the periportal lesion with minimal so-called ductular proliferation; preservation of the bile ducts, particularly in the small portal tracts, in which they are generally absent in PSC; the presence of intra-acinar hepatitis; absence of, or the presence of only minimal amounts of, copper-associated protein demonstrable on the orcein stain in periportal or periseptal hepatocytes.

Cirrhosis is, in the majority of cases, a sequel to PSC but in some it may represent progression from CAH. Non-caseating granulomas are usually seen in association with Crohn's disease and have been shown to resolve after colectomy[28]. Hepatic amyloidosis has been reported almost exclusively in association with Crohn's disease and here again regression may follow colectomy[29].

Primary sclerosing cholangitis (PSC)

The true incidence of PSC as a complication of chronic inflammatory bowel disease is uncertain; it is not justifiable, on ethical grounds, to carry out routine ERCP and/or liver biopsy in a series of patients with chronic inflammatory bowel disease. Most of the clinical studies have been carried out on patients with ulcerative colitis and an association with Crohn's disease has been questioned. However, recent reports have indicated that in a series of patients with PSC and inflammatory bowel disease, 10% will have Crohn's disease[30,31], usually colonic and with total eolonic involvement[31].

Primary sclerosing cholangitis may affect any part of the biliary tree. The important observations of the Mayo Clinic group have confirmed this, and they have reported that small duct involvement (in which ERCP will be negative) may be the earliest lesion in many cases[32,33]. This progresses to involve larger ducts (resulting in positive ERCP findings). Where there is large duct involvement, small duct involvement is always present, and in the later stages of the disease involvement of the extrahepatic biliary tract is an almost invariable occurrence. It is now generally accepted that so-called pericholangitis represents small duct involvement by PSC and the use of this inaccurate term is therefore no longer appropriate.

Morphologically there is a chronic progressive fibro-obliterative destruction of the bile ducts. This is characterized by periductal fibrosis, degeneration and ulceration of the ductal epithelium, progressive narrowing of the bile duct lumen and replacement of the duct by fibrous tissue (Figure 4). There

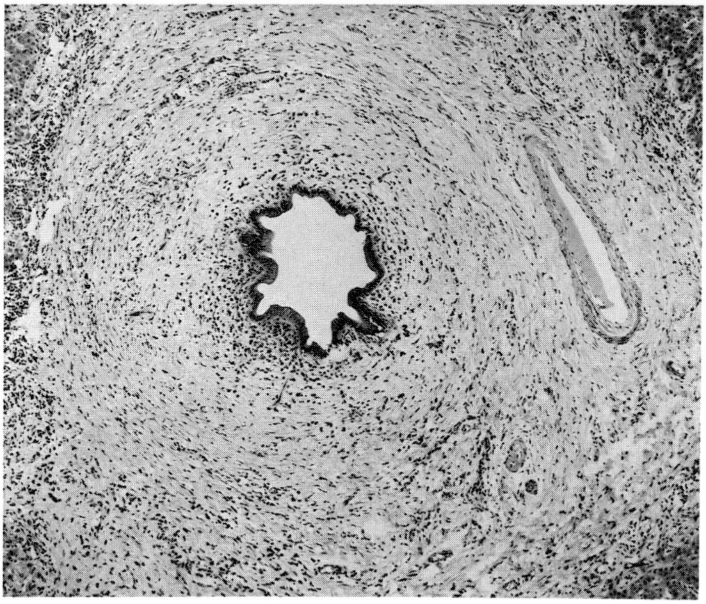

(a)

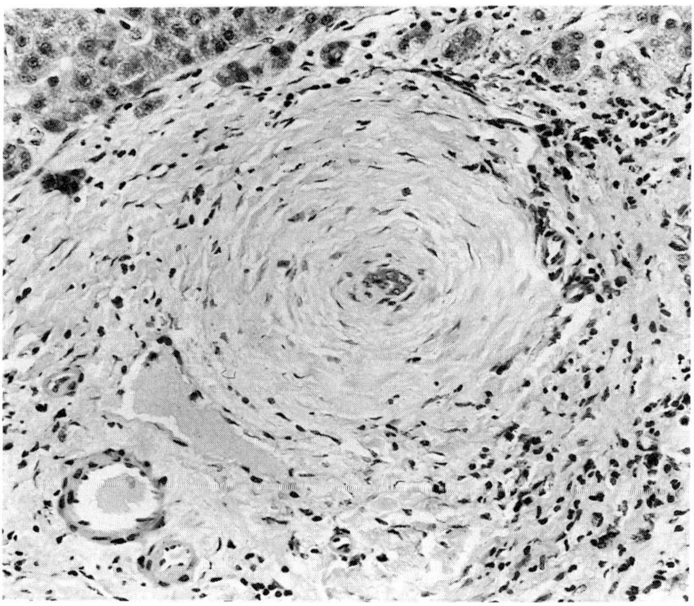

(b)

Figure 4 Primary sclerosing cholangitis in a patient with ulcerative colitis. (**a**) Bile duct showing periductal fibrosis; there is a chronic inflammatory cell infiltrate, moderately intense, immediately periductal and less marked in the peripheral fibrous tissue (H&E ×80). (**b**) This bile duct is almost obliterated by the fibrous tissue and only epithelial remnants remain within narrowed lumen (H&E ×80). (**c**) Total obliteration of a bile duct with the formation of a whorled fibrous scar (H&E ×160). (**d**) Fibrous obliteration of a small bile duct; note the periductal fibrosis (arrowed), the degenerate biliary epithelium and the considerable narrowing of the lumen (H&E ×110)

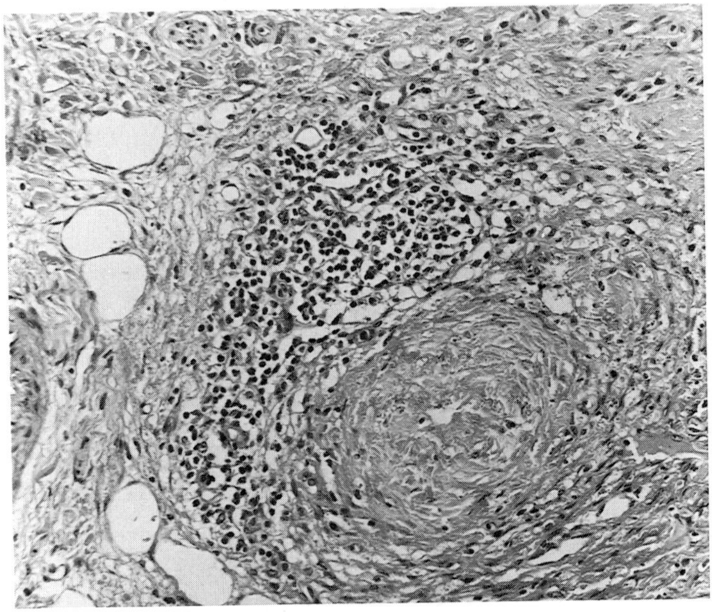

(c)

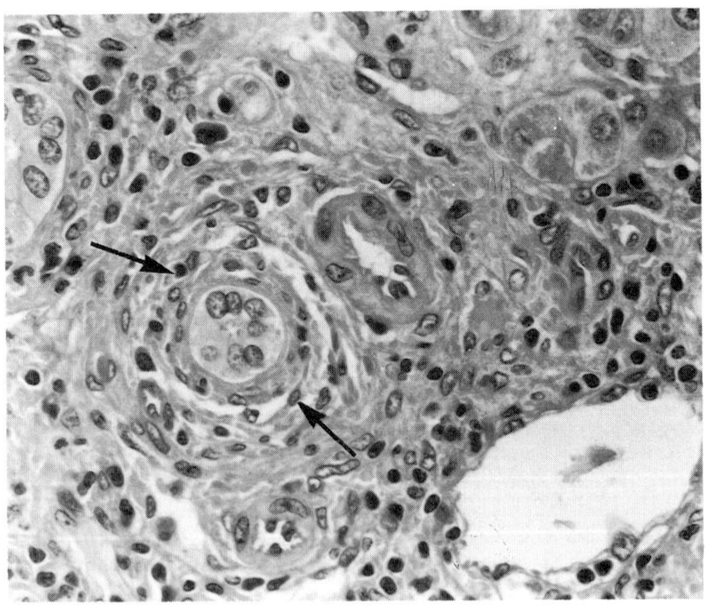

(d)

Figure 4 *continued*

is a chronic inflammatory cell infiltrate, lymphocytic and plasma cell, in the interstices of the periductal fibrous tissue and sometimes throughout the portal tract; there may be periductal oedema and sometimes there is a superimposed cholangitis (presumably due to bile retention) when neutrophil polymorphs may be present or even predominant. These features may be present to a variable degree: in some cases there is predominantly a periductal mononuclear cell infiltrate with features which may be difficult to distinguish from primary biliary cirrhosis (Figure 5a); in others there is an exuberant fibrotic reaction producing prominent fibrous whorls within the portal tracts (Figure 5b); in others the acute cholangitis may be marked and the background fibro-obliterative lesion affecting the ducts can be overlooked. The changes affecting the small ducts are similar (Figure 4d) but the lesions can readily be overlooked. With small bile ducts such as those illustrated in Figure 4d, there is normally no periductal fibrous tissue. The PAS/diastase stain is useful in identifying these smaller affected bile ducts; their basement mem-

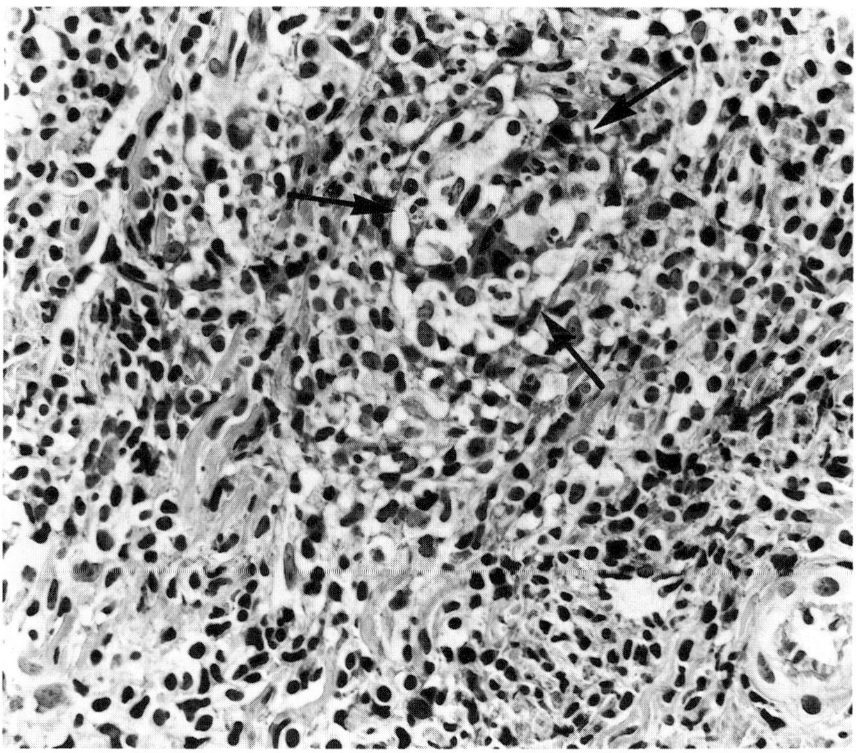

(a)

Figure 5 Primary sclerosing cholangitis. (**a**) In this biopsy from a patient with ulcerative colitis and ERCP-proven sclerosing cholangitis there was an intense mononuclear cell infiltrate in the portal tracts; the remains of the bile duct are outlined by the arrows; note the degenerate epithelial cells filling the lumen. (H&E × 500). (**b**) Fibrotic scars in an autopsy liver in which the destructive lesions of the bile duct were characterized by the presence of dense fibrous tissue with abundant elastic fibres (elastica van Gieson × 27)

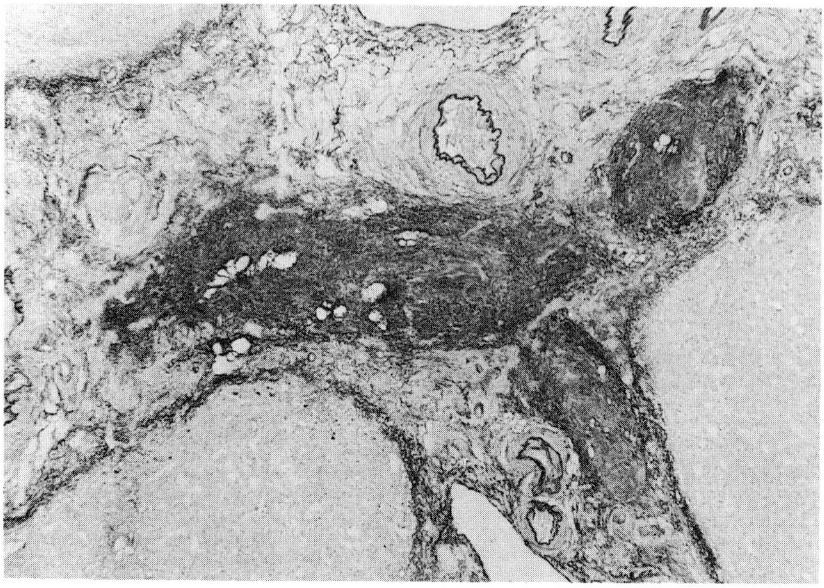

Figure 5 *continued*

brane remains intact and also appears thickened.

It must be emphasized that these virtually diagnostic bile duct lesions may be seen in only 50% of cases. In the others the bile ducts disappear, sometimes without trace, and sometimes with only a light mononuclear/histiocytic cell reaction or a lymphoid aggregate marking their previous site. In these cases the histopathologist must remember that in each normal portal tract the hepatic artery branch is accompanied by a bile duct of approximately the same diameter. An unaccompanied hepatic artery or arteries suggests there is a disappearing bile duct syndrome and the differential diagnoses then include PSC, primary biliary cirrhosis, Alagille's syndrome[34], and idiopathic adulthood ductopenia[35]. These topics have been recently reviewed[36]. The definitive diagnosis is dependent on a careful clinical, biochemical, immunological and morphological assessment of the patient.

With progressive loss of intrahepatic bile ducts and increasing cholestasis, periportal hepatitis develops with a pattern of biliary piecemeal necrosis in which so-called ductular proliferation is prominent. There is loss of some periportal hepatocytes, and in surviving ones features of cholate stasis occur – swelling, a hydropic appearance of the cytoplasm, Mallory body formation retention of copper and accumulation of copper-associated protein. Portal–portal necroinflammatory and then fibrous linkages are formed. Regenerative activity is evident; this may be of a nodular pattern from an early stage of the disease producing non-cirrhotic portal hypertension (Figure 6). There is eventual progression to an established biliary cirrhosis. In my opinion these periportal and parenchymal changes are secondary to the bile duct loss and

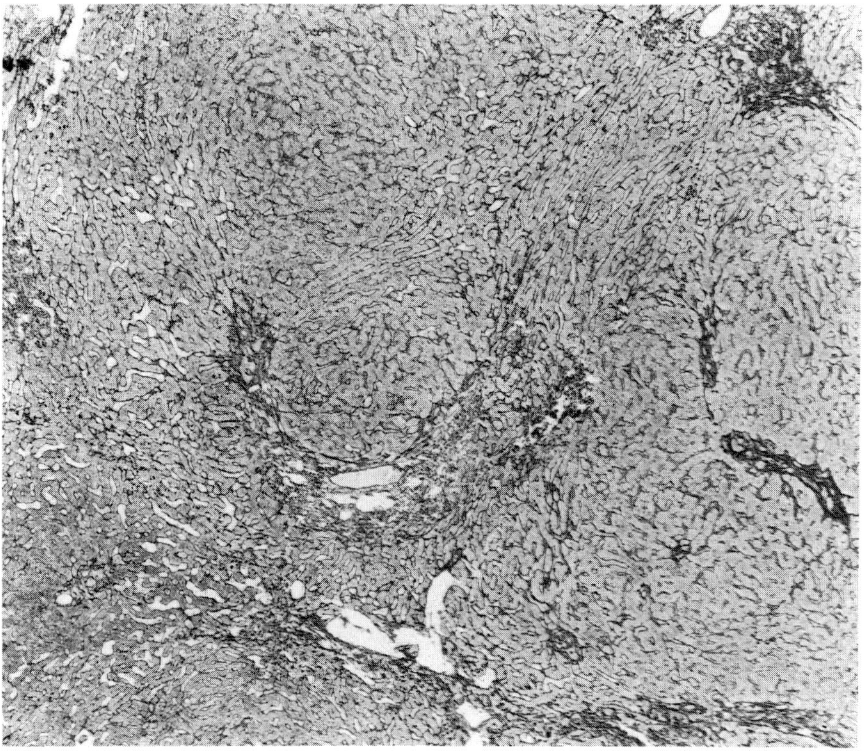

Figure 6 Wedge biopsy of liver from same case as illustrated in Figure 4. Regenerative nodules are producing architectural disturbance with compression of adjacent liver cells and sinusoidal dilatation (Gordon and Sweets' reticulin ×45)

the consequent cholestasis. Similar changes are seen, albeit to varying degrees, in all chronic cholestatic syndromes and there are no morphological features in these secondary changes which allow the histopathologist to distinguish one syndrome from the others.

The association between PSC and chronic inflammatory bowel disease is an intriguing one. As has already been mentioned, in 20–30% of patients with PSC there is no association with inflammatory bowel disease. Less commonly reported clinical associations[37] include retroperitoneal and mediastinal fibrosis, Reidel's thyroiditis, pseudotumour of the orbit, Peyronie's disease, porphyria cutanea tarda, submandibular gland fibrosis and others; histiocytosis X and immunodeficiency states are often seen in children[38]. In a third group the PSC occurs on its own. The questions which arise, therefore, are whether in these three broad groups of patients the same pathogenetic mechanisms are involved, and whether the liver disease is completely similar.

The strong association between PSC and chronic inflammatory bowel disease plausibly suggests that a similar aetiological agent or agents is responsible for the two disparate diseases. In patients with both diseases the ulcerative colitis frequently develops before the age of 20, the entire colon is usually involved, and the bowel disease may often be mild[39,40]. In a small number of cases the liver disease may be symptomatic and may be diagnosed before the bowel disease, and in others the liver disease presents some time after colectomy. The liver disease is slowly but variably progressive[30,31]. The asymptomatic patient may not necessarily have a good outlook and when hepatic symptoms develop the median survival time has been estimated to be 17 years[31]. However, careful prospective studies have shown that the two diseases progress virtually independent of each other[41,42]. This independent behaviour of the two diseases could be adduced as evidence that they are of different aetiology. Nevertheless, as La Russo *et al.*[41] have observed, the existence of a common cause but with a variable organ response may explain why the disorders may occur alone, together or in any time sequence.

The aetiology and pathogenesis of PSC are unknown but postulated factors include disturbances in bile acid metabolism, immunological mechanisms, portal bacteraemia and viral infection. Disturbances in bile acid metabolism secondary to colonic inflammation could result in the enterohepatic circulation of metabolites toxic to biliary epithelium. This hypothesis merits further investigation.

The association of PSC with the HLA-B8/DR3 haplotype[43] and reports of familial cases[44] suggest that immunological and genetic factors may be significant. Immunological investigations have shown: abnormalities of cellular immunity[45]; increased serum and bile immunoglobulin levels and the presence of circulating immune complexes and of immune complexes in bile[46,47]; and an increased prevalence of some serum autoantibodies[48]. The presence of an autoantibody unusual in its reactivity with neutrophil nuclear antigen (ANNA) in over 80% each of patients with PSC and of patients with chronic inflammatory bowel disease alone, provides circumstantial evidence that there may be immunological disturbances which are common to the two diseases[49]. However, as previously discussed, it remains unclear whether the immunological disturbances which have been described in PSC are secondary rather than primary phenomena, secondary that is to the gastrointestinal and/or liver disease.

Evidence for a microbial agent being significantly involved in either or both diseases has not been provided. In PSC patients the prevalence of antibodies to reovirus type 3 (previously associated with neonatal biliary disease) is not significantly different from a normal population[50].

Thus, the intriguing enigmas of primary sclerosing cholangitis and its close association with chronic inflammatory bowel disease remain unexplained, and present a considerable investigative challenge.

Bile duct carcinoma

This complication of chronic inflammatory bowel disease is now well recognized. It has been estimated that its prevalence in ulcerative colitis patients is 0.5%, and the relative risk of its development is 30-fold as compared with a normal population[51]. The carcinoma invariably develops against a background of PSC, occurring as a complication in 10–15% of cases, possibly more common where there is large duct involvement[31,40,52,53]. This complication may result from the chronic inflammatory process affecting the bile ducts, together with bile stasis and the possible production of carcinogenic metabolites, postulates which have also been advanced in respect of cholangiocarcinoma complicating other intrahepatic bile duct lesions characterized by infection and bile stasis[54]. There are a few reports of hepatocellular carcinoma complicating ulcerative colitis[52,53] including one recent case of the fibrolamellar variant[55].

References

1. Thomas, H. C., MacSween, R. N. M. and White, R. G. (1973). Role of the liver in controlling the immunogenicity of commensal bacteria in the gut. *Lancet*, **1**, 1288–91
2. Thomas, H. C., Singer, C. R. J., Tilney, N. L., Folch, H. and MacSween, R. N.M. (1976). The immune response in cirrhotic rats. Antigen distribution, humoral immunity, cell-mediated immunity and splenic suppressor cell activity. *Clin. Exp. Immunol.*, **26**, 574–82
3. Triger, D. R., Alp, M. H. and Wright, R. (1972). Bacterial and dietary antibodies in liver diseases. *Lancet*, **1**, 60–3
4. Nolan, J. P. (1981). Endotoxin, recituloendothelial function, and liver injury. *Hepatology*, **1**, 458–65
5. Billiar, T. R., Maddaus, M. A., West, M. A., Curran, R. D., Wells, C. A. and Simmons, R. L. (1988). *Ann. Surg.*, **208**, 532–40
6. Popper, H. and Schaffner, F. (1957). *Liver: Structure and Function.* (New York: McGraw-Hill)
7. MacSween, R. N. M. (1987). Liver pathology associated with diseases of other organs. In MacSween, R. N. M., Anthony, P. P. and Scheuer, P. J. (eds), *Pathology of the Liver*, 2nd edn, pp. 646–88. (Edinburgh: Churchill Livingstone)
8. Zimmerman, H. J. (1979). Clinical conference: jaundice due to bacterial infection. *Gastroenterology*, **77**, 362–74
9. Banks, J. G., Foulis, A. K., Ledingham, I. McA. and MacSween, R. N. M. (1982). Liver function in septic shock. *J. Clin. Pathol.*, **35**, 1249–52
10. Lefkowitch, J. H. (1982). Bile ductular cholestasis: an ominous histopathologic sign related to sepsis and 'cholangitis lenta'. *Hum. Pathol.*, **13**, 19–24
11. Utili, R., Abernathy, C. O. and Zimmerman, H. J. (1976). Cholestatic effects of *Escherichia coli* endotoxin on the isolated perfused rat liver. *Gastroenterology*, **70**, 248–53
12. Olesen, L. L., Ejlertsen, T., Paulsen, S. M. and Knudsen, P. R. (1989). Liver abscesses due to *Yersinia enterocolitica* in patients with haemochromatosis. *J. Intern. Med.*, **225**, 351–4
13. Simson, I. W. and Gear, J. H. S. (1987). Other viral and infectious diseases. In MacSween, R. N. M., Anthony, P. P. and Scheuer, P. J. (eds), *Pathology of the Liver*, 2nd edn, pp. 224–264. (Edinburgh: Churchill Livingstone)
14. Seel, D. J. and Park, Y. K. (1983). Oriental infestational cholangitis. *Am. J. Surg.*, **146**, 366–70
15. Saint-Marc Girardin, M.-F., Zafrani, E. S., Chaumette, M.-T., Delchier, J. C., Metreau, J. M. and Dheumeaux, D. (1984). Hepatic granulomas in Whipple's disease. *Gastroenterology*, **86**, 753–6
16. Sieracki, C. and Fine, G. (1959). Whipple's disease – observations on systemic involvement. II. Gross and histologic observations. *Arch. Pathol.*, **67**, 81–93
17. Misra, O. S., Lebwohl, P. and Laufer, H. (1981). Hepatic and appendiceal Whipple's disease with negative jejunal biopsies. *Am. J. Gastroenterol.*, **75**, 302–6
18. Margulis, S. J., Honig, C. L., Soave, R., Govoni, A. F., Mouradian, J. A. and Jacobson, I. M. (1986). Biliary tract obstruction in the acquired immunodeficiency syndrome. *Ann. Intern. Med.*, **105**, 207–10
19. Schneiderman, D. J., Cello, J. P. and Laing, F. C. (1987). Papillary stenosis and sclerosing cholangitis in the acquired immunodeficiency syndrome. *Ann. Intern. Med.*, **106**, 546–9
20. Davis, J. J., Heyman, M. B., Ferrell, L., Kerner, J., Kerlan, R. Jr and Thaler, M. M. (1987).

Sclerosing cholangitis associated with chronic cryptosporidiosis in a child with a congenital immunodeficiency disorder. *Am. J. Gastroenterol.*, **82**, 1196–1202

21. Roberts-Thomson, I. C., Anders, R. F. and Bhathal, P. S. (1982). Granulomatous hepatitis and cholangitis associated with giardiasis. *Gastroenterology*, **83**, 480–3
22. Daly, J. J. and Baker, G. F. (1984). Pinworm granuloma of the liver. *Am. J. Trop. Med. Hyg.*, **33**, 62–4
23. Everett, G. D. and Mitros, F. A. (1980). Eosinophilic gastroenteritis with hepatic eosinophilic granulomas. *Am. J. Gastroenterol.*, **74**, 519–21
24. Hagander, B., Brandt, L., Sjolung, K., Berg, N. O., Norden, A. and Stenstam, M. (1977). Hepatic injury in adult coeliac disease. *Lancet*, **2**, 270–2
25. Logan, R. F. A., Ferguson, A., Finlayson, N. D. C. and Weir, D. G. (1978). Primary biliary cirrhosis and coeliac disease. *Lancet*, **1**, 230–3
26. Hay, J. E., Wiesner, R. H., Shorter, R. G., LaRusso, N. F. and Baldus, W. P. (1988). Primary sclerosing cholangitis and coeliac disease. *Ann. Intern. Med.*, **109**, 713–17
27. Wee, A. and Ludwig, J. (1985). Pericholangitis in chronic ulcerative colitis: primary sclerosing cholangitis of the small bile ducts? *Ann. Intern. Med.*, **102**, 581–7
28. Eade, M. N., Cooke, W. T., Brooke, B. N. and Thompson, H. (1971). Liver disease in Crohn's colitis. *Ann. Intern. Med.*, **74**, 518–28
29. Fitchen, J. H. (1975). Amyloidosis and granulomatous ileocolitis. *N. Engl. J. Med.*, **292**, 352–3
30. Wiesner, R. H. and La Russo, N. F. (1980). Clinicopathological features of the syndrome of primary sclerosing cholangitis. *Gastroenterology*, **79**, 200–6
31. Aadland, E., Schrumpf, E., Fausa, O., Elgjo, K., Heilo, A., Aakhus, T. and Gjone, E. (1987). Primary sclerosing cholangitis: a long-term follow-up study. *Scand. J. Gastroenterol.*, **22**, 655–64
32. Ludwig, J., Barham, S. S., La Russo, N. F., Elveback, L. R., Wiesner, R. H. and McCall, J. T. (1981). Morphologic features of chronic hepatitis associated with primary sclerosing cholangitis or chronic ulcerative colitis. *Hepatology*, **1**, 632–40
33. Wee, A. and Ludwig, J. (1985). Pericholangitis in chronic ulcerative colitis: primary sclerosing cholangitis of the small bile ducts? *Ann. Intern. Med.*, **102**, 581–7
34. Alagille, D., Estrada, A., Hadchouel, M., Gautier, M., Odievre, M. and Dommergues, J. P. (1987). Syndromatic paucity of interlobular bile ducts (Alagille syndrome or arteriohepatic dysplasia) Review of 80 cases. *J. Paediatr.*, **110**, 195–200
35. Ludwig, J. (1987). New concepts in biliary cirrhosis. *Semin. Liver Dis.*, **7**, 293–301
36. MacSween, R. N. M. and Burt, A. D. (1989). Pathology of the intrahepatic bile ducts. In Anthony, P. P. and MacSween, R. N. M. (eds), *Recent Advances in Histopathology*, pp. 161–84. (Edinburgh: Churchill Livingstone)
37. MacSween, R. N. M. (1984). Aspects of liver disease: Primary sclerosing cholangitis. In Anthony, P. P. and MacSween, R. N. M. (eds), *Recent Advances in Histopathology*, pp. 158–67. (Edinburgh: Churchill Livingstone)
38. Sisto, A., Feldman, P., Garel, L., Seidman, E., Brochu, P., Morin, C. L., Weber, A. M. and Roy, C. C. (1987). Primary sclerosing cholangitis in children: study of 5 cases and review of the literature. *Pediatrics*, **80**, 918–23
39. Schrumpf, E., Elgjo, K., Fausa, O., Gjone, E., Kolmannskig, F. and Ritland, S. (1980). Sclerosing cholangitis in ulcerative colitis. *Scand. J. Gastroenterol.*, **15**, 689–97
40. Chapman, R. W. G. *et al.* (1980). Primary sclerosing cholangitis: a review of its clinical features, cholangiography, and hepatic histology. *Gut*, **21**, 870–7
41. La Russo, N. F., Wiesner, R. H., Ludwig, J. and MacCarty, R. L. (1984). Primary sclerosing cholangitis. *N. Engl. J. Med.*, **310**, 899–903
42. Cangemi, J. R., Wiesner, R. H., Beaver, S. J., Ludwig, J., MacCarty, R. L., Dozois, R. R., Zinsmeister, A. R. and La Russo, N. F. (1989). Effect of proctocolectomy for chronic ulcerative colitis on the natural history of primary sclerosing cholangitis. *Gastroenterology*, **96**, 790–4
43. Chapman, R. W., Varghese, Z., Gaul, R., Patel, G., Kokinon, N. and Sherlock, S. (1980). Association of primary sclerosing cholangitis with HLA-B8. *Gut*, **24**, 38–41
44. Quigley, E. M. M., La Russo, N. F., Ludwig, J., MacSween, R. N. M., Birnie, G. G. and Watkinson, G. (1983). Familial occurrence of primary sclerosing cholangitis and ulcerative colitis. *Gastroenterology*, **85**, 1160–5

45. Mieli-Vergani, G., Lobo-Yeo, A., McFarlane, B. M., McFarlane, I. G., Mowat, A. P. and Vergani, D. (1989). Different immune mechanisms leading to autoimmunity in primary sclerosing cholangitis and autoimmune chronic active hepatitis of childhood. *Hepatology*, **9**, 198–203
46. Bodenheimer, H. C. Jr, La Russo, N. F., Thayer, W. R. Jr, Charland, C., Staples, P. and Ludwig, J. (1983). Elevated circulating immune complexes in primary sclerosing cholangitis. *Hepatology*, **3**, 150–4
47. Alberti-Flor, J. J., De Medina, M., Jeffers, L., Schultz, D. R. and Schiff, E. R. (1986). Elevated levels of immunoglobulins and immune complexes in the bile of patients with primary sclerosing cholangitis. *Am. J. Gastroenterol.*, **81**, 325–8
48. Zauli, D., Schrumpf, E., Crespi, C., Cassani, F., Fausa, L. and Aadland, E. (1987). An autoantibody profile in primary sclerosing cholangitis. *J. Hepatol.*, **5**, 14–18
49. Snook, J. A., Chapman, R. W., Fleming, K. and Jewell, D. P. (1989). Anti-neutrophil nuclear antibody in ulcerative colitis, Crohn's disease and primary sclerosing cholangitis. *Clin. Exp. Immunol.*, **86**, 30–3
50. Minuk, G. Y., Paul, R. W. and Lee, P. W. K. (1985). The prevalence of antibodies to reovirus type 3 in adults with idiopathic cholestatic liver disease. *J. Med. Virol.*, **16**, 55–60
51. Mir-Madjlessi, S. H., Farmer, R. G. and Sivak, M. V. (1987). Bile duct carcinoma in patients with ulcerative colitis. Relationship to sclerosing cholangitis: report of six cases and review of the literature. *Dig. Dis. Sci.*, **32**, 145–54
52. Ritchie, J. K., Allan, R. N., MacCartney, J., Thompson, H., Hawley, P. R. and Cooke, W. T. (1974). Biliary tract carcinoma associated with ulcerative colitis. *Quart. J. Med.*, **43**, 263–79
53. Wee, A., Ludwig, J., Coffey, R. J., La Russo, N. F. and Wiesner, R. H. (1985). Hepatobiliary carcinoma associated with primary sclerosing cholangitis and chronic ulcerative colitis. *Hum. Pathol.*, **16**, 719–26
54. Anthony, P. P. (1987). Tumours and tumour-like lesions of the liver and biliary tract. In MacSween, R. N. M., Anthony, P. P. and Scheuer, P. J. (eds), *Pathology of the Liver*, 2nd edn, pp. 574–645. (Edinburgh: Churchill Livingstone)
55. Snook, J. A., Kelly, P., Chapman, R. W. and Jewell, D. P. (1989). Fibrolamellar hepatocellular carcinoma complicating ulcerative colitis with primary sclerosing cholangitis. *Gut*, **30**, 243–5

12
The liver in chronic inflammatory bowel disease: clinical findings

A. HOLSTEGE, J. SCHÖLMERICH and W. GEROK

INTRODUCTION

Ulcerative colitis is two to three times as common as Crohn's disease with an incidence of 5 to 8 cases/100 000 per year[1]. In Germany 49 cases/100 000 people are affected by ulcerative colitis[2]. Chronic inflammatory bowel disease is often associated with hepatobiliary disturbances. Prevalence data of liver disease in these patients differ considerably, ranging from 3%[3,4] to 95%[5,6] (Table 1). Abnormal liver findings by ultrasound were detected in about 25% of patients with Crohn's disease or ulcerative colitis[7]. Selection bias, as well as a more widespread and earlier use of better diagnostic tools, may be the reason for this wide range of variation. True epidemiological data could be obtained only from serial liver biopsies in every patient with chronic inflammatory bowel disease, which of course cannot be done since the associated liver disease is usually clinically of minor importance. However, the clinician should be aware of a few clinically relevant exceptions.

Table 1 Prevalence of hepatobiliary disease in chronic inflammatory bowel disease

Diagnosis	*Prevalence (percentages)*
Liver abscesses	0.3 (CD)[a]
Secondary amyloidosis	1–8 (CD)
Cholelithiasis	25–35 (CD)
Fatty liver	4–45 (CD)
Granulomatous hepatitis	1 (CD)
Pericholangitis[c]	20–35 (UC)[b]
Primary sclerosing cholangitis	5 (UC)
Cholangiocarcinoma	0.5 (UC)
Cirrhosis	2–5 (UC > CD)

[a]CD = Crohn's disease
[b]UC = ulcerative colitis
[c]'Small-duct' primary sclerosing cholangitis presumably identical with pericholangitis

Despite our increased knowledge of the prevalence of hepatobiliary lesions in bowel disease, the aetiology and pathogenesis of this relationship remain obscure. Three different types of association between bowel and liver disease can be differentiated. The relationship may be incidental with completely separate aetiologies of both diseases (Figure 1). Such an occasional association can be provoked by medical treatment of ulcerative colitis or Crohn's disease (Table 2)[8,9]. Most of the drugs used in chronic inflammatory bowel disease may cause a wide variety of liver lesions. Primary biliary cirrhosis in ulcerative colitis probably is a similar incidental finding[10,11].

A second type of association between liver and bowel abnormalities involves a causal relationship (Figure 2). A prerequisite for such an association is that liver disease exclusively depends on the presence of bowel disease. Improvement in intestinal disease will usually be followed by an amelioration of hepatic disturbances. Examples for such causally related diseases are secondary amyloidosis, liver abscesses, and, presumably, the formation of

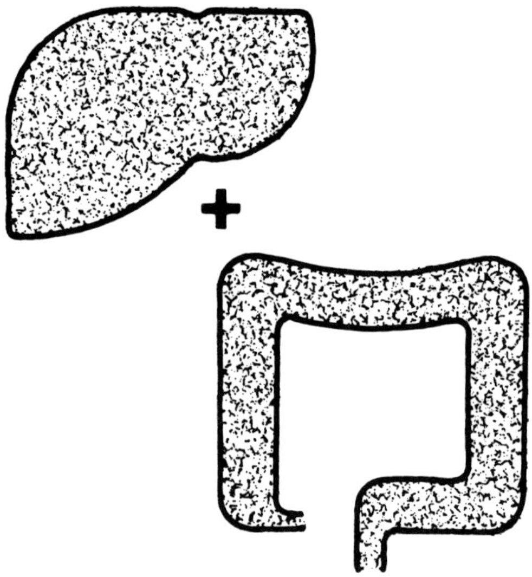

Figure 1 Independent liver and bowel disease (incidental association)

Table 2 Drug-induced liver lesions and chronic inflammatory bowel disease

Therapy	*Complications*
Steroids	fatty liver
Sulfasalazine	liver cell necrosis, hepatitis
Azathioprine/6-mercaptopurine	cholestasis
	veno-occlusive disease
	peliosis hepatis
Total parenteral nutrition	liver cell necrosis
	cholestasis
	fatty liver

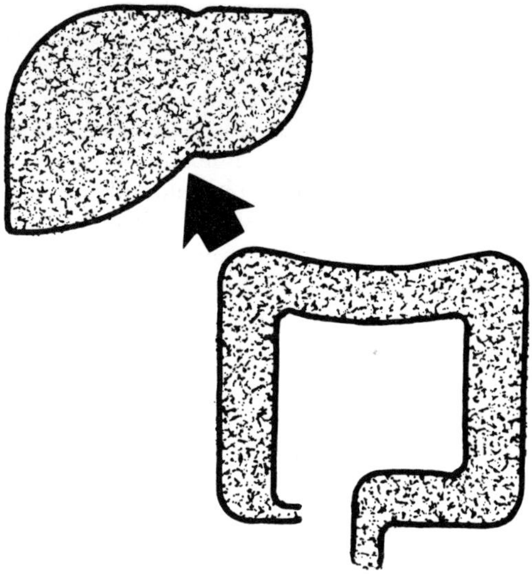

Figure 2 Chronic inflammatory bowel disease causes liver lesions (causal relationship)

new gallstones.

In a third type of association involvement of both organs is thought to be due to a common pathogenetic pathway representing two different targets of a common and as yet unknown pathogen (Figure 3). Such an association is suggested for coexisting primary sclerosing cholangitis and ulcerative

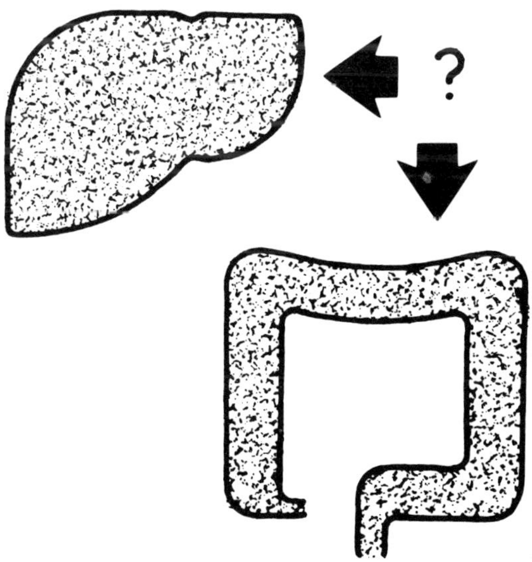

Figure 3 Liver and bowel disease are targets of a common unknown pathogen

colitis. The aetiology of both diseases is unknown, although common immunological abnormalities, viral agents, or a genetic predisposition have been suggested[12]. Either disease may develop independently, preceding or following the other[13–15]. Primary sclerosing cholangitis is not influenced by duration and severity of ulcerative colitis or prior resection of the diseased colon[13].

Our knowledge of the aetiology and pathogenesis of both chronic inflammatory bowel disease and hepatobiliary lesions is limited and in most cases does not allow discrimination between different types of association. Fatty liver can be directly related to the severity of colitis[6] but may have many other causes in these patients independent from bowel disease. Similarly, granulomatous hepatitis and Crohn's disease may be causally linked. Liver granulomas, however, may be an incidental finding in ulcerative colitis due to treatment with sulfasalazine[9]. In many other coexisting disease manifestations the relationship cannot be classified, and remains obscure.

SECONDARY AMYLOIDOSIS OF THE LIVER

Secondary amyloidosis of the liver is a rare event in inflammatory bowel disease. Histological examination of liver biopsies in 103 patients led to the detection of only one case of hepatic amyloidosis[16]. In a prospective study of 177 patients with inflammatory bowel disease of more than 5 years' duration no new cases were found[17]. Amyloidosis appears not to be over represented in ulcerative colitis[17–20], whereas amyloid depositions were detected in 2 of 20 biopsies of patients with Crohn's disease[6], in 7 of 85 patients submitted to intestinal resection[21], and in 12 of 214 patients with this disease seen in a medical department[22].

Secondary amyloidosis is characterized by the extracellular accumulation of a degradation product, amyloid A (AA), of a serum acute-phase protein called serum amyloid A (SAA)[23]. The key site of SAA synthesis is the liver, which far outweighs its production by any other tissue. The kinetics of SAA are similar to those of C-reactive protein. Both are acute-phase proteins which can be induced in human hepatocytes by interleukin-6, and with much less efficiency by interleukin-1 or a recombinant human tumour necrosis factor[24]. Interleukin-1, however, may synergistically enhance the effects of interleukin-6. All three are hormone-like cytokines which are released from monocytes and regulate the synthesis of acute-phase proteins in hepatocytes through induction of transcription of their genes[25]. Chronic inflammatory bowel disease may lead to persistent stimulation of monocytes via release of endotoxins or other as yet unknown mediators. Subsequent formation of cytokines by monocytes may induce a sustained release of serum amyloid A followed by amyloid A formation and precipitation in the liver and other tissues. Great variations have been shown in the ability of monocytes[26] and polymorphonuclear leucocytes to degrade the SAA to amyloid A[27], which might explain why not all people with elevated SAA develop secondary amyloidosis[28]. A hypothetical model of pathogenesis of secondary amyloidosis in Crohn's disease is depicted in Figure 4.

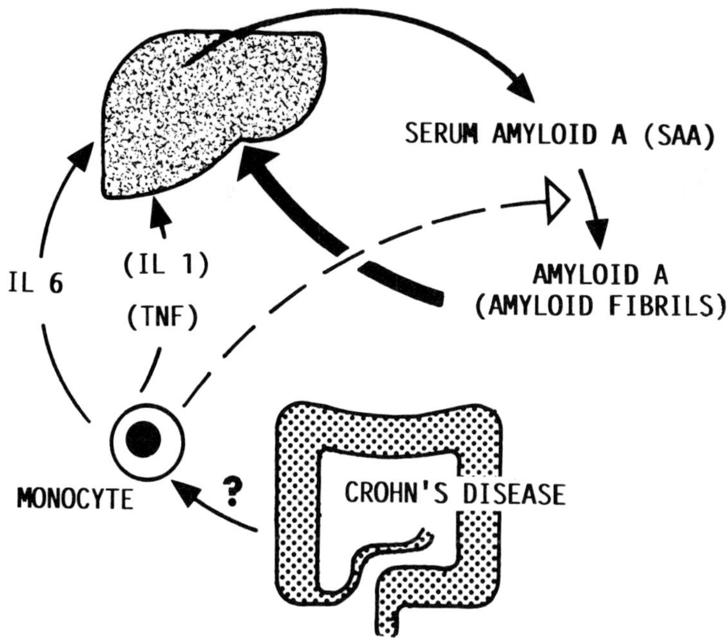

Figure 4 Hypothetical model of the pathogenesis of secondary amyloidosis in Crohn's disease

The occurrence of amyloidosis in Crohn's disease appears to be not strictly correlated to the localization and expansion of the underlying inflammatory bowel disease[17,21]. The amyloid deposition is found in the media of portal blood vessels and in the sinusoidal walls, leading to atrophy and disappearance of hepatocytes. Clinical symptoms and signs of hepatic amyloidosis are non-specific[29,30]. Hepatomegaly may be the only positive physical finding. Liver function abnormalities are unusual and occur late in the disease. The most common pathological findings in a series of 47 cases of hepatic amyloid unrelated to chronic inflammatory bowel disease were hypoalbuminaemia, elevated BSP retention, alkaline phosphatase, and cholesterol[31]. Others[32] noted occasional mild hypoprothrombinaemia, rare elevations in serum lactic acid dehydrogenase and glutamic-oxaloacetic transaminase levels, and mild elevations in bilirubin. However, these parameters did not correlate well with the extent of hepatic disease.

The diagnosis is confirmed by liver biopsy and histological examination of the collected specimen using the Congo red stain on formalin-fixed tissues and polarization microscopy. Liver puncture in amyloid liver is somewhat more often complicated by haemorrhage, particularly in patients with massive hepatomegaly, who are often in the terminal stages of their liver disease. A technetium-99m-pyrophosphate scan can be helpful to delineate soft tissue amyloidosis[33]. An increased awareness and high degree of suspicion with regular examination of the urine for proteinuria might result in earlier and more frequent diagnosis in long-standing Crohn's disease[17]. Proteinuria and renal dysfunction indicate a late stage of the disease and a poor prognosis. It remains to be established whether the measurement of serum amyloid A protein and amyloid A degrading activity, together with serum albumin or C-reactive protein[34,34a,35] will allow earlier detection of secondary liver amyloidosis.

Steroid treatment of Crohn's disease presumably does not improve liver amyloidosis or prevent its development[21,22]. Regression may be seen after surgical excision of the inflamed bowel[17,21]. However, contradictory observations have been published[36]. Liver transplantation may be a therapeutic option in selected cases[26]. Progressive deterioration of renal function will lead to death in more than half of the patients with secondary amyloidosis and Crohn's disease[37].

LIVER ABSCESS IN CROHN'S DISEASE

Pyogenic liver abscess is a serious clinical problem which is a rare event in Crohn's disease[38] and even less often a complication of ulcerative colitis[39]. However, the incidence of liver abscess in patients with Crohn's disease (114–297 per 100 000) appears to be higher than that of liver abscess in the general population (8–16 per 100 000)[38]. The patients present with fever, chills, sweats, right upper abdominal pain, weight loss, nausea and vomiting[38]. The clinical manifestations of liver abscess can be mistaken for a reactivation of Crohn's disease leading to a treatment with increased doses of corticosteroids or even surgical resection of the inflamed bowel[38a,39–41]. Involvement of the liver is associated with polymorphonuclear leucocytosis and increased levels of serum alkaline phosphatase[38]. Other liver function tests are of less diagnostic value (serum albumin, glutamic oxaloacetic transaminase, total bilirubin). Diagnosis is best made by ultrasonographic examination, CT scanning, or radioisotopic liver scanning[38,42–45].

Abscess formation is favoured in patients with active chronic inflammatory disease under steroid treatment and subsequent to abdominal operations. Ulcerations and loss of integrity of the normal mucosal barrier may predispose to microbial invasion of the portal venous system with seeding of the liver[38,46,46a]. Streptococci, especially *Streptococcus milleri*, have been shown to be the most frequent cause of liver abscess in patients with Crohn's disease[38]. A prerequisite for rational treatment is the identification of the responsible pathogen by aerobic and anaerobic cultures of material from the liver accompanied by Gram-stained smears of aspirates. In one study blood cultures were also helpful in about half of the patients[38].

Therapy of liver abscess is initiated by the administration of appropriate antibiotics. Medical treatment is usually followed by percutaneous aspiration and drainage of the abscess under CT or ultrasonic guidance[43,44,47].

GALLSTONES IN CROHN'S DISEASE

Bile salt synthesis from cholesterol in the liver is repressed to low levels by the high flux of bile salts returning to the liver in the enterohepatic circulation.

Synthesis appears to be sensitive to the magnitude of this flux. Malabsorption of bile acids interrupts this enterohepatic circulation and leads to increased hepatocellular bile acid synthesis. A small bile salt pool with its high cycling frequency affects not only *de novo* bile salt synthesis but also faecal loss, to a slight degree. Absorption efficiency is lower in the presence of small bile acid pools[48], increasing the loss of bile acids due to ileal dysfunction. This mechanism is operative in patients with ileal resection or presumably Crohn's disease interfering with the patient's capacity to solubilize cholesterol in bile (Figure 5). The biliary consequences of ileal dysfunction are an increased cholesterol saturation associated with an increased prevalence of gallstones in Crohn's disease[7,49–57]. Moreover, gall bladder motility may be impaired in chronic inflammatory bowel disease[58]. Depletion of bile acids might be magnified by cholestyramine treatment of bile acid diarrhoea occasionally complicating Crohn's disease.

Gallstones were found in 31.9% of patients with disorders of the terminal ileum[54]. Lower figures were reported from a series of patients operated on for Crohn's disease (17%)[49] or from an ultrasound study in 74 patients with Crohn's disease (19%; mean age 35 years)[7]. In contrast to findings in the normal population[59], the incidence of gallstones was not related to age in the presence of ileal dysfunction but correlated best with the duration of the disease[49,51,54]. The cumulative probability of developing gallbladder disease approached 50% during a 20-year period of distal ileopathy[50]. The prevalence in males was 22.2% and in females 34.8%[51]. Gallstones were more often detected in patients with more than 100 cm diseased or resected ileum (35%) but only in 9% of those with less extended resections[49].

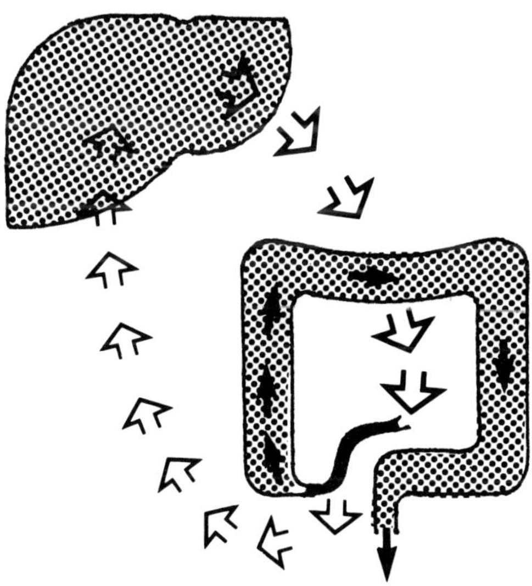

Figure 5 Pathogenesis of cholesterol cholelithiasis in Crohn's disease. Bile acid malabsorption due to ileal dysfunction is followed by a reduced excretion of bile acids into bile and subsequent biliary cholesterol supersaturation. This increases the risk for gallstone formation. Arrows indicate bile acid flow

A more recent survey of gallstones in patients with Crohn's disease using ultrasound[60] revealed similar prevalence data when compared to age-matched controls included into a Norwegian large population study[61,62]. According to these observations, further studies confirming a true over-representation of gallstones in Crohn's disease are warranted[62]. In addition, we do not know whether the incidence of symptomatic stones or complications is higher in patients with inflammatory bowel disease (Figure 6).

LIVER GRANULOMAS

Epithelioid cell granulomas with occasional multinucleated giant cells, lymphocytes and granulocytes can be detected in liver biopsies from patients with Crohn's disease[6,16,51,63–67]. Of 20 consecutive liver biopsies performed in patients undergoing colectomy for Crohn's disease affecting the entire colon, 15% revealed hepatic granulomas. An almost identical prevalence of granulomas (9 of 132) was reported from a similar study in patients with

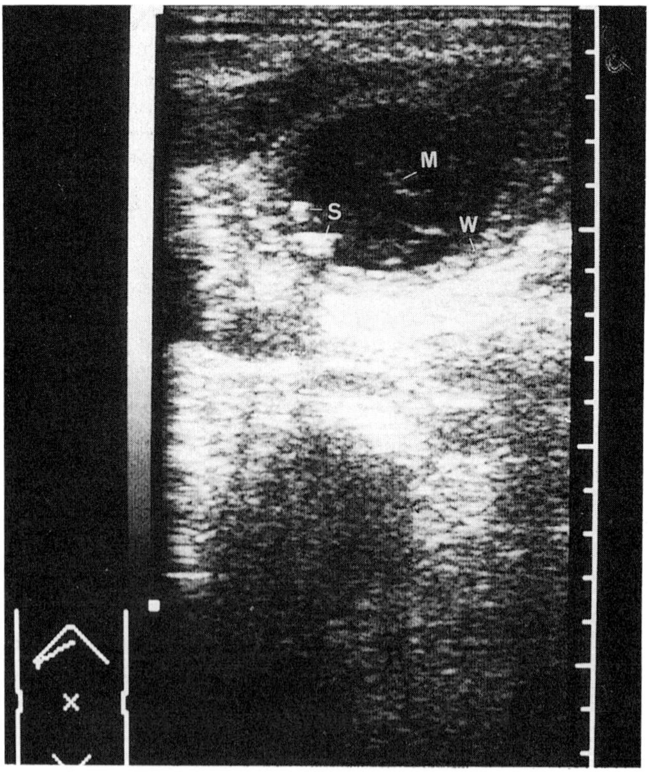

Figure 6 Cholecystolithiasis and cholecystitis in a patient with Crohn's disease: ultrasound study. A thickened gallbladder wall (W), the presence of stones (S) and echogenic floating material (M) within the lumen are positive indicators of cholecystitis

ulcerative colitis[5].

Hepatomegaly may be the only clinical sign in patients with granulomatous hepatitis and Crohn's disease[63]. Elevations of serum alkaline phosphatase and of 5′-nucleotidase have been measured in patients with liver granulomas as well as with other liver manifestations of chronic inflammatory bowel disease[6,65]. Accordingly, liver biopsy is the only way to diagnose granulomatous hepatitis.

The granulomas may disappear without scarring after removal of the inflamed bowel[66]. An association between hepatic granulomas and ulcerative colitis has been questioned, since further examination of such patients often disclosed Crohn's disease[68]. A causal role of sulfasalazine treatment for development of hepatic granulomas in ulcerative colitis cannot be excluded[9].

FATTY LIVER

Fatty infiltration is the most frequent finding in patients with chronic inflammatory bowel disease[5,6,16,69]. In one-third of biopsies taken at colectomy from 20 consecutive patients with Crohn's disease a periportal or perilobular fatty infiltration has been detected[6]. Similar data are available for patients with ulcerative colitis[5]. Probably due to differences in selection of patients the incidence of fatty liver in chronic inflammatory bowel disease varies from 4 to 45%[5,6,16,62,69,70]. No clear correlation was found between severity of bowel disease and histological changes in liver biopsies[6,69–71]. Follow-up examinations in fatty liver indicated complete reversibility of the lesion with no progression to cirrhosis[6,16,71]. Fatty liver is often associated with total parenteral nutrition or steroid treatment[8,9]. Symptoms are absent, and hepatomegaly may be the only clinical sign.

PRIMARY BILARY CIRRHOSIS

Primary biliary cirrhosis has been described in patients with ulcerative colitis[10,11]. All the patients revealed positive antimitochondrial antibody tests and displayed normal cholangiographic appearances when endoscopic retrograde cholangiopancreatography was performed[10]. Ulcerative colitis predated the development of primary biliary cirrhosis, which had a mild course with prolonged remissions in all patients. However, whether this represents a new hepatobiliary involvement or a chance association remains to be evaluated prospectively in a large series of patients with ulcerative colitis.

CHRONIC ACTIVE HEPATITIS

Histological evidence for chronic active hepatitis has been obtained from liver biopsies from patients with ulcerative colitis and/or primary sclerosing cholangitis[15,71–76]. Of patients with primary sclerosing cholangitis (PSC) confirmed either by histology or cholangiography 66% showed piecemeal necrosis, suggesting a possible diagnosis of chronic active hepatitis[72]. In these cases necrosis was believed to represent one of the many different histological features of PSC[72–74,74a]. Morphological features of liver specimens from patients with primary sclerosing cholangitis were strikingly similar to those specimens taken from patients who had chronic hepatitis associated with chronic inflammatory bowel disease alone[74]. From these data a common cause of both conditions has been delineated[74]. Reports of liver biopsy diagnoses in patients with PSC or ulcerative colitis unfortunately are hampered by obscure terminology[77]. The term pericholangitis has been rejected as a disease designation for chronic hepatitis in chronic inflammatory bowel disease[78]. No terminology exists to differentiate between chronic hepatitis and cirrhosis in PSC or chronic ulcerative colitis. However, in most cases the liver diseases associated with both conditions presumably represent one distinct entity[74]. Inflammatory changes including both inflammatory cellular infiltration and the increased fibrosis that may develop subsequently were detected in 12 of 20 liver biopsy specimens from patients with severe Crohn's colitis[6].

PRIMARY SCLEROSING CHOLANGITIS

Epidemiology

There is a striking association between primary sclerosing cholangitis and chronic inflammatory bowel disease, since about 50–75% of patients with PSC suffer from concurrent ulcerative colitis (Table 3)[15,72,76,79–82]. Crohn's disease was present in only 4–13% of the cases with hepatobiliary disease. The increased prevalence of asymptomatic PSC rising from 10% in 1980 to 33% in 1988 reflects an earlier and more widespread use of ERCP in patients with ulcerative colitis and laboratory signs of hepatobiliary disease. Conversely, 2–7.5% of all patients with ulcerative colitis were diagnosed to have PSC[4,62,83]. Usually patients with PSC are under the age of 40[15,72,83] and the mean ratio of males to females is 2:1 (Table 3).

Table 3 Epidemiological and clinical features of primary sclerosing cholangitis

n	*M/F*	*Symptomatic*	*Asymptomatic*	*Ulcerative colitis*	*Crohn's disease*	*Reference*
29	2/1	93%	7%	72%	?[a]	72
50	2.3/1	90%	10%	48%	6%	15
53	1.4/1	75%	25%	58%	4%	79
38	1.5/1	76%	24%	47%	13%	80
46	2.1/1	67%	33%	78%	4%	76
70	1.9/1	76%	24%	?[a]	?[a]	81
174	1.9/1	79%	21%	71%	?[a]	82, 84
460	1.9/1	79%	21%	62%	7%	Total/Mean

[a] = data not given

Aetiology and pathogenesis

PSC is a syndrome of unknown aetiology. An immunological hypothesis has been invoked which originates from the following observations.

The frequency of anticolon antibodies was markedly increased in PSC with ulcerative colitis (62.5%) as compared with patients with ulcerative colitis (17%) and Crohn's colitis (16%) without hepatobiliary involvement[85]. Serum anticolon antibodies crossreacted with portal tracts, a reaction detected in 8 of 15 patients with PSC[85]. A colonic protein has been characterized which acts as an autoantigen that may initiate a specific IgG antibody response in ulcerative colitis[86]. Antibodies against a cross-reactive epitope on this protein which is shared by human colon and bile duct epithelia were present in sera of 5 of 8 patients with sclerosing cholangitis[87]. Sera from patients with other liver diseases, ulcerative colitis or healthy controls apparently failed to show a negative reaction in an inhibition immunoperoxidase assay indicative of antibody presence. Circulating immune complexes were detected by at least one of two different techniques in 80% (16/20) of the patients with PSC[88]. Levels by each assay were higher in sera from patients with PSC than in sera from patients with inflammatory bowel disease alone or healthy controls. In PSC, but not in control patients with other liver disease, there was a delayed clearance of radiolabelled immune complexes[89].

Primary sclerosing cholangitis and autoimmune chronic active hepatitis in childhood have many similarities. In both conditions there are increased levels of IgG and circulating non-organ specific autoantibodies, in particular antinuclear antibody and smooth muscle antibody[23]. A variety of regulatory and/or effector immune mechanisms, including liver-specific autoantibody production, number and function of suppressor T cells and T lymphocyte activation were studied in eight children with PSC and compared to the findings in 14 children with autoimmune chronic active hepatitis[90]. From these data it was suggested that liver-damaging mechanisms are similar in PSC and autoimmune chronic active hepatitis but the factors leading to autoimmunity probably differed. Autoimmunity in PSC could result from B lymphocyte activation bypassing T cells, whereas in autoimmune chronic active hepatitis autoimmunity presumably derives from defective T-dependent immune regulation. Different results concerning the helper/suppressor ratio are obtained from typing and enumeration of T lymphocytes in hepatic tissues from patients with PSC[91]. No suppressor cells were detected in and around bile ducts, whereas there was an increase in the number of these lymphocytes in the portal triads. The opposite was seen in biopsies from patients with primary biliary cirrhosis. Moreover, autoreactive suppressor T lymphocytes were reported to be increased in PSC[92], which is in contrast to the findings in a more recent study[90]. Anti-neutrophil nuclear antibodies were found in the serum of 84% of patients with primary sclerosing cholangitis as well as in 86% of patients with inflammatory bowel disease alone[93].

A close relationship was found between primary sclerosing cholangitis and the human leucocyte antigens, HLA-B8 and HLA-DR3[4,94–97], being closely associated with other organ-specific autoimmune diseases. HLA-B8 could be detected in 80% of patients with PSC and ulcerative colitis compared with 32% in inflammatory bowel disease without hepatobiliary involvement and 25% in controls[95]. The class II major histocompatibility complex (MHC) antigens (HLA-DR) are glycoproteins inserted into the cell membrane which play an important role in presenting antigens. An aberrant expression of HLA-DR antigens was always detected in primary sclerosing cholangitis at an early stage of histological liver damage[98]. However, a similar aberrant expression was found in patients with primary biliary cirrhosis and extrahepatic biliary obstruction.

Inhibition of leucocytes in response to biliary antigen[99] and an increased metabolism of complement C3[100] provide further support for the role of an abnormal immune regulation in PSC. The familial occurrence of both PSC and ulcerative colitis supports the hypothesis that genetic factors may play a role in the aetiology of primary sclerosing cholangitis[101]. In addition, a viral aetiology of the disease has been discussed[92].

Clinical features

The relative frequency of symptoms (reasons for referral) and clinical signs in 53 patients with PSC is given in Table 4 and Table 5, respectively[79]. Jaundice was one of the most common subjective symptoms in patients with PSC from other studies[15,26,81,83]. Symptomatic as compared to

Table 4 Reasons for referral (A) and symptoms (B) in primary sclerosing cholangitis ($n = 53$)[79]

(A)	*Percentage*	*(B)*	*Percentage*
Abnormal liver chemistry	32	Malaise, fatigue	64
Jaundice	30	Jaundice	51
Cholangitis (fever, jaundice, pain)	13	Abdominal pain	43
Abdominal pain (no cholangitis)	9	Weight loss	42
Pruritus	8	Fever	42
Fatigue	4	Pruritus	40
Fever	2	Nausea, vomiting	23
Ascites	1	Cholangitis	13

Table 5 Physical findings in primary sclerosing cholangitis[79]

Clinical signs	*Percentage*
Hepatomegaly	58
Jaundice	43
Splenomegaly	23
Spider telangiectasia	19
Palmar erythema	15
Ascites	11
Encephalopathy	8
Peripheral oedema	6
Muscular wasting	4
Dupuytren's contracture	2

asymptomatic patients more often presented with hepatomegaly, an elevated serum bilirubin (more than 1.5 mg/dl), and a liver biopsy specimen with bridging fibrosis or cirrhosis[79]. There was no difference in the prevalence of inflammatory bowel disease or in the cholangiographic pattern of bile duct involvement. A minority of patients will present with gross hepatic lobar atrophy at surgery[102].

Alkaline phosphatase is usually elevated in most patients with PSC, although 3% of reported cases present with a normal enzyme activity[79,103,104]. Normal values were measured even in patients who were either symptomatic or who presented with advanced hepatobiliary disease. Accordingly a normal alkaline phosphatase activity should not preclude further investigation for PSC in chronic inflammatory bowel disease when other symptoms or signs suggest liver disease. Cholestasis is further indicated by an elevated serum bilirubin in about 50% of patients with PSC[79]. Of these cases 92% had enhanced transaminase activities in blood serum[79] which may be the only symptom at routine blood donation in patients with PSC[105]. In serum, anti-mitochondrial antibodies are always absent[76,79]. In a few cases smooth muscle antibodies and antinuclear antibodies may be detected. Eosinophilia is a rare finding[106].

Patients with PSC reveal considerable abnormalities in tests of copper metabolism[15,72,107,108]. Histological examination of liver biopsy specimens demonstrated substantial amounts of copper pigment and copper-associated protein in 77% of patients[72]. Hepatic copper levels ranged from 38 to 700 μg/g liver dry weight[15,108] which are quite similar to those seen in Wilson's disease or primary biliary cirrhosis[107,108]. Elevated 24-h urinary copper levels were detected in 64%[107]. Serum caeruloplasmin was usually in the upper normal range associated with increased serum copper concentrations[107,108].

Radiological features

Confirmation of PSC in patients with chronic inflammatory bowel disease usually necessitates either retrograde or percutaneous transhepatic cholangiography. Intravenous cholangiography resulted in poor or no visualization[15]. The main diagnostic criteria involve generalized beading and irregular multifocal strictures of intra- and extrahepatic bile ducts in the absence of choledocholithiasis or a history of bile duct surgery[109–111] (Figures 7 and 8). Involvement of both intra- and extrahepatic bile ducts was a more frequent finding (94%) as compared to changes restricted to the extrahepatic duct (3%)[84]. Only 3% of these cases (n = 131) presented with intrahepatic duct involvement alone. However, contrary findings were reported from other studies which detected exclusive intrahepatic involvement in up to 30% of cases[4,81]. Intra- and extrahepatic duct abnormalities have been classified according to the extent of narrowing of bile ducts, severity of narrowing, contour abnormalities, and presence of poststenotic dilatation[110].

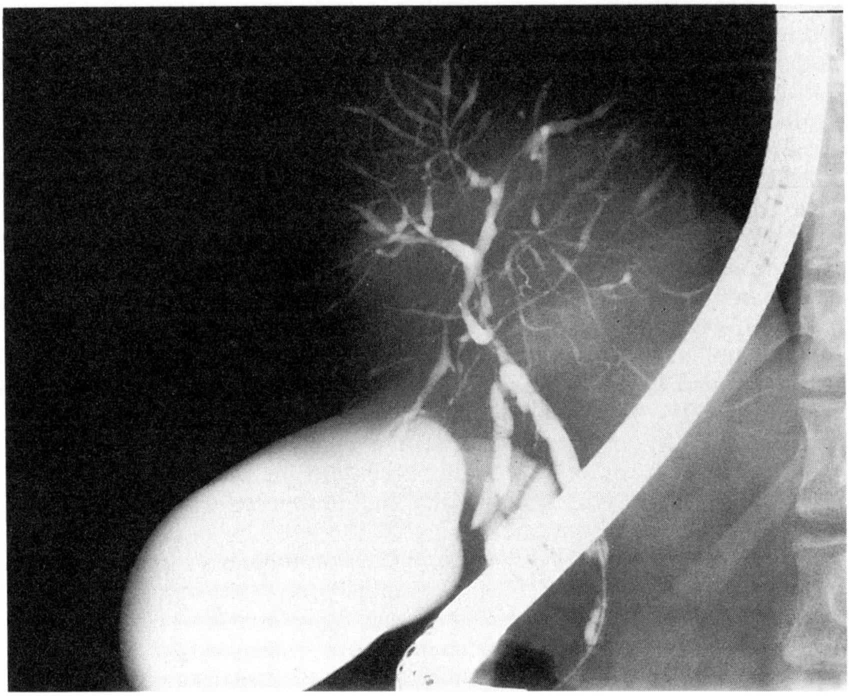

Figure 7 Cholangiographic appearance of the biliary tract in a patient with primary sclerosing cholangitis with multifocal stenoses of intra- and extrahepatic bile ducts

Prognosis

The natural history of patients with primary sclerosing cholangitis remains poorly defined. Ten-year survival was found to range from 55% to more than 80%[79–81,83,112] and even asymptomatic patients had a decreased survival as compared to a control population matched for age, race and sex[82,83]. In the latter study, independent high-risk factors of dying were age, serum bilirubin, haemoglobin, presence or absence of inflammatory bowel disease, and histological stage on liver biopsy. In addition, higher hepatic and urinary copper levels at initial evaluation were associated with decreased survival: patients with hepatic copper above 250 μg/g dry weight and urinary copper excretion above 200 μg/24 h had an 18-month survival of 60%[107]. A poor outcome can probably be predicted from a bilirubin value four times above the upper normal limit: 50% of these patients died within 2.5 years of the initial observation of this abnormal bilirubin value[80]. Asymptomatic presentation, the presence or absence of bowel disease, and age were not considered prognostically important[80]. In another series of patients a multivariate analysis of clinical features at disease onset demonstrated that hepatomegaly as well as serum bilirubin ($>$1.5 mg/dl) were independent discriminators of poor prognosis[80]. Age, the presence of cirrhosis or fibrous bridging on liver biopsy, presence or absence of bowel disease, and the

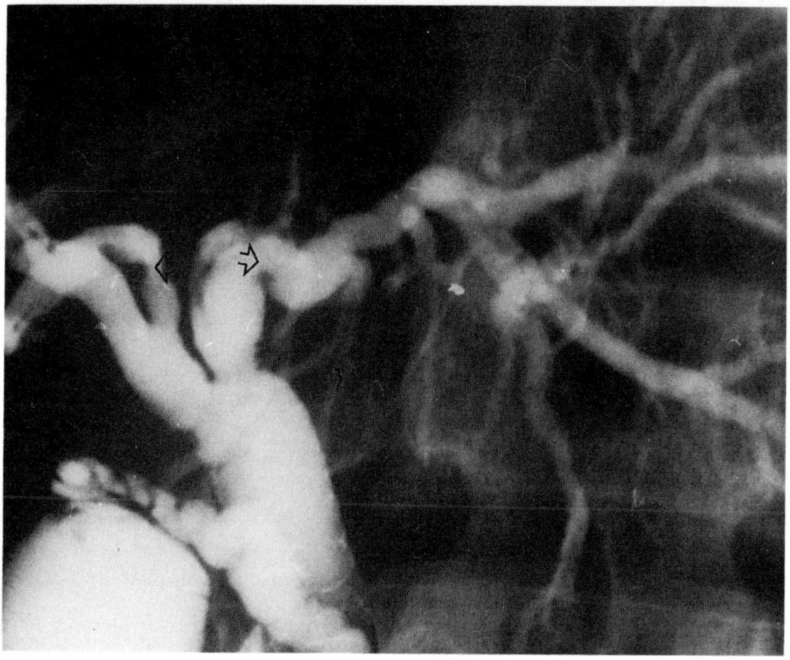

Figure 8 Endoscopic retrograde cholangiography reveals narrowing (arrows) and beading of intrahepatic bile ducts in a patient with primary sclerosing cholangitis

pattern of duct involvement did not correlate significantly with survival[29]. The latter finding was in contrast to a more recent study indicating that combined intra- and extrahepatic duct involvement was associated with a considerably worse prognosis[81]. Ten-year survival for intrahepatic duct disease was about 90% as compared to 50% for diffuse duct involvement (Table 6).

The course of primary sclerosing cholangitis is very variable. Some patients develop jaundice and liver failure and die within a few months, whereas others remain asymptomatic for many years. Prognostic factors may help in patient counselling and in selection and proper timing of liver transplantation in patients with end-stage liver disease. However, more studies are warranted to precisely define prognosis in individual patients.

Table 6 Discriminators of poor prognosis in primary sclerosing cholangitis

Prognostic sign	*Survival*	*Reference*
Hepatic copper > 250 μg/g dry weight		
Urinary copper > 200 μg/24 h	1.5 years: 60%	107
Serum bilirubin ⩾ 4 × normal	2.5 years: 50%	80
Intra- + extrahepatic duct involvement	10 years: 50%	81

Treatment

There are three different principal treatment modalities in primary sclerosing cholangitis: (1) drug treatment, (2) endoscopic or percutaneous interventions, and (3) surgical therapy. In spite of these treatment options, several questions remain to be answered. It remains to be defined more precisely at which time point the patient will benefit from treatment of primary sclerosing cholangitis and which therapy should be initiated.

Because of the cupruretic, antifibrogenic, and immunosuppressive effects of D-penicillamine, its therapeutic efficacy in primary sclerosing cholangitis was evaluated in a randomized, prospective, double-blind trial with 39 patients receiving penicillamine and 31 placebo[113]. Drug treatment was without any beneficial effect on disease progression or survival associated with considerable toxicity. Methotrexate treatment showed improvement in symptoms as well as biochemical and histological parameters in a total of seven patients with hepatobiliary disease[114,115]. Preliminary results from three different centres using ursodeoxycholic acid point to a dramatic improvement of clinical and biochemical parameters[116–118]. No side-effects were observed in a total of 32 patients including 20 with chronic inflammatory bowel disease, except for diarrhoea in two patients[118]. Clinical and enzymatic relapse was seen after withdrawal of ursodeoxycholic acid in five patients[116,117]. No change in the activity of inflammatory bowel disease was noted[116,118]. No data are available showing whether the biochemical and clinical improvement is accompanied by a histological amelioration. In addition, the future will tell whether there will be a prolonged survival of treated patients.

Corticosteroids presumably have no effect[15,72,83,119–123]. However, impressive improvements in bilirubin, alkaline phosphatase, and aspartate aminotransferase values were seen when steroids were administered in combination with colchicine[124,125]. The combination of colchicine with corticosteroids, and the use of cyclosporine or azathioprine cannot at present be sufficiently assessed due to lack of controlled trials, which are under way[92].

Endoscopic[126,127] or percutaneous transhepatic approaches[128–133] represent palliative treatments in primary sclerosing cholangitis which may be useful in postponing the date of liver transplantation. Endoscopic treatment includes balloon dilatation of strictures, placement of an endoprosthesis, or insertion of a nasobiliary tube with subsequent perfusion of bile ducts with steroids, antibiotics, or saline[119,122,127]. A topical application of steroids via an endoscopically placed nasobiliary tube was either not effective[119] or of minor benefit[122]. Some cases responded to this topical treatment with a re-established undisturbed bile flow[122,127], others were complicated by septicaemia[119,122].

Endoscopic treatment of strictures by balloon dilatation and/or placement of endoprostheses resulted in a decrease in serum bilirubin of approximately 80%[126,127]. Other biochemical parameters also improved. The success of endoscopic intervention persisted during a mean follow-up of 3.5 years[127]. The frequency of hospitalization was reduced in these patients. Moreover, the advantage of endoscopic over surgical intervention is in the consideration and acceptance of a patient for liver transplantation since prior surgery of the biliary tract may severely complicate the transplantation procedure[134,135]. A multicentre, randomized trial would be required to comment definitively on endoscopic procedures in primary sclerosing cholangitis[126].

Operative treatment for the severe ductal obstruction caused by primary sclerosing cholangitis includes choledochoenterostomy[136], intrahepatic cholangiojejunostomy[137], cholecystoenterostomy[138], transduodenal sphincterotomy, or intraoperative placement of biliary stents[139] with concurrent hepaticojejunostomy[140]. The surgical procedures may provide effective palliation in selected patients[136–140] with increasing survival but considerably enhancing the risk of a subsequent liver transplantation[135].

A prospective study in 45 patients with both primary sclerosing cholangitis and ulcerative colitis indicated that proctocolectomy did not influence biochemical alterations, clinical signs and symptoms, histological progression on liver biopsies, or the natural course of the hepatobiliary disease[13].

Orthotopic liver transplantation is the best treatment option in end-stage liver disease. Fifty-five consecutive liver replacements for primary sclerosing cholangitis resulted in 71% and 57% survival rates after 1 and 2 years, respectively[141]. The results from four other centres, however, indicated lower survival rates amounting to a survival probability of only 25% after 1 year[142]. Associated intestinal disease was usually minimally symptomatic after transplantation but colonoscopic findings never became totally normal[141]. Recently evidence has been presented for recurrence of the disease in the graft in a minority of patients[141,143]. Unrecognized cholangiocarcinoma was found in five of 55 transplanted patients (9.9%)[141], indicating that a prior aggressive diagnostic approach is necessary to exclude malignant disease in the liver of transplant candidates[144,145].

CIRRHOSIS

Cirrhosis is a common finding in 17–36% of patients with primary sclerosing cholangitis[72,76,79] and in 20% of patients with laboratory signs of a hepatic lesion and chronic inflammatory bowel disease[16,84]. The incidence of liver cirrhosis was lower in patients hospitalized for ulcerative colitis, amounting to 1%[16]. Others reported 2.5% and 1.5% cases of cirrhosis in 624 and 720 patients with ulcerative colitis, respectively[146,147]. Only 3 (0.6%) cases were found in 517 patients with Crohn's disease[148]. Conversely, 5% of 519 patients with liver cirrhosis suffered from ulcerative colitis[83]. Also in the absence of 'large-duct PSC', the cholangiographically identifiable PSC, patients with ulcerative colitis develop liver cirrhosis[75,77]. However, it cannot be excluded that some of the reported cases of liver cirrhosis reflect the end stage of 'small-duct PSC'[74a,75,77] indicating a progression from 'pericholangitis' to cirrhosis[95]. The cause and pathogenesis of cirrhosis in chronic inflammatory bowel disease remains obscure. Alcoholism and viral hepatitis are rarely present.

In patients with PSC with and without proctocolectomy, new onset of splenomegaly, oesophageal varices, and ascites did not differ, reflecting no effect of proctocolectomy on progression of liver disease and survival[13]. Accordingly no relationship appears to exist between the natural history of hepatobiliary disease and extent or duration of colonic involvement in ulcerative colitis[13]. Both the liver and the large bowel presumably represent different targets, resulting in different expressions of the same disease. In approximately half the patients with ulcerative colitis and PSC who undergo proctocolectomy and ileostomy, peristomal varices will develop and can result in serious and life-threatening bleeding[148].

Sixty per cent of the patients with PSC who died during a prolonged follow-up examination had cirrhosis, as compared to 30% of the living patients[15,72,79]. Late complications include portal hypertension and oesophageal varices[72,79,149]. Therapy follows established principles for the treatment of cirrhosis. When end-stage liver disease has developed, liver transplantation is a therapeutic option[141,150,151].

CHOLANGIOCARCINOMA

The prevalence of bile duct carcinoma is increased in patients with ulcerative colitis[152]. Six cases of cholangiocarcinoma were detected in 1207 patients with this disease, indicating a prevalence rate of 0.5% which was considerably higher compared to the general population with 0.0045%[153] to 0.0008%[154]. The relative risk of bile duct carcinoma was calculated to be 31.3[152,155]. In four patients with cholangiocarcinoma small-duct and large-duct PSC preexisted[152]. PSC must be regarded as a premalignant lesion since 13% of 60 patients[156] and 9.9% of 55 removed liver specimens[141] from transplanted patients with this disease revealed cholangiocarcinoma. Accordingly, causes of death in PSC often include bile duct carcinoma in addition to the more frequent liver failure[15,72,79,81]. The relationship between PSC and bile duct carcinoma associated with ulcerative colitis is not clear.

The mean age at diagnosis was lower with 38 years than in other patients with cholangiocarcinoma[152,157]. The mean interval between onset of ulcerative colitis and diagnosis of bile duct carcinoma was 23 years[152]. The bile duct carcinoma in ulcerative colitis is frequently preceded by a history of PSC[15,22,79,81,152,154–157], which is probably also a prerequisite for its development in Crohn's disease[62,156] (Figure 9).

Patients with cholangiocarcinoma usually present with painless progressive obstructive jaundice of relatively short duration[152]. Diagnosis may be difficult, because the symptoms of extrahepatic obstruction are the same as those of sclerosing cholangitis. ERC or percutaneous transhepatic cholangiography (PTC) will lead to the diagnosis of bile duct carcinoma when cholangiography reveals marked dilatation of bile ducts, an abrupt cutoff, or a localized stricture of the bile duct with irregular margin; the latter, however, will be less diagnostic in PSC. Occasionally, cholangiocarcinoma is an incidental finding in patients with PSC during liver transplantation. Mean survival is only 11–12 months, reflecting the extremely poor prognosis of this malignant disease[152]. The medical[152] and surgical[13] treatment of

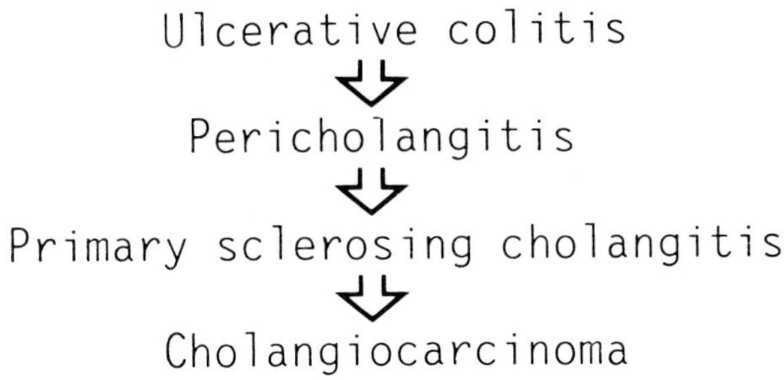

Figure 9 Ulcerative colitis and primary sclerosing cholangitis may lead to the development of cholangiocarcinoma: sequence of events

colitis presumably does not influence the development of bile duct carcinoma. A prophylactic cancer surveillance programme in patients with PSC and ulcerative colitis is hard to perform in the absence of a diagnostic tool sensitive enough to detect early biliary cancer development. Results of transplantation for bile duct cancers are discouraging since a survival beyond 2 years is extremely rare. An aggressive diagnostic protocol including surgical exploration may improve identification of possible candidates amenable to surgical palliation, resection, or transplantation[144,145]. Non-surgical biliary drainage procedures can be used for palliative treatment of patients with advanced biliary malignant disease[158].

References

1. Mayberry, J. F. (1985). Some aspects of the epidemiology of ulcerative colitis. *Gut*, **26**, 968–74
2. Brandes, J. W. and Lorenz-Meyer, H. (1983). Epidemiologische Aspekte zur Enterocolitis regionalis, Crohn and Colitis ulcerosa in Marburg/Lahn (FRG) zwischen 1962 und 1975. *Z. Gastroenterol.*, **21**, 69–78
3. Christophi, C. and Hughes, E. R. (1985). Hepatobiliary disorders in inflammatory bowel disease. *Surg. Gynecol. Obstet.*, **160**, 187–93
4. Shepherd, H. A., Selby, W. S., Chapman, R. W. G., Nolan, D., Barbatis, C., McGee, J.O'D and Jewell, D. P. (1983). Ulcerative colitis and persistent liver dysfunction. *Quart. J. Med.*, **52**, 503–13
5. Eade, M. N. (1970). Liver disease in ulcerative colitis. I. Analysis of operative liver biopsy in 138 consecutive patients having colectomy. *Ann. Intern. Med.*, **72**, 475–82
6. Eade, M. N., Cooke, W. T., Brooke, B. N. and Thompson, H. (1971). Liver disease in Crohn's colitis. *Ann. Intern. Med.*, **74**, 518–28
7. Schölmerich, J., Braun, G., Volk,, B. A., Spamer, C., Hoppe-Seyler, P. and Gerok, W. (1987). Detection of extraintestinal and intestinal abnormalities in inflammatory bowel disease by ultrasound. *Dig. Surg.*, **4**, 82–7
8. Dolz, C., Xiol, X., Abad, A., Cabré, E., Gonzaléz-Huix, F., Giné, J. J. and Gassull, M. A. (1989). Changes in liver function tests in patients with inflammatory bowel disease on

enteral nutrition. *J. Parent. Nutr.*, **13**, 401–5
9. Stricker, B. H. C. and Spoelstra, P. (1985). *Drug-induced Hepatic Injury*. (Amsterdam: Elsevier)
10. Bush, A., Mitchison, H., Walt, R., Baron, J. H., Boylston, A. W. and Summerfield, J. A. (1987). Primary biliary cirrhosis and ulcerative colitis. *Gastroenterology*, **92**, 2009–13
11. Kato, Y., Morimoto, H., Unoura, M., Kobayashi, K., Haltori, N. and Nakanuma, Y. (1985). Primary biliary cirrhosis and chronic pancreatitis in a patient with ulcerative colitis. *J. Clin. Gastroenterol.*, **7**, 425–7
12. Lindor, K. D., Wiesner, R. H., LaRusso, N. F. and Homburger, H. A. (1987). Enhanced autoreactivity of T-lymphocytes in primary sclerosing cholangitis. *Hepatology*, **7**, 884–8
13. Cangemi, J. R., Wiesner, R. H., Beaver, S. J., Ludwig, J., MacCarty, R. L., Dozois, R. R., Zinsmeister, A. R. and LaRusso, N. F. (1989). Effect of proctocolectomy for chronic ulcerative colitis on the natural history of primary sclerosing cholangitis. *Gastroenterology*, **96**, 790–4
14. Steckmann, M., Drossman, D. A. and Lesesne, H. R. (1984). Hepatobiliary disease that precedes ulcerative colitis. *J. Clin. Gastroenterol.*, **6**, 425–8
15. Wiesner, R. H. and LaRusso, N. F. (1980). Clinicopathologic features of the syndrome of primary sclerosing cholangitis. *Gastroenterology*, **79**, 200–6
16. Dordal, E., Glagov, S. and Kirsner, J. B. (1967). Hepatic lesions in chronic inflammatory bowel disease. *Gastroenterology*, **52**, 239–53
17. Lowdell, C. P., Shousha, S. and Parkins, R. A. (1986). The incidence of amyloidosis complicating inflammatory bowel disease: a prospective survey of 177 patients. *Dis. Col. Rect.*, **29**, 351–4
18. Edwards, P., Cooper, D. A., Turner, J., O'Connor, T. J. and Byrnes, D. J. (1988). Resolution of amyloidosis (AA type) complicating chronic ulcerative colitis. *Gastroenterology*, **95**, 810–15
19. Greenstein, A. J., Janowitz, H. D. and Sachar, D. B. (1976). The extra-intestinal complications of Crohn's disease and ulcerative colitis: a study of 700 patients. *Medicine* (*Baltimore*), **55**, 401–12
20. Shorvon, P. J. (1977). Amyloidosis and inflammatory bowel disease. *Am. J. Dig. Dis.*, **22**, 209–13
21. Fausa, O., Nygaard, K. and Elgjo, K. (1977). Amyloidosis and Crohn's disease. *Scand. J. Gastroenterol.*, **12**, 657–62
22. Lind, E., Fausa, O., Elgjo, K. and Gjone, E. (1985). Crohn's disease. Clinical manifestations. *Scand. J. Gastroenterol.*, **20**, 665–70
23. Benson, M. D. and Wallace, M. R. (1989). Amyloidosis. In Scriver, C. R., Beaudet, A. I., Sly, W. S. and Valle, B. (eds) *The Metabolic Basis of Inherited Disease*, 6th edn, Vol. II, 2439–60 (McGraw-Hill, New York)
24. Castell, J. V., Gómez-Lechón, M. J., David, M., Andus, T., Geiger, T., Trullenque, R., Fabra, R. and Heinrich, P. C. (1989). Interleukin-6 is the major regulator of acute phase protein synthesis in adult human hepatocytes. *FEBS Lett.*, **242**, 237–9
25. Ramadori, G., Sipe, J. D., Dinarello, C. A., Mizel, S. B. and Colten, H. R. (1985). Pretranslational modulation of acute phase hepatic protein synthesis by murine recombinant interleukin-1 and purified human IL-1. *J. Exp. Med.*, **162**, 930–42
26. Franklin, E. C. (1979). Some unsolved problems in the amyloid diseases. *Am. J. Med.*, **66**, 365–7
27. Lavie, G. *et al.* (1978). The degradation of serum amyloid A protein by peripheral blood monocytes. *J. Exp. Med.*, **148**, 1020
28. Kedar, I., Sohar, E. and Ravid, M. (1982). Degradation of amyloid by a serum component and inhibition of degradation. *J. Lab. clin. Med.*, **99**, 693–700
29. Kleckner, M. S. and Magidson, J. (1955). Amyloidosis of the liver: Correlation of clinical and pathologic features. *Gastroenterology*, **29**, 56–63
30. Levy, M., Polliack, A., Lender, M. and Eliakim, M. (1974). The liver in amyloidosis. *Digestion*, **10**, 40–51
31. Levine, R. A. (1962). Amyloid disease of liver: Correlation of clinical, functional and morphologic features in 47 patients. *Am. J. Med.*, **33**, 349
32. Brandt, K., Cathcart, S. and Cohen, A. S. (1968). A clinical analysis of the course of forty-two patients with amyloidosis. *Am. J. Med.*, **44**, 955–69

33. Yood, R. A., Skinner, M., Cohen, A. S. and Lee, V. W. (1981). Soft tissue uptake of bone seeking radionuclide in amyloidosis. *J. Rheumatol.*, **8**, 760–6
34. DeBeer, F. C., Mallya, R. K., Fagan, E. A., Lanham, J. G., Hughes, G. R. and Pepys, M. B. (1982). Serum amyloid-A protein concentration in inflammatory diseases and its relationship to incidence of reactive systemic amyloidosis. *Lancet*, **2**, 231–4
34a. Falck, H. M., Maury, C. P., Teppo, A. M. and Wegelius, O. (1983). Correlation of persistently high serum amyloid A protein and C-reactive protein concentrations with rapid progression of secondary amyloidosis. *Br. Med. J.*, **286**, 1391–3
35. Maury, C. P. and Teppo, A. M. (1982). Mechanisms of reduced amyloid-A degrading activity in serum of patients with secondary amyloidosis. *Lancet*, **2**, 234–7
36. Mir-Madjlessi, S. H., Brown, C. H. and Hawk, W. J. (1977). Amyloidosis associated with Crohn's disease. *Am. J. Gastroenterol.*, **58**, 563–77
37. Gries, E., Singer, M. V. and Goebell, H. (1989). Amyloidose bei Morbus Crohn. *Med. Klin.*, **84**, 65–71
38. Mir-Madjlessi, S. H., McHenry, M. C. and Farmer, R. G. (1986). Liver abscess in Crohn's disease. *Gastroenterology*, **91**, 987–93
38a. Greenstein, A. J., Sachar, D. B., Lowenthal, D., Goldofsky, E. and Aufses, A. H. (1985). Pyogenic liver abscess in Crohn's disease. *Quart. J. Med.*, **56**, 505–18
39. MacDonald, P. H. and Mercer, C. D. (1989). Hepatic abscess associated with subclinical ulcerative colitis. *Can. J. Gastroenterol.*, **3**, 123–5
40. Sparberg, M., Gottschalk, A. and Kirsner, J. B. (1965). Liver abscess complicating regional enteritis: report of two cases. *Gastroenterology*, **49**, 548–51
41. Weinberg, R. J., Klish, W. J., Brown, M. R., Smalley, J. R. and Emmens, R. W. (1983). Hepatic abscess as a complication of Crohn's disease. *J. Pediatr. Gastroenterol. Nutr.*, **2**, 171–4
42. Denison, H. and Wallersteldt, S. (1989). Diagnosis of pyogenic liver abscess via liver scanning with indium-111 labelled granulocytes. *Scand. J. Infect. Dis.*, **21**, 345–8
43. Kandel, G. and Marcon, N. E. (1984). Pyogenic liver abscess: new concepts of an old disease. *Am. J. Gastroenterol.*, **79**, 65–71
44. Reynolds, T. B. (1982). Medical treatment of pyogenic liver abscess. *Ann. Intern. Med.*, **96**, 373–4
45. Steinson, W. F., Eckert, T. and Avioli, L. A. (1983). Pyogenic liver abscess. *Arch. Intern. Med.*, **143**, 126–8
46. Eade, M. N. and Brooke, B. N. (1969). Portal bacteremiae in cases of ulcerative colitis submitted to colectomy. *Lancet*, **1**, 1008–9
46a. Brooke, B. N. and Slaney, G. (1958). Portal bacteremia in ulcerative colitis. *Lancet*, **1**, 1206–7
47. Herbert, D. A., Rothman, J., Simmons, F., Fogel, D. A., Wilson, S. and Ruskin, J. (1982). Pyogenic liver abscesses: successful non-surgical therapy. *Lancet*, **1**, 134–6
48. Mok, H. Y. I., Bergmann, K. and Grundy, S. M. (1977). Regulation of pool size of bile acids in man. *Gastroenterology*, **73**, 684–90
49. Andersson, H., Bosaeus, I., Fasth, S., Hellberg, R. and Hultén, L. (1987). Cholelithiasis and urolithiasis in Crohn's disease. *Scand. J. Gastroenterol.*, **22**, 253–6
50. Baker, A. L., Kaplan, M. M., Norton, R. A. and Patterson, J. F. (1975). Gallstones in inflammatory bowel disease. *Am. J. Dig. Dis.*, **19**, 109–12
51. Cohen, S., Kaplan, M., Gottlieb, L. and Patterson, J. (1971). Liver disease and gallstones in regional enteritis. *Gastroenterology*, **60**, 237–45
52. Dowling, R. H., Bell, G. D. and White, J. (1972). Lithogenic bile in patients with ileal dysfunction. *Gut*, **13**, 415–20
53. Heaton, K. W., Austad, W. I., Lack, L. and Tyor, M. P. (1968). Enterohepatic circulation of C^{14}-labeled bile salts in disorders of the distal small bowel. *Gastroenterology*, **55**, 5–16
54. Heaton, K. W. and Read, A. E. (1969). Gall stones in patients with disorders of the terminal ileum and disturbed bile salt metabolism. *Br. Med. J.*, **3**, 494–6
55. Marks, J. W., Conley, D. R., Capretta, T. L., Bonorris, G. G., Chung, A., Coyne, M. J. and Schoenfield, L. J. (1977). Gallstone prevalence and biliary lipid composition in inflammatory bowel disease. *Am. J. Dig. Dis.*, **22**, 1097–1100
56. Meihoff, W. E. and Kern, F. (1968). Bile salt malabsorption in regional ileitis, ileal resection, and mannitol-induced diarrhea. *J. Clin. Invest.*, **47**, 261–7

57. Pellerin, D., Bertin, P., Nihoul-Fekete, C. I. and Ricour, C. I. (1975). Cholelithiasis and ileal pathology in childhood. *J. Pediatr. Surg.*, **10**, 35–41
58. Maurer, P., Kuder, C., Schölmerich, J. and Gerok, W. (1989). Gallenblasenkontraktion nach Reizmahlzeit bei Patienten mit Morbus Crohn. (Abstr.) *Ultraschall Klin. Prax.*, Suppl. 1, 136
59. Barbara, L., Sama, C., Morselli Labate, A. M., Taroni, F., Rusticali, A. G., Festi, D., Sapio, C., Roda, E., Banterle, C., Puci, A., Formentini, F., Colasanti, S. and Naardin, F. (1987). A population study on the prevalence of gallstone disease: the Sirmione study. *Hepatology*, **7**, 913–17
60. Whorwell, P. J., Hawkins, R., Dewbury, K. and Wright, R. (1984). Ultrasound survey of gallstones and other hepatobiliary disorders in patients with Crohn's disease. *Dig. Dis. Sci.*, **29**, 930–3
61. Glambek, I., Kvaale, G., Arnesjø, B. and Søreide, O. (1987). Prevalence of gallstones in a Norwegian population. *Scand. J. Gastroenterol.*, **22**, 1089–94
62. Schrumpf, E., Fausa, O., Elgjo, K. and Kolmannskog, F. (1988). Hepatobiliary complications of inflammatory bowel disease. *Sem. Liver Dis.*, **8**, 201–9
63. Braunsdorf, A. and Heuchel, G. (1986). Granulomatöse Leberveränderungen bei Morbus Crohn. *Zentralbl. Allg. Pathol. Pathol. Anat.*, **132**, 37–40
64. Chapin, L. E., Scudamore, H. H., Baggenstoss, A. H. and Bargen, J. A. (1956). Regional enteritis: associated visceral changes. *Gastroenterology*, **30**, 404–15
65. Maurer, L., Hughes, R. W., Folley, J. H. and Mosenthal, W. T. (1967). Granulomatous hepatitis associated with regional enteritis. *Gastroenterology*, **53**, 301–5
66. Mörl, M. (1975). Hepatische Mitreaktionen bei Colitis ulcerosa und Morbus Crohn. *Med. Klin.*, **70**, 670–3
67. Warren, S. and Sommers, S. C. (1948). Cicatrizing enteritis (regional ileitis) as a pathologic entity. Analysis of 120 cases. *Am. J. Pathol.*, **24**, 475–501
68. Mistilis, S. P. (1965). Pericholangitis and ulcerative colitis. I. Pathology, etiology and pathogenesis. *Ann. Intern. Med.*, **63**, 17–26
69. Perrett, A. D., Higgins, G., Johnston, H. H., Massarella, G. R., Truelove, S. C. and Wright, R. (1971). The liver in Crohn's disease. *Quart. J. Med.*, **40**, 187–209
70. Perrett, A. D., Higgins, G., Johnston, H. H., Massarella, G. R., Truelove, S. C. and Wright, R. (1971). The liver in ulcerative colitis. *Quart. J. Med.*, **40**, 211–38
71. Lloyd-Still, J. D. and Cahan, J. (1987). Liver disease associated with childhood inflammatory bowel disease (IBD). (Abstr.) *Hepatology*, **7**, 1088
72. Chapman, R. W., Marborgh, B. Å., Rhodes, J. M., Summerfield, J. A., Dick, R., Scheuer, P. J. and Sherlock, S. (1980). Primary sclerosing cholangitis: a review of its clinical features, cholangiography, and hepatic histology. *Gut*, **21**, 870–7
73. El-Shabrawi, M., Wilkinson, M. L., Portmann, B., Mieli-Vergani, G., Chong, S. K. F., Williams, R. and Mowat, A. P. (1987). Primary sclerosing cholangitis in childhood. *Gastroenterology*, **92**, 1226–35
74. Ludwig, J. (1979). Some names hang on like leeches (editorial). *Dig. Dis. Sci.*, **24**, 967–9
74a. Wee, A. and Ludwig, J. (1985). Pericholangitis in chronic ulcerative colitis: primary sclerosing cholangitis of the small bile ducts? *Ann. Intern. Med.*, **102**, 581–7
75. Schrumpf, E. and Gjone, E. (1982). Hepatobiliary disease in ulcerative colitis. *Scand. J. Gastroenterol.*, **17**, 961–4
76. Stockbrügger, R. W., Olsson, R., Jaup, B. and Jensen, J. (1988). Forty-six patients with primary sclerosing cholangitis: radiological bile duct changes in relationship to clinical course and concomitant inflammatory bowel disease. *Hepato-gastroenterology*, **35**, 289–94
77. Ludwig, J., Barham, S. S., LaRusso, N. F., Elveback, L. R., Wiesner, R. H. and McCall, J. T. (1981). Morphologic features of chronic hepatitis associated with primary sclerosing cholangitis and chronic ulcerative colitis. *Hepatology*, **1**, 632–40
78. Leevy, C. M., Popper, H. and Sherlock, S. (1976). Diseases of the liver and biliary tract: standardization of nomenclature, diagnostic criteria, and diagnostic methodology. *Fogarty Int. Center Proc.*, **22**, 1–212
79. Helzberg, J. H., Petersen, J. M. and Boyer, J. L. (1987). Improved survival with primary sclerosing cholangitis. A review of clinicopathologic features and comparison of symptomatic and asymptomatic patients. *Gastroenterology*, **92**, 1869–75

78. Leevy, C. M., Popper, H. and Sherlock, S. (1976). Diseases of the liver and biliary tract: standardization of nomenclature, diagnostic criteria, and diagnostic methodology. *Fogarty Int. Center Proc.*, **22**, 1–212
79. Helzberg, J. H., Petersen, J. M. and Boyer, J. L. (1987). Improved survival with primary sclerosing cholangitis. A review of clinicopathologic features and comparison of symptomatic and asymptomatic patients. *Gastroenterology*, **92**, 1869–75
80. Lebovics, E., Palmer, M., Woo, J. and Schaffner, F. (1987). Outcome of primary sclerosing cholangitis. *Arch. Intern. Med.*, **147**, 729–31
81. Herrmann, R., Dooley, J. S., Sherlock, S. and McIntyre, N. (1988). Natural history and mortality in primary sclerosing cholangitis. (Abstr.) *Gut*, **29**, A1430
82. Hunter, E. B., Wiesner, R. H., LaRusso, N. F., Dickson, E. R. and Grambsch, P. B. (1989). Primary sclerosing cholangitis: Natural history, prognostic factors, and survival analysis. (Abstr.) *Gastroenterology*, **96**, A111
83. Schrumpf, E., Elgjo, K., Fausa, O., Gjone, E., Kolmannskog, F. and Ritland, S. (1980). Sclerosing cholangitis in ulcerative colitis. *Scand. J. Gastroenterol.*, **15**, 689–97
84. Wiesner, R. H., Grambsch, P. M., Dickson, E. R., Ludwig, J., MacCarty, R. L., Hunter, E. B., Fleming, T. R., Fisher, L. D., Beaver, S. J. and LaRusso, N. F. (1989). Primary sclerosing cholangitis: natural history, prognostic factors and survival analysis. *Hepatology*, **10**, 430–6
85. Chapman, R. W., Cottone, M., Selby, W. S., Shepherd, H. A., Sherlock, S. and Jewell, D. P. (1986). Serum autoantibodies, ulcerative colitis and primary sclerosing cholangitis. *Gut*, **27**, 86–91
86. Takahashi, F. and Das, K. M. (1985). Isolation and characterization of a colonic autoantigen specifically recognized by colon tissue-bound immunoglobulin G from idiopathic ulcerative colitis. *J. Clin. Invest.*, **76**, 311–18
87. Das, K. M., Jeffers, L., Squillante, L., Hyder, S., Reddy, R. and Schiff, E. (1989). The presence of circulating antibodies in patients with sclerosing cholangitis against an epitope(s) on MR 40,000 protein shared by colon and bile duct epithelial cells. (Abstr.). *Gastroenterology*, **96**, A590
88. Bodenheimer, H. C., LaRusso, N. F., Thayer, W. R., Charland, C., Staples, P. J. and Ludwig, J. (1983). Elevated circulating immune complexes in primary sclerosing cholangitis. *Hepatology*, **3**, 150–4
89. Minuk, G. Y., Angus, M., Brickman, C. M., Lawley, T. J., Frank, M. M., Hoofnagle, J. H. and Jones, E. A. (1988). Abnormal clearance of immune complexes from the circulation of patients with primary sclerosing cholangitis. *Gastroenterology*, **88**, 166–70
90. Mieli-Vergani, G., Lobo-Yeo, A., McFarlane, B. M., McFarlane, I. G., Mowat, A. P. and Vergani, D. (1989). Different immune mechanisms leading to autoimmunity in primary sclerosing cholangitis and autoimmune chronic active hepatitis of childhood. *Hepatology*, **9**, 198–203
91. Si, L., Whiteside, T. L., Schade, R. R., Starzl, T. E. and van Thiel, D. H. (1984). T-lymphocyte subsets in liver tissues of patients with primary biliary cirrhosis (PBC), patients with primary sclerosing cholangitis (PSC), and normal controls. *J. Clin. Immunol.*, **4**, 262–72
92. Lindor, K. D., Wiesner, R. H. and LaRusso, N. F. (1987). Recent advances in the management of primary sclerosing cholangitis. *Sem. Liver Dis.*, **7**, 322–7
93. Snook, J. A., Chapman, R. W., Fleming, K. and Jewell, D. P. (1989). Anti-neutrophil nuclear antibody in ulcerative colitis, Crohn's disease and primary sclerosing cholangitis. *Clin. Exp. Immunol.*, **76**, 30–3
94. Chapman, R. W., Varghese, Z., Gaul, R., Kokkinson, N. and Sherlock, S. (1983). Association of primary sclerosing cholangitis with HLA-B8. *Gut*, **24**, 38–41
95. Hopf, U., Riecken, E.-O., Zeitz, M., Eckhardt, R., Lobeck, H., Malchus, R. and Möller, B. (1983). Immunologische Parameter bei Pericholangitis und primär sklerosierender Cholangitis mit und ohne Colitis ulcerosa. *Dtsch. Med. Wochenschr.*, **108**, 1515–21
96. Schrumpf, E., Fausa, O., Førre, Ø., Dobloug, J. H., Ritland, S. and Thorsby, E. (1982). HLA-antigens and immunoregulatory T-cells in ulcerative colitis associated with hepatobiliary disease. *Scand. J. Gastroenterol.*, **17**, 187–91
97. Schrumpf, E., Fausa, O., Kolmannskog, F., Elgjo, K., Ritland, S. and Gjone, E. (1982). Sclerosing cholangitis in ulcerative colitis. *Scand. J. Gastroenterol.*, **17**, 33–9

98. Chapman, R. W., Kelly, P. M. A., Heryet, A., Jewell, D. P. and Fleming, K. A. (1988). Expression of HLA-DR antigens on bile duct epithelium in primary sclerosing cholangitis. *Gut*, **29**, 422–7
99. McFarlane, J. G., Woicicka, B. M., Tsantoolas, D. C., Portmann, B. G., Eddleston, A. L. W. F. and Williams, R. (1979). Leukocyte migration inhibition in response to biliary antigens in primary biliary cirrhosis, sclerosing cholangitis, and other chronic liver diseases. *Gastroenterology*, **76**, 1333–40
100. Brinch, L., Teisberg, P., Schrumpf, E. and Åkesson, I. (1982). The in vivo metabolism of C3 in hepatobiliary disease associated with ulcerative colitis. *Scand. J. Gastroenterol.*, **17**, 523–7
101. Quigley, E. M. M., LaRusso, N. F., Ludwig, J., MacSween, R. N. M., Birnie, G. G. and Watkinson, G. (1983). Familial occurrence of primary sclerosing cholangitis and ulcerative colitis. *Gastroenterology*, **85**, 1160–5
102. Hadjis, N. S., Adam, A., Blenkharn, I., Hatzis, G., Benjamin, I. S. and Blumgart, L. H. (1989). Primary sclerosing cholangitis associated with liver atrophy. *Am. J. Surg.*, **158**, 43–7
103. Balasubramaniam, K., Wiesner, R. H. and LaRusso, N. F. (1988). Primary sclerosing cholangitis with normal serum alkaline phosphatase activity. *Gastroenterology*, **95**, 1395–8
104. Cooper, J. F. and Brand, E. B. (1988). Symptomatic sclerosing cholangitis in patients with a normal alkaline phosphatase: two case reports and a review of the literature. *Am. J. Gastroenterol.*, **83**, 308–11
105. Keeffe, E. B. (1989). Diagnosis of primary sclerosing cholangitis in a blood donor with elevated serum alanine aminotransferase. *Gastroenterology*, **96**, 1358–9
106. Balzer, K., Hotz, J. and Goebell, G. (1980). Eosinophilie als Leitsymptom der primär sklerosierenden Cholangitis. *Z. Gastroenterol.*, **18**, 89–93
107. Gross, J. B., Ludwig, J., Wiesner, R. H., McCall, J. T. and LaRusso, N. F. (1985). Abnormalities in tests of copper metabolism in primary sclerosing cholangitis. *Gastroenterology*, **89**, 272–8
108. Wiesner, R. H., LaRusso, N. F., Ludwig, J. and Dickson, E. R. (1985). Comparison of the clinicopathologic features of primary biliary cirrhosis. *Gastroenterology*, **88**, 108–14
109. Cameron, J. L., Gayler, B. W., Sanfey, H., Milligan, F., Kaufman, S., Maddrey, W. C. and Herlong, F. (1984). Sclerosing cholangitis. Anatomical distribution of obstructive lesions. *Ann. Surg.*, **200**, 54–60
110. Li-Yeng, C. and Goldberg, H. I. (1984). Sclerosing cholangitis: broad spectrum of radiographic features. *Gastrointest. Radiol.*, **9**, 39–47
111. McCarty, R. L., LaRusso, N. F., Wiesner, R. H., and Ludwig, J. (1983). Primary sclerosing cholangitis: findings on cholangiography and pancreatography. *Radiology*, **149**, 39–44
112. Aadland, E., Schrumpf, E., Fausa, O., Elgjo, K., Heilo, A., Aakhus, T. and Gjone, E. (1987). Primary sclerosing cholangitis: a long-term follow-up study. *Scand. J. Gastroenterol.*, **22**, 655–64
113. LaRusso, N. F., Wiesner, R. H., Ludwig, J., MacCarty, R. L. and Beaver, S. J. (1988). Prospective trial of penicillamine in primary sclerosing cholangitis. *Gastroenterology*, **95**, 1036–42
114. Kaplan, M. M., Arora, S. and Pincus, S. H. (1987). Primary sclerosing cholangitis and low-dose oral pulse methotrexate therapy. *Ann. Intern. Med.*, **106**, 231–5
115. Knox, T. A. and Kaplan, M. M. (1989). Methotrexate treatment of primary sclerosing cholangitis. (Abstr.) *Gastroenterology*, **96**, A614
116. Chazouillères, O., Poupon, R., Capron, J. P., Metman, E. H., Dhumeaux, D., Amourelli, M., Couzlgou, P., Labayle, D. and Trinchet, J. C. (1989). Is ursodeoxycholic acid an effective treatment for primary sclerosing cholangitis? (Abstr.) *Gastroenterology*, **96**, A583
117. O'Brien, C., Senior, J. R., Batta, A. K., Arora, R., Tint, G. S. and Salen, G. (1989). Ursodeoxycholic acid treatment produces marked clinical and biochemical amelioration of primary sclerosing cholangitis. (Abstr.) *Gastroenterology*, **96**, A640
118. Stiehl, A., Raedsch, R., Rudolph, G., Galle, P. and Theilmann, L. (1989). Ursodesoxycholsäure (Urso) in der Behandlung der primär sklerosierenden Cholangitis (PSC). (Abstr.) *Z. Gastroenterol.*, **9**, 527
119. Allison, M. C., Burroughs, A. K., Noone, P. and Summerfield, J. A. (1986). Biliary lavage with corticosteroids in primary sclerosing cholangitis. A clinical, cholangiographic and bacteriological study. *J. Hepatol.*, **3**, 118–22

120. Brown, B. P., LaBrecque, D. R. and Anuras, S. (1981). Response of sclerosing cholangitis (SC) to long-term steroid therapy. (Abstr.) *Gastroenterology*, **80**, 1117
121. Burgert, S. L., Brown, B. P., Kirkpatrick, R. B. and LaBrecque, D. R. (1984). Positive corticosteroid response in early primary sclerosing cholangitis. (Abstr.) *Gastroenterology*, **86**, 1037
122. Grijm, R., Huibregtse, K., Bartelsman, J., Mathus-Vliegen, E. M. H., Dekker, W. and Tytgat, G. N. (1986). Therapeutic investigations in primary sclerosing cholangitis. *Dig. Dis. Sci.*, **31**, 792–8
123. Myers, R. N., Cooper, J. H. and Padis, N. (1970). Primary sclerosing cholangitis. Complete gross and histologic reversal after long-term steroid therapy. *Am. J. Gastroenterol.*, **53**, 527–38
124. LaRusso, N. F., Wiesner R. H. and Beaver, S. J. (1987). Combined antifibrogenic and immunosuppressive therapy in primary sclerosing cholangitis. (Abstr.) *Gastroenterology*, **92**, 1493
125. Leiser, A. and Kadish, U. (1986). Beneficial effect of colchicine in a case of sclerosing cholangitis. *Am. J. Med. Sci.*, **291**, 416–18
126. Johnson, G. K., Geenen, J. E., Venu, R. P. and Hogan, W. J. (1987). Endoscopic treatment of biliary duct strictures in sclerosing cholangitis: follow-up assessment of a new therapeutic approach. *Gastrointest. Endosc.*, **33**, 9–12
127. Siegel, J. H. (1989). Endoscopic management of benign biliary strictures, biliary tract fistulae, and sclerosing cholangitis. In Jacobson, I. M. (ed.), *ERCP, Diagnostic and Therapeutic Applications*, pp. 171–88. (New York, Amsterdam, London: Elsevier)
128. Martin, E. C., Fankuchen, E. I., Schultz, R. W. and Casarella, W. J. (1981). Percutaneous dilation in primary sclerosing cholangitis: two experiences. *Am. J. Radiol.*, **137**, 603–5
129. McLean, G. K., Ring, E. J. and Freiman, D. B. (1982). Therapeutic alternatives in the treatment of intrahepatic biliary obstruction. *Diagn. Radiol.*, **145**, 289–95
130. Molnar, W. and Stockum, A. E. (1974). Relief of obstructive jaundice through percutaneous transhepatic catheter – a new therapeutic method. *Am. J. Radiol.*, **122**, 356–67
131. Solkin, M. D., Alspaugh, J. P., Casarella, W. J., Chuang, V. P. and Galambos, J. T. (1989). Sclerosing cholangitis: palliation with percutaneous cholangioplasty. *Radiology*, **170**, 199–206
132. Vogel, S. B., Howard, R. J., Caridi, J. and Hawkins, J. F., Jr. (1985). Evaluation of percutaneous transhepatic balloon dilation of benign biliary strictures in high risk patients. *Am. J. Surg.*, **149**, 73–9
133. Wood, R. A. and Cuschieri, A. (1980). Is sclerosing cholangitis complicating ulcerative colitis a reversible condition? *Lancet*, **2**, 716–18
134. LaRusso, N. F., Wiesner, R. H., Ludwig, J. and MacCarty, R. L. (1984). Primary sclerosing cholangitis. *N. Engl. J. Med.*, **310**, 899–903
135. Starzl, T. E., Demetris, A. J. and van Thiel, D. (1989). Liver transplantation. (First of two parts). *N. Engl. J. Med.*, **321**, 1014–22
136. Pitt, H. A., Thompson, H. H., Tompkins, R. K. and Longmire, W. P., Jr. (1982). Primary sclerosing cholangitis: results of an aggressive approach. *Ann. Surg.*, **196**, 259–68
137. Goldenring, J. R. and Cahow, C. E. (1989). Intrahepatic cholangiojejunostomy as a palliative procedure in primary sclerosing cholangitis. *Arch. Surg.*, **124**, 565–7
138. Miller, R. T. (1927). Benign stricture of the bile ducts. *Ann. Surg.*, **86**, 296–303
139. Cameron, J. L., Gayler, B. W., Herlong, H. F. and Maddrey, W. C. (1983). Sclerosing cholangitis: biliary reconstruction with Silastic transhepatic stents. *Surgery*, **94**, 324–30
140. Krige, J. E. J., Terblanche, J., Harries-Jones, E. P. and Bornman, P. C. (1987). Primary sclerosing cholangitis: biliary drainage and duct dilatation. *Br. J. Surg.*, **74**, 54–7
141. Marsh, J. W., Iwatsuki, S., Makowka, L., Esquivel, C. O., Gordon, R. D., Todo, S., Tzakis, A., Miller, C., van Thiel, D. and Starzl, T. E. (1988). Orthotopic liver transplantation of primary sclerosing cholangitis. *Ann. Surg.*, **207**, 21–5
142. Scharschmidt, B. F. (1984). Human liver transplantation: analysis of data on 540 patients from four centers. *Hepatology*, **4** (Suppl. 1), 95S–101S
143. Hunter, E. B., Wiesner, R. H., MacCarty, R. L., LaRusso, N. F., Porayko, M. K., Eid, A. and Krom, R. A. F. (1989). Does primary sclerosing cholangitis recur after liver transplantation? (Abstr.) *Gastroenterology*, **96**, A610
144. Pichlmayr, R. (1988). Is there a place for liver grafting for malignancy? *Transplant. Proc.*,

20 (Suppl. 1), 478–82
145. Pichlmayr, R., Ringe, B., Lauchart, W. and Bechstein, W. O. (1988). Radical resection and liver grafting as the two main components of surgical strategy in the treatment of proximal bile duct cancer. *World J. Surg.*, **12**, 68–77
146. Dew, M. J., Thompson, H. and Allain, R. A. (1979). The spectrum of hepatic dysfunction in inflammatory bowel disease. *Quart. J. Med.*, **48**, 113–21
147. Edwards, F. C. and Truelove, S. C. (1964). The course and prognosis of ulcerative colitis: III. Complications. *Gut*, **5**, 1–4
148. Wiesner, R. H., LaRusso, N. F., Dozois, R. R. and Beaver, S. J. (1986). Peristomal varices after proctocolectomy in patients with primary sclerosing cholangitis. *Gastroenterology*, **90**, 316–22
149. Cameron, A. D. and Fone, D. J. (1970). Portal hypertension and bleeding varices after colectomy and bleeding varices after colectomy and ileostomy for chronic ulcerative colitis. *Gut*, **11**, 755–7
150. Jenkins, R. L. and Fairchild, R. B. (1989). The role of transplantation in liver disease. *Surg. Clin. N. Am.*, **69**, 371–82
151. Vierling, J. M. (1984). Epidemiology and clinical course of liver diseases: identification of candidates for hepatic transplantation. *Hepatology*, **4** (Suppl. 1), 84S–94S
152. Mir-Madjlessi, S. H., Farmer, R. G. and Sivak, M. V. (1987). Bile duct carcinoma in patients with ulcerative colitis. *Dig. Dis. Sci.*, **32**, 145–54
153. Ritchie, J. K., Allan, R. N., Macartney, J., Thompson, H., Hawley, P. R. and Cooke, W. T. (1974). Biliary tract carcinoma associated wtih ulcerative colitis. *Quart. J. Med.*, **43**, 263–79
154. Roberts-Thompson, I. C., Strickland, R. G. and Mackay, I. B. (1973). Bile duct carcinoma in chronic ulcerative colitis. *Aust. NZ J. Med.*, **3**, 264–7
155. Prior, P., Gyde, S. N., Macartney, J. C., Thompson, H., Waterhouse, J. A. H. and Allan, R. N. (1982). Cancer morbidity in ulcerative colitis. *Gut*, **23**, 490–7
156. Schrumpf, E. and Fausa, O. (1989). The frequency of cholangiocarcinoma (CC) in primary sclerosing cholangitis (PSC). (Abstr.) *J. Hepatol.*, **9** (Suppl. 1), S83
157. Converse, C. F., Reagan, J. W. and De Cosse, J. J. (1971). Ulcerative colitis and carcinoma of the bile ducts. *Am. J. Surg.*, **121**, 39–45
158. Classen, M., Geenen, J. and Kawai, J. (1984). *Nonsurgical Biliary Drainage*. (Springer-Verlag, Berlin, Heidelberg, New York, Tokyo)

Section III: The Liver in Protozoal and Parasitic Infections

13
Amoebic abscess of the liver

J. P. ACKERS

Entamoeba histolytica is in many ways a typical amoeba – a single-celled protozoan organism which moves and ingests food with the aid of pseudopodia. As is usual amongst parasitologists we refer to the motile, feeding, reproducing stage as the trophozoite, and the resistant and metabolically quiescent stage as the cyst. A typical trophozoite (Figure 1) has a single nucleus and actively extends pseudopodia; the typical size range is 10–30 μm. The newly formed cyst is also uninucleate but the mature infective cyst

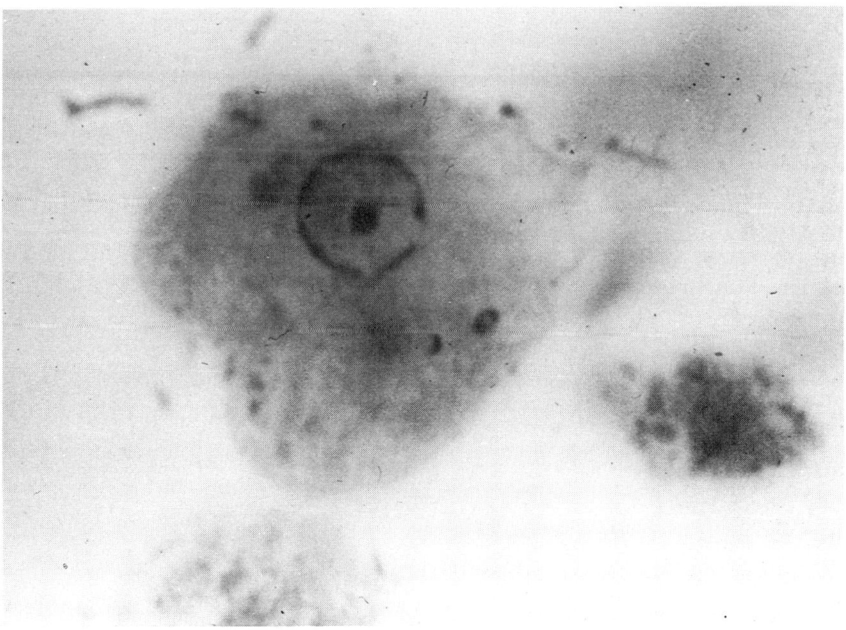

Figure 1 Trophozoite of *Entamoeba histolytica* showing nuclear morphology and pseudopodia (× 2550)

usually has four smaller nuclei and chromidial bars – ribosomal aggregates revealed only by certain stains and of unknown function. Cysts are normally spherical and 10–15 μm in diameter (Figure 2). The life cycle is simple and begins by the ingestion of the cyst which passes unscathed through the acidic contents of the stomach and excysts in the small intestine. A rapid division yields eight small amoebas, which pass into the large bowel where they feed and divide. Unknown stimuli cause certain members of the population to round up, expel ingested material and form a resistant coat. Two cycles of nuclear division produce the mature, infective quadrinucleate cyst.

It is always assumed (probably correctly) that only the cyst can survive exposure to gastric acidity, and that trophozoites play no part in the transmission of *E. histolytica*, but it is not known whether cysts need to be exposed to low pH to trigger excystation (as seems to be the case with *Giardia lamblia*[1]). The shed cyst is resistant to oxygen (and to the normal concentrations of halogens used for water purification[2]) and can survive for months if kept moist, but is rapidly killed by heat (probably 65 °C is sufficient) and drying.

Human infections with *E. histolytica* are amongst the commonest of those detected, with at least 500 million new cases every year[3]. The vast majority of these are, however, wholly asymptomatic and are only detected by the finding of cysts in their faeces. They are therefore frequently referred to as 'asymptomatic cyst-passers' and this is the term which I shall use here. It is important to note, however, that the approved World Health Organization

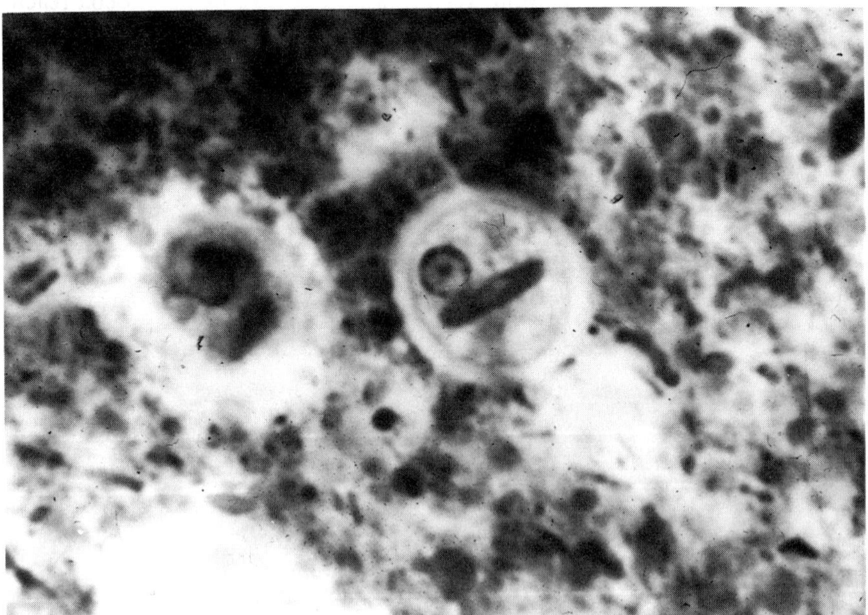

Figure 2 Cyst of *Entamoeba histolytica* showing one nucleus (of four; the others are out of focus) and a chromidial bar (× 2550)

definition of amoebiasis refers simply to the presence of infection with *E. histolytica*[4], and that symptoms need not be present to satisfy it. All asymptomatic cyst-passers therefore count as cases of amoebiasis; they seem to remain infected for weeks or months before spontaneously losing the parasite. It appears that totally non-invasive infections do not induce any serum antibody response.

There are several other large-bowel protozoa which lead equally harmless lives and which are in fact much more common than *E. histolytica* – *Entamoeba coli* and *Endolimax nana* are reported many times more often in routine stools surveys than is *E. histolytica.* Their only medical importance, however, appears to be their correct differentiation from *E. histolytica*, and the reason for this, of course, is that on occasions *E. histolytica* can and does disseminate outside the colon, producing severe and sometimes fatal cases of invasive amoebiasis. Classically, invasive amoebiasis consists of invasive intestinal disease ('amoebic dysentery') and hepatic amoebiasis ('amoebic liver abscess'), although dissemination to other sites (for example the brain or the skin) also occurs. Dissemination is not a frequent occurrence – reliable figures are simply not available, but it is estimated that there are 1–2 million cases of invasive amoebiasis, causing at least 40 000 deaths, world-wide each year[3]. Intestinal disease is possibly ten times more common than hepatic, while hepatic disease is by far the most common extraintestinal manifestation. The reason *why* invasion may occur will be discussed later, after the clinical aspects of hepatic amoebiasis have been briefly described.

It is assumed that *E. histolytica* always reaches the liver from the intestine by way of the portal circulation. We do not know how often amoeba reach the liver but are unable to establish themselves, or how many small abscesses develop and resolve spontaneously without causing any symptoms or being detected, but both events may be quite frequent. On the other hand, many lesions enlarge relentlessly. Although described as an 'abscess' containing 'pus', in fact, in the absence of secondary bacterial infection, the host's cellular response is modest, and no granuloma forms. Trophozoites of *E. histolytica* possess a formidable array of mechanisms for lysing target cells[5], and the sterile, odourless fluid contents of an hepatic abscess consist largely of the remains of liquefied hepatocytes – hence the specific name '*histolytica*'. Trophozoites are rarely found within the body of the abscess, but are largely confined to the margins where they are busy destroying fresh tissue.

Clinically, the commonest symptoms of amoebic liver abscess are pain (usually in the right upper quadrant, since right-side lesions are many times more common than left), fever and weight loss[6]. On examination, 80% will have extreme tenderness and about half hepatomegaly; dullness and rales at the right base of the lung are common. Eighty-five per cent of acutely ill patients (those with symptoms for less than 10 days) had fever and abdominal pain, while with more chronic cases (2–12 weeks of symptoms) the proportion with fever and pain fell to one-third, but two-thirds had hepatomegaly and weight loss[6]. Although hepatic amoebiasis can occur at any age it is most common in young adults; the sex ratio is also very unequal, with cases in males outnumbering those in females by up to seven to one[7]. Most, but not all, authors claim the sex ratio in *intestinal* invasive amoebiasis is approximately equal. The greatly enhanced incidence in males seems to be due to more than greater exposure to the risk of infection; higher iron and alcohol intake have been suggested as possible causes, but the true reason is not known.

The diagnosis is usually made by a combination of clinical signs and symptoms (which are fairly characteristic), imaging techniques, and serology.

The various imaging techniques now in use have recently been the subject of a comprehensive and well-illustrated review[8], which should be consulted for further details. Plain X-ray films of the chest are not diagnostic, but usually show smooth elevation of the right hemi-diaphragm; abdominal films are less often positive, but may show liver enlargement. More modern imaging techniques can actually detect and characterize hepatic parenchymal lesions. The first method to be employed involved scintiscans after administration of ^{99}Tc-labelled colloids. Hepatic amoebic abscesses show up as regions of reduced isotope uptake; unfortunately using this technique they cannot be distinguished from pyogenic or echinococcal abscesses or tumours. The method is, however, very sensitive and can find early lesions before they are detectable by other imaging techniques. Computerized tomography (CT) is very efficient in assessing the size of hepatic and abdominal abscesses; amoebic abscesses typically appear as well-defined, rounded low-density lesions. Because of its relatively low cost and completely non-invasive nature, diagnostic sonography was soon tested; the method proved to be both sensitive and specific, and using grey-scale techniques five image characteristics have been established[8]: (1) round or oval shape; (2) no significant wall echoes; (3) lower-than-normal echo intensity within the lesion, with faint homogeneous echoes seen on high gain; (4) peripheral location, contiguous to the liver capsule and (5) enhancement of echoes behind the lesion, due to increased through transmission.

One-third of hepatic amoebic abscesses show all five of these characteristics, and 90% at least three[8]. Particularly consistent features are peripheral location (found in 97%), distal sonic enhancement (93%) and round or oval shape (82%). Nearly 10% show some bizarre and uncharacteristic features. At present a combination of lowest cost (particularly important in the developing countries where amoebiasis is common), high diagnostic accuracy and non-invasiveness make sonography the imaging technique of choice for diagnosing hepatic amoebiasis.

Finally, antibody test results are strongly positive in almost 100% of well-developed amoebic abscesses[9], and are of considerable value in making the diagnosis. Recent work in San Diego, where travellers from Mexico have been examined by CT scanning very early in their illness have, however, shown that patients with very small abscesses may be seronegative[10], although virtually all ultimately convert.

It is important to note that, although all cases of hepatic amoebiasis must presumably have begun with an intestinal infection, trophozoites or cysts are demonstrable in the faeces in only about one-third of cases. It is generally agreed also that at least half of amoebic liver abscess patients will not be able to recall an attack of dysentery, although one report claims that such a history can eventually be obtained from a large proportion of patients[11].

With early diagnosis and effective therapy, the mortality from uncomplicated amoebiasis is less than 1%. Untreated, however, many lesions continue relentlessly to increase in size, and ultimately to rupture. Extension into the chest is the most common complication, occurring in 20–35% of patients and ranging from a small, almost symptomless, serous effusion to rupture of the abscess into the pleural cavity with formation of an empyema.

This complication has the highest mortality (15–36%). Second in frequency is intraperitoneal rupture, which has been reported in 2–7.5% of cases. Sometimes a localized abscess forms, but otherwise peritonitis occurs. The mortality used to be extremely high but improved techniques of surgical drainage and more effective chemotherapy has reduced this from over 80% to 14%. The rarest complication is extension to the pericardium which, as with the other two conditions described above, may be gradual or abrupt; before 1950 the mortality rate was greater than 90% but is now about 40% even in cases of acute rupture.

The 5-nitroimidazole drugs, particularly metronidazole, are probably the most widely used at the present time; the standard course of treatment (750 mg orally three times a day for 5–10 days) will cure more than 90% of patients. Single-dose therapy with 2.4 g has also been effective. Parenteral emetine is still used in some cases of imminent rupture as it is felt to act more rapidly, but the drug produces significant gastrointestinal and cardiovascular side-effects. Any extra efficacy of combinations of metronidazole and emetine has not been firmly established. It is usual to complete the course of treatment with a lumenal amoebicide such as diloxanide furoate to eradicate the parasite from the bowel, since metronidazole is too well absorbed to be completely effective in this role. The role of aspiration is not finally established, but a general consensus seems to be that the procedure is necessary only if rupture is imminent; up to 10% of lesions may be secondarily infected with bacteria following repeated aspiration or open drainage. Because of the almost complete absence of a granulomatous response by the host, hepatic amoebic abscesses, even large ones, usually heal without scarring.

The fact that only a few patients with amoebiasis go on to develop the invasive disease while most remain as asymptomatic cyst-passers has intrigued parasitologists for many years. For a long while it was assumed that all strains of *E. histolytica* had the *ability* to invade and were either prevented from doing so by the host's defence mechanisms, or (the so-called 'Promethean' hypothesis) the parasites were always destroying the gut epithelium but that normally the host was able to repair the damage faster than it was being caused. In either case there was not expected to be any difference in the *parasites* isolated from asymptomatic cyst-passers or patients with invasive amoebiasis. Anecdotal evidence for a role for the immune system came from reports of serious or even fatal exacerbations of unapparent amoebiasis in patients who were given corticosteroids[12] or who were pregnant[13]. In 1972, however, the first indications appeared of inherent differences between isolates of *E. histolytica* from asymptomatic cyst-passers and patients, when the latter were shown to be much more readily agglutinated by the lectin concanavalin-A, even after being grown for some time in *in vitro* culture[14]. Subsequently it was shown that such parasites had distinctive isoenzyme patterns with the enzymes hexokinase and phosphoglucomutase[15]; reacted with certain invasive specific monoclonal antibodies[16] and DNA probes[17]; could be cultivated *in vitro* without needing the presence of bacteria or other living organisms ('axenic culture'); were resistant to lysis following activation of complement by the alternative pathway[18], and were more tolerant of the presence of oxygen than non-invasive strains[19] (data also from Ackers, unpublished observations). Most of these properties must be regarded as markers, whose relevance to the invasive process is not clear, but the last three attributes are clearly necessary for a parasite which intends to survive in the bloodstream or liver.

There are further anomalies. Amoebiasis, as would be expected from its mode of transmission, is much more common in developing countries than in western Europe or the United States of America. Nevertheless it is locally common in both these areas in groups of patients in whom faecal–oral transmission of pathogens is likely – for example severely mentally handicapped people living in institutions (particularly in overcrowded wards with few staff), and male homosexuals. There seem, however, to be virtually no cases of indigenous hepatic amoebiasis amongst these people, and surveys amongst both groups have shown only the presence of non-invasive zymodemes[20,21]. It is also reported[22] that although asymptomatic cyst-passers are common in the Gambia, hepatic amoebiasis is almost unknown (Bray, personal communication), whereas in Mexico City it is a leading cause of death amongst young adult males.

From an evolutionary point it is very hard to see what advantage *E. histolytica* obtains from disseminating outside the gut, since this either reduces (intestinal invasive disease) or abolishes (hepatic amoebiasis) the production of cysts, which are almost certainly the only infectious form of the parasite. (Trophozoites, rather than exclusively cysts, appear in the faeces not only during amoebic dysentery, but also whenever diarrhoea occurs due to infection with another enteric pathogen, because the reduced transit time does not allow time for encystment to occur. The diagnosis of invasive intestinal amoebiasis should be made only when trophozoites are found containing ingested erythrocytes, since this occurs only when the parasite invades the tissues.) Not only is non-invasive *E. histolytica* a very successful parasite, judged by world-wide incidence rate, but the totally non-invasive gut protozoa are, if anything, even more successful. Therefore it seems to me that either invasion confers some advantage on the parasite which we cannot yet appreciate, or that maybe transmission of invasive strains does not occur at all! This second possibility is suggested by some very recent work of Mirelman, who has shown that under certain (admittedly very artificial) conditions non-invasive isolates may be transformed into strains with the zymodeme markers of invasive strains[23], and that these strains appear to be genuinely pathogenic in *in vitro* cytopathogenicity assays and in animal models[24]. Within the community of those who study this parasite there is intense argument at present as to whether these results are significant or simply a laboratory artifact. If, however, they do represent a model of a process that can and does take place inside the human gut, then it is possible that invasive strains arise *de novo* inside every patient with clinical amoebiasis, the change being triggered by some changes in the conditions inside the gut whose nature we can only guess at. There would therefore be no need to postulate any selective advantage to the parasite from this change, since onward transmission would not need to occur. However, in removing one difficulty we have replaced it by another: if the differences between invasive and non-invasive isolates of *E. histolytica* are phenotypic rather than genotypic, then we now have to explain why the non-invasive organisms possess a whole group of metabolic and other functions (as listed above) which are apparently coordinately expressed but which, we have suggested above, confer no benefit on the organism. There is clearly a great deal about this fascinating parasite that we still do not understand.

References

1. Bingham, A. K. and Meyer, E. A. (1979). *Giardia* excystation can be induced *in vitro* in acidic solutions. *Nature (London)*, **277**, 301–2
2. Jarrol, E. L., Bingham, A. K. and Meyer, E. A. (1980). *Giardia* cyst destruction: effectiveness of six small-quantity water disinfection methods. *Am. J. Trop. Med. Hyg.*, **29**, 8–11
3. Walsh, J. A. (1988). Prevalence of *Entamoeba histolytica* infection. In Ravdin, J. I. (ed.), *Amebiasis: Human Infection by* Entamoeba histolytica, pp. 93–105. (New York: John Wiley)
4. World Health Organisation (1969). Amoebiasis. *Tech. Rep. Ser.* No. 421.
5. Ravdin, J. I. (1986). Pathogenesis of disease caused by *Entamoeba histolytica*: studies of adherence, secreted toxins, and contact-dependent cytolysis. *Rev. Infect. Dis.*, **8**, 247–60
6. Reed, S. L. and Braude, A. I. (1988). Extraintestinal disease: clinical syndromes, diagnostic profile and therapy. In Ravdin, J. I. (ed.), *Amebiasis: Human Infection by* Entamoeba histolytica, pp. 511–22. (New York: John Wiley)
7. Sepulveda, B. and Martinez-Palomo, A. (1984). Amebiasis. In Warren, K. S. and Mahmoud, A. F. (eds.), *Topical and Geographic Medicine*, (New York: McGraw-Hill)
8. Ralls, P. W., Colletti, P. M. and Halls, J. M. (1988). Imaging in hepatic amebic abscess. In Ravdin, J. I. (ed.), *Amebiasis: Human Infection by* Entamoeba histolytica, pp. 664–704 (New York: John Wiley)
9. Salata, R. A. (1988). The role of antibody in the host defence against *Entamoeba histolytica.* In Ravdin, J. I. (ed.), *Amebiasis: Human Infection by* Entamoeba histolytica, pp. 446–52. (New York: John Wiley)
10. Katzenstein, D., Rickerson, V. and Braude, A. (1982). New concepts of amebic liver abscess derived from hepatic imaging, serodiagnosis and hepatic enzymes in 67 consecutive cases in San Diego. *Medicine*, **61**, 237–46
11. Petri, W. A. and Ravdin, J. I. (1989). *Entamoeba histolytica.* In Walzer, P. D. and Genta, R. M. (eds.), *Parasitic Infections in the Compromised Host*, pp. 385–438. (New York: Marcel Dekker)
12. Eisert, J., Hannibal, J. E. and Sanders, S. L. (1959). Fatal amebiasis complicating corticosteroid management of pemphigus vulgaris. *N. Engl. J. Med.*, **261**, 843–5
13. Lewis, E. A. and Anita, A. U. (1969). Amoebic colitis: review of 295 cases. *Trans. Roy. Soc. Trop. Med. Hyg.*, **63**, 633–8
14. Martinez-Palomo, A., Gonzales-Robles, A. and de la Torre, M. (1972). Selective agglutination of pathogenic strains of *Entamoeba histolytica* induced by Con, A. *Nature New Biol.*, **245**, 186–7
15. Sargeaunt, P. G., Williams, J. E. and Green, J. D. (1978). The differentiation of invasive and non-invasive *Entamoeba histolytica* by isoenzyme electrophoresis. *Trans. Roy. Soc. Trop. Med. Hyg.*, **72**, 519–21
16. Strachan, W. D., Chiodini, P. L., Spice, W. M., Moody, A. H. and Ackers, J. P. (1988). Immunological differentiation of pathogenic and non-pathogenic isolates of *Entamoeba histolytica. Lancet*, **1**, 561–3

17. Garfinkel, L. I., Gilada, M., Huber, M., Gitler, C., Mirelman, D., Revel, M. and Rozenblat, S. (1989). DNA probes specific for *Entamoeba histolytica* possessing pathogenic and non-pathogenic zymodemes. *Infect. Immun.*, **57**, 926–31
18. Reed, S. R., Sargeaunt, P. G. and Braude, A. (1983). Resistance to lysis by immune serum of pathogenic *Entamoeba histolytica. Trans. Roy. Soc. Trop. Med. Hyg.*, **77**, 248–53
19. Ghadirian, E., Somerfield, S. D. and Kongshavn, P. A. L. (1986). Susceptibility of *Entamoeba histolytica* to oxidants. *Infect. Immun.*, **51**, 263–7
20. Sargeaunt, P. G. and Williams, J. E. (1982). A study of intestinal protozoa including non-pathogenic *Entamoeba histolytica* from patients in a group of mental hospitals. *Am. J. Publ. Hlth.*, **72**, 178–80
21. Sargeaunt, P. G., Oates, K. J., Maclenna, I., Oriel, J. D. and Goldmeier, D. (1983). *Entamoeba histolytica* in male homosexuals. *Br. J. Vener. Dis.*, **59**, 193–5
22. Bray, R. S. and Harris, W. G. (1977). The epidemiology of infection with *E. histolytica* in the Gambia, West Africa. *Trans. Roy. Soc. Trop. Med. Hyg.*, **71**, 401–7
23. Mirelman, D., Bracha, R., Wexler, A. and Chayen, A. (1986). Changes in isoenzyme patterns of a cloned culture of non-pathogenic *Entamoeba histolytica* during axenization. *Infect. Immun.*, **54**, 827–32
24. Mirelman, D. and Sargeaunt, P. G. (1987). The pathogenicity of *Entamoeba histolytica. Parasitol. Today*, **3**, 37–43

14
Hepatic structure and function in experimental and human malaria

G. C. COOK

INTRODUCTION

Throughout his long and varied history, *Homo sapiens* has been subject to the ravages of infections caused by *Plasmodium* sp.; there is no doubt that this protozoan parasite was present in the 'cradle of civilization' in Africa[1]. Available facts on the early history of human malaria have been reviewed[2]; it is likely that *Plasmodium* sp. evolved from the coccidia (luminal protozoa involving the small intestine) many millions of years ago – their appearance in the bloodstream would have facilitated transmission by blood sucking arthropods. Laveran first visualized the parasite of the human disease in infected erythrocytes while working in Algeria[3], and Sir Ronald Ross elucidated the man–mosquito cycle in India[4,5]; Sir Patrick Manson, who had predicted this discovery, finally clinched the saga by infecting a non-immune volunteer – his elder son – with *P. vivax* malaria via a mosquito bite[6]. In a world context a vast amount of morbidity and mortality remains associated with malaria, especially *P. falciparum* infection. This is very largely because control and prevention strategies have failed, and the *P. falciparum* parasite has become, and continues to develop increasing resistance to the currently available chemoprophylactic and chemotherapeutic agents[7–9].

Human malaria is a multisystem disease, and when death occurs it usually results from cerebral or renal involvement. The liver has in the past been the subject of much interest and research; however, present-day texts devoted to tropical medicine pay only scant attention to its role in this disease[10–12]. Writing in 1898, Manson described liver involvement in human malaria[13]:

> Under the influence of a succession of acute attacks, hepatic congestion may gradually acquire a more or less permanent character. [This he considered, brought about] various kinds and degrees of chronic hepatitis with hypertrophy of the interlobular connective tissues, and in time leads to hypertrophic, or to different forms of atrophic, cirrhosis,

> [and further, that as this progresses] irremediable organic disease of the liver, portal obstruction, and ascites may ensue.

Today few, if any, investigators would agree with many of Manson's conclusions. There are, however, very few recent reviews on this subject, although the present state of knowledge on the role of the hepatocyte in this disease has lately been summarized[14]; much of the interest at the molecular level lies in work on a possible sporozoite (or merozoite) vaccine.

ROLE OF THE HEPATOCYTE IN THE LIFE CYCLE OF *PLASMODIUM* SP.

The hepatocyte plays a crucial part in the human component of the *Plasmodium* sp. life cycle. Following a mosquito bite the sporozoite travels rapidly to the hepatocyte (via the bloodstream); entry then occurs equally quickly, but the mechanism of this crucial event is poorly understood[14]; the presence of surface receptors on hepatocytes is well documented. In man the time required for this event was shown by Fairley[15] to be less than 60 min. In the rat, numerous sporozoites can be demonstrated in hepatocytes within 2 min after intravenous inoculation of *P. berghei*[16]. Uptake of *P. yoellii nigeriensis* sporozoites by isolated and perfused rat liver has also been shown to be extremely rapid and efficient[17]; 67% of the initial load was removed (by mechanical trapping) from the perfusion fluid during the first passage through the liver, and 95% after 15 min of perfusion. Demonstration of transformation of intrahepatocytic sporozoites into pre-erythrocytic forms (merozoites) has been demonstrated in *P. berghei* infections in the rat[18,19]; development of the hepatic stage of *P. ovale* has also been studied *in vitro* in a model using a human hepatoma cell line[20]. Whether or not sporozoites also penetrate other cells is less clear. Using an immunofluorescence technique, phagocytosis by Kupffer cells has been demonstrated; however, most of these organisms probably die rapidly and do *not* contribute to the continuation of the parasite cycle[21]. Working with *P. berghei* infection in the rat, pre-erythrocytic merozoites were demonstrated in Kupffer cells within the hepatic sinusoids[22]; although the possibility still exists that their development occurs there, these authors considered that it merely represented a host defence mechanism. Some evidence has, however, been presented (also using the *P. berghei* infected rat) which indicates that some merozoites do escape to, and survive in, surrounding hepatocytes[23,24].

Monoclonal antibody to the species-specific circumsporozoite[25] protein antigen of *P. berghei* blocks sporozoite attachment to, and invasion of, human hepatoma (HepG2–A16) cells *in vitro*; it seems likely therefore that the CS protein constitutes the ligand which recognises the hepatocyte receptor[14].

Within the hepatocyte, schizogony takes place during a time span which varies from species to species; in human malaria the mean time in *P. falciparum* infection is 5.5 days, and in *P. malariae* 15 days. Large numbers of merozoites are liberated as the schizont ruptures into the hepatic sinusoid, and the resultant merozoites enter the sinusoidal blood. Although similar to the erythrocytic merozoite, the intrahepatocytic merozoite is a more elongated structure[25]; it also contains more micronemes, and the rhoptries are more elongated; none of the pre-erythrocytic stages contains typical mitochondria. At this point the hepatocyte has completed its role in the *Plasmodium* sp. life cycle in all except the *P. vivax* group of primate malarias (which includes *P. ovale*).

Awareness of the pre-erythrocytic, or hepatocytic, part of the cycle was in fact first demonstrated by Shortt and Garnham and their colleagues in 1948[26,27]; this discovery has subsequently been described in detail[28–30] and more recent work reviewed[31]. The dormant stage within the hepatocyte in the *P. vivax* group which accounts for relapses (which was not identified until 1980 by Krotoski *et al.*[21]) has been termed the hypnozoite[28]; this measures 5–6 μm in length[29] but its ultrastructure has not yet been determined[25]. Growth of the exoerythrocytic stages of *P. vivax* has now been accomplished in a human hepatoma cell line[14,32]; the changes parallel closely those of other *Plasmodium* spp.

EXPERIMENTAL MALARIA: STRUCTURAL HEPATIC ABNORMALITIES

Early observations on human liver structure at post-mortem (see below) convinced many physicians that severe abnormalities, and subsequent hepatocellular dysfunction, were clinically important. Following upon this, a great deal of experimental work was carried out to determine the nature and cause of this morphological change.

Many investigators considered that a 'toxic' factor, possibly malaria pigment itself (see below), was aetiologically important[33,34]. Manson considered this to be melanin (see below)[13]. Two distinct types of pigment were recognized: (1) an iron-containing pigment – directly derived from haemoglobin, and (2) a parasite-derived form ferrihaemic acid or haematin, which was considered to be a metabolic product of haemoglobin ingested by *Plasmodium* sp. The nature of this substance was studied in Pekin ducks infected with *P. lophurae*[35]; this author suggested that it was slowly oxidized by endothelial cells to iron pigment. Ferrihaemate, rather than the pigment itself, was also considered to exert a direct toxic action, especially on the kidneys[34]. Maegraith[36] concluded that the amount, shape and colour of the pigment granules – demonstrable as fine granules in Kupffer cells and sinusoidal macrophages – varied with the clinical history and species of *Plasmodium* together with other factors. The search for a malarial toxic factor was pursued until relatively recently[37]; a serum factor in both mice and monkeys infected with *P. berghei* and *P. knowlesi*, respectively, was postulated to produce a permeability change within the mitochondrial membrane, which allowed the escape of certain oxidative enzymes.

Vascular occlusion, superimposed upon severe anaemia, with resultant anoxia, was also considered a possible explanation for the hepatic changes[34]; this was supported by work on monkeys infected with *P. knowlesi*.

These two concepts involving malaria 'toxin', and 'blockage' were, however, subsequently replaced as a result of a great deal of work carried out by Maegraith and his co-workers at the Liverpool School of Tropical Medicine[36]. Experiments using *P. knowlesi*-infected rhesus monkeys had clearly shown that the major hepatic lesions consisted of sinusoidal dilatation around the central veins with necrosis of hepatocytes in the centrilobular region[38]. Figure 1 shows an example of centrilobular congestion in a monkey dying of a *P. knowlesi* infection in one of the Liverpool studies; these changes are compared with those from a patient who died as a result of *P. falciparum* infection (see below).

Working on the possibility that these histological changes represented anoxia which resulted from reduced blood flow, portal angiography was carried out in monkeys (*Macaca mulatta*) infected with *P. knowlesi*[39,40]; a

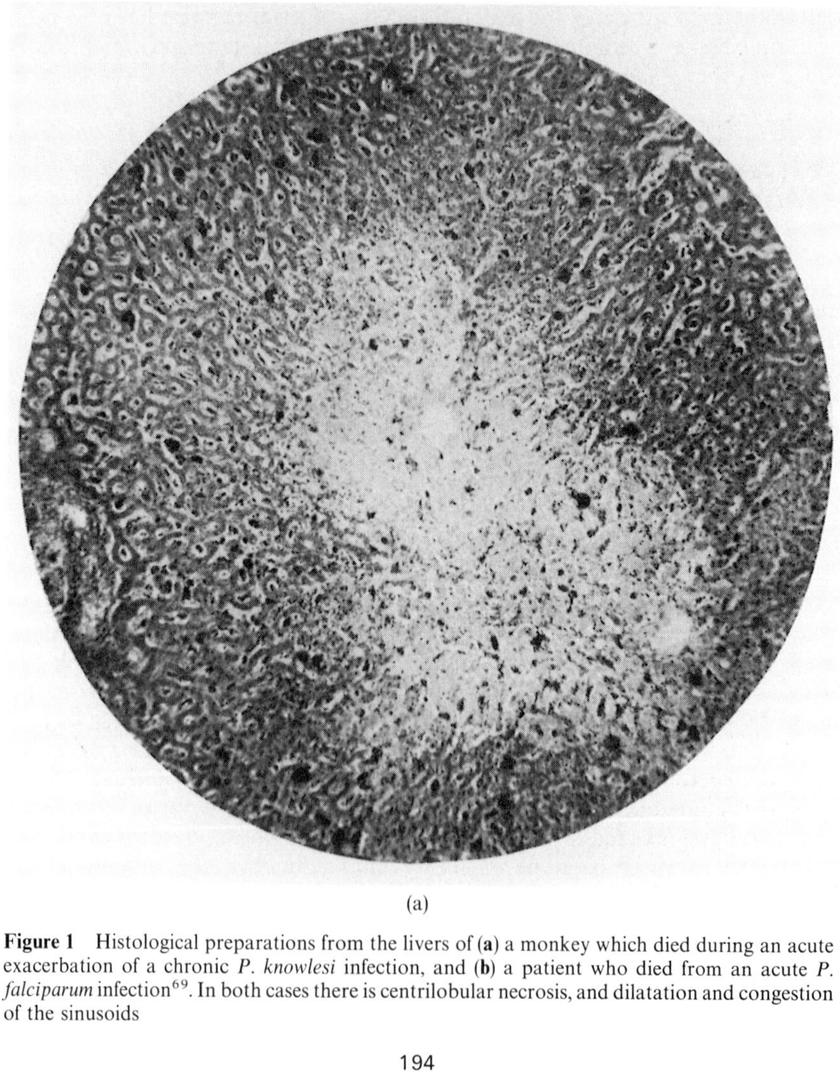

(a)

Figure 1 Histological preparations from the livers of (**a**) a monkey which died during an acute exacerbation of a chronic *P. knowlesi* infection, and (**b**) a patient who died from an acute *P. falciparum* infection[69]. In both cases there is centrilobular necrosis, and dilatation and congestion of the sinusoids

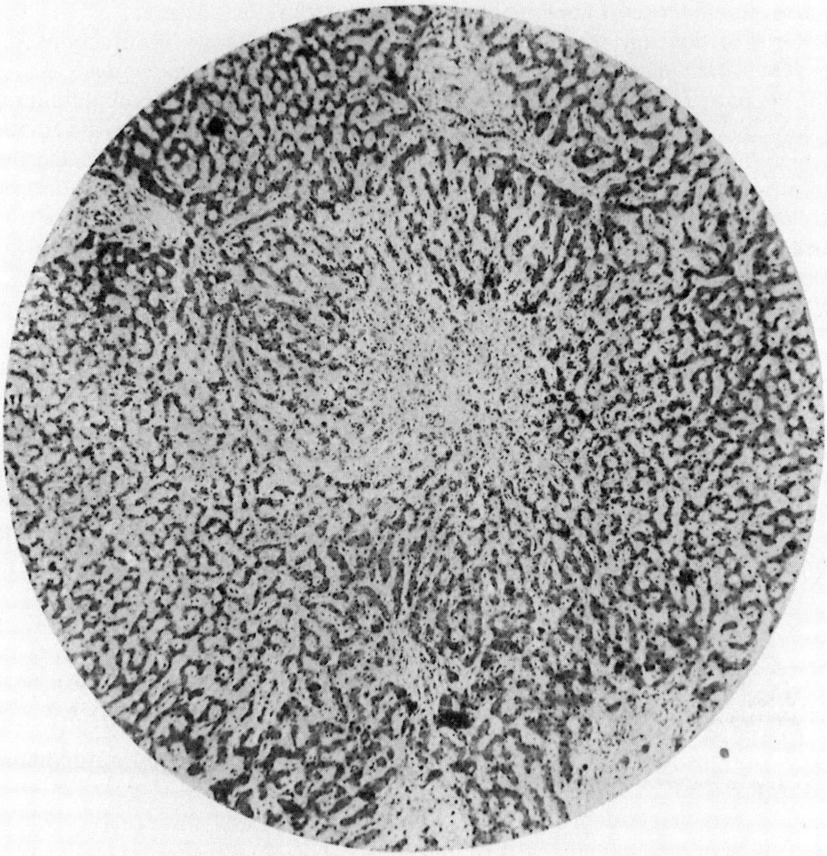

(b)

Figure 1 *continued*

constriction was demonstrated in all of the branches of the portal vein, together with a reduction in sinusoidal perfusion (and portal hypertension); furthermore, these changes were shown to be mediated via sympathetic activity and reversed by adrenergic blockade[41]. However, the factor(s) involved in the initiation of these 'shock'-like changes still remain undetermined.

EXPERIMENTAL MALARIA: FUNCTIONAL HEPATIC ABNORMALITIES

Much of the older literature on malaria-induced hepatic abnormalities is difficult to evaluate, largely because techniques used for assessment of hepatocellular function were far from perfect and often non-specific. By measuring blood transaminase concentrations in *P. berghei*-infected mice, however, evidence of hepatocyte damage has been demonstrated[42,43]; in the latter investigation, serum ornithine carbamoyltransferase – a mitochondrial enzyme – was used as a marker of hepatocellular damage. A decrease in intrahepatic transaminases which coincided with their elevation in peripheral blood has also been demonstrated in *P. berghei*-infected mice[44]. The South American owl monkey (*Aotus trivirgatus*), which is susceptible to *P. falciparum* infection, has been used as an experimental model by two groups of workers. Using Ugandan and Vietnamese strains of the parasite (with erythrocyte infection rates varying from 1.6% to 83.8%), serum transaminase concentrations were elevated, but did not correlate with the level of parasitaemia[45]. Comparable results were obtained using the Camp strain of *P. falciparum* (with a parasitaemia ranging from 13% to 78%)[46].

It seems likely that these elevated enzyme concentrations result from areas of parenchymal necrosis, and this has been shown to be associated with severe loss of intracellular glycogen[47].

Following up the evidence for mitochondrial damage (see above), which has been confirmed in mice acutely infected with *P. berghei*, and also rhesus monkeys infected with *P. knowlesi*[48,49], Fletcher and Maegraith[50] demonstrated the release of oxidative enzymes from the damaged mitochondrial membrane; a concurrent elevation of alkaline phosphatase led them to conclude that the lysosomal membrane was also damaged.

HUMAN MALARIA: STRUCTURAL HEPATIC ABNORMALITIES

Many of the existing studies on hepatic change in human malaria originated from three sources: (1) 'therapeutic' malaria (which was used in psychiatry, and in the treatment of neurosyphilis and certain other neurological conditions), and which was produced by a *P vivax* infection; (2) infections (many of them caused by *P. falciparum*) in British soldiers who were serving in tropical and subtropical countries during the Second World War (1939–45); and (3) similar infections in US servicemen during the Korean and Vietnam wars.

Manson[13] was fully aware of the presence of *siderosis* in human malaria. This was, he considered:

> a condition resulting from chemical changes undergone by the yellow pigment with which the various cells of the organ (the liver) are charged. [Furthermore, he wrote], As the deposit becomes older... the ochre pigment is no longer in minute grains, as when first deposited, but in blocks and globules as large as, or even larger than, blood corpuscles. This pigment is, of course, something quite apart from the parasite-derived melanin deposited in the same organs.

It is clearly important to distinguish between the hepatic morphological changes in the liver of an individual indigenous to a malarious area, and those in a 'non-immune' person with an acute attack which has been either naturally or experimentally induced.

Endemic malaria

Histologically, three chronological phases can be delineated in individuals in hyper- or meso-endemic areas[51]; these coincide with developmental stages in the immune response of the host:

1. First 3–6 months of life: maternal immunity produces relatively effective protection, and the changes are consequently minimal.
2. After 6 months (the phase of waning passive immunity): this is associated with a high parasitaemia, significant clinical symptoms (fever and splenomegaly), and a varying degree of morbidity and mortality. There is hypertrophy and hyperplasia of the hepatic (and splenic) macrophages, and the Kupffer cells contain large amounts of malaria (haemozoin) pigment; however, significant hepatocyte damage is very unusual[52,53].
3. The phase of increased immunity (from the middle of the first decade of life): the malarial antibody concentration increases, the parasitaemia is coincidentally lower and the splenomegaly rate reduced. Haemozoin production is diminished markedly, and as this declines the pigment slowly clears from the Kupffer cells; this process begins in the centre of the liver lobule and spreads slowly to the periportal areas (pigment is never present in hepatocytes). It is transported to the portal areas, cleared by lymphatic drainage and deposited in the upper abdominal lymph nodes; this series of events closely parallels clearance of *iron* from the liver lobule. However, Kupffer cell hypertrophy and hyperplasia does not completely resolve. With the development of humoral immunity hepatic sinusoidal lymphocytes and plasma cells proliferate, and in a small proportion of cases hepatic sinusoidal lymphocytosis becomes dense. This latter event is usually associated with a grossly enlarged spleen, a markedly raised malarial antibody concentration, and an elevated serum IgM concentration; this clinical syndrome, which is considered to result from an aberrant immunological response to all of the human *Plasmodium* sp., is termed *hyperreactive malarious splenomegaly*[54,55].

Therefore the major impact on the liver of a resident of an endemic area is upon the reticuloendothelial components – Kupffer cells, and sinusoidal and portal macrophages – and significant hepatocyte damage is very unusual; if the latter does occur it probably results from a complicating factor such as anoxia[51,56] (see below).

Acute *P. falciparum* infection

Following an acute attack in a non-immune individual, the liver (at post-mortem) appears congested, tense, blunt-edged, and has a chocolate or slate-grey coloration[56]; the cut surface may lose its distinct lobular pattern and exhibit marked flaccidity; there is, however, no evidence of gross necrosis or haemorrhage.

The relative dearth of available data on hepatic morphology in an acute

P. falciparum infection largely reflects the ethical restrictions involved in obtaining needle-liver biopsy specimens in *severe* acute disease. Most existing histological data relate to uncomplicated disease. The reticuloendothelial changes seem to be comparable to those described above in experimental studies. In a study carried out in Sri Lanka, 90% and 80% of 65 patients with a primary acute attack of *P. falciparum* or *P. vivax* infection had evidence of Kupffer cell activity and deposition of malaria pigment, respectively[57]; 40% had lymphocytic collections within the sinusoids. Pigment deposits are demonstrable within Kupffer cells and sinusoidal macrophages within 6 days of an acute attack[58]; they disappear within 6 months and this rate depends on the amount of pigment originally present. The intensity of pigment deposition does *not*, however, directly correlate with the height of parasitaemia (or in fact with the degree of hepatocellular dysfunction)[56]; pigment may in consequence be scanty following a fatal *P. falciparum* infection, but plentiful after a prolonged chronic infection. Hyperplasia of Kupffer cells (which exhibit active phagocytosis) is striking; as the infection proceeds this follows a centripetal direction[59]. Pigment, together with parasitized and non-parasitized erythrocytes, are phagocytosed by Kupffer cells and macrophages circulating in the sinusoids, the latter being congested with infected erythrocytes and inflammatory cells.

Adhesive properties of *P. falciparum*-infected erythrocytes (cells containing young trophozoites are important in the pathogenesis of cerebral vascular occlusion in the acute disease, and are in large part responsible for the potentially lethal disease – cerebral malaria[60–63]) have probably evolved evolutionarily as a parasite-survival mechanism to escape the scavenging events within the liver (and spleen).

Numerous accounts document some degree or other of centrilobular hepatocyte damage in acute *P. falciparum* malaria[64,65]; in fatal blackwater fever this is considered to be a frequent event (only the cells around the portal triads surviving) (Figure 1)[65]; however, unlike pigment deposition and Kupffer cell and macrophage activity this does *not* show a direct correlation with the height of the parasitaemia. Not all investigators have detected evidence of *necrosis* of hepatocytes[66]; these authors, for example, examined needle liver-biopsy specimens from 38 American soldiers infected with *P. falciparum* and only found (in addition to Kupffer cell hyperplasia and mononuclear infiltration) evidence of increased hepatocyte nuclear and cytoplasmic activity. Spitz[67] recorded small, round, deeply acidophilic, hyaline-like bodies in hepatocytes (and Kupffer cells) in severe *P. falciparum* infection, which were associated with hepatocellular necrosis; he compared these structures with cytoplasmic inclusion-bodies, which were regarded as evidence of degeneration, in yellow fever. Other investigators have likened them to the Councilman bodies of yellow fever[68]. In a well-established case the histological picture is of centrilobular degeneration and necrosis with preservation of intact hepatocytes at the periphery of the lobule[69]; the central vein and sinusoids are filled with erythrocytes, many of which contain parasites. These erythrocytes, unlike those in cerebral vessels, retain their form – a fact which was appreciated 60 years ago[70].

While several earlier writers had referred to 'malarial hepatitis'[17,66,68,72,73], few presented compelling evidence for this. There is certainly no evidence of progression to chronic hepatitis[74].

Ultrastructural studies have also been carried out in acute *P. falciparum* infection. Hypertrophy of Kupffer cells and sinusoidal macrophages go hand in hand. In severe disease, hepatocyte swelling, changes in the endoplasmic reticulum and mitochondria, and loss of microvilli at the sinusoidal pole were demonstrated; these might be related to impaired biliary transport[75]. These authors concluded that the abnormalities in the endoplasmic reticulum were more striking than the mitochondrial damage; this contrasts with some of the experimental studies (see above). Figure 2 shows electron micrographs in a human *P. falciparum* infection; abnormalities within the reticulo-endothelial components and hepatocyte are demonstrated[75]. Pigment granules have been shown in another electron microscopic study to consist of rectangular crystalline structures[74]. Figure 3 shows parasitized erythrocytes in hepatic sinusoids. In an ultrastructural study of material obtained 15 min post-mortem, from a case of *P. falciparum* infection accompanied by blackwater fever, damage to the hepatocyte plasma membrane, together with abnormalities in the bile capillary microvilli, were noted[76]; however, some of these changes might have resulted from autolysis.

The overall interpretation of these morphological findings has received a great deal of attention. Although focal necrosis and fatty degeneration have been ascribed by some to obliteration of bile flow, impaired blood flow with resultant anoxia seems more likely to be important[68,77]; the spatial configuration of the lesions certainly supports this concept[59]. This is also in keeping with the experimental findings of Maegraith and his colleagues (see above), who were of the opinion that the changes resulted chiefly from stasis in the central regions of the lobules which arose from obstruction to the venous outflow, and that this probably has a reflex origin[36,78]. Andrews[69] likened these changes to the anoxic ones observed in right-sided cardiac failure and in the Budd–Chiari syndrome.

The other human malarias

As with an acute *P. falciparum* infection, the liver subjected to *P. vivax* or one of the other infections may be enlarged, congested, and either normal in colour or tinged with slate grey[56,74]. Kupffer cell activity, changes in circulating sinusoidal macrophages, and the degree of malaria-pigment deposition are, however, all less prominent[58,66]. Increased mitotic activity within the hepatocyte has been stressed by several authors[68,72]; while the former attributed this to a regenerative phase, older workers considered it to be caused either by a direct irritative effect of *P. vivax* or its metabolic products[72]. The overall extent of the pathological change was considered by McMahon *et al.*[73] to show a lack of correlation with the severity of hepatocellular dysfunction. Non-specific granulomas have also been recorded by some investigators[57,66,72]; however, these have been demonstrated in a minority of cases only, being most prominent in the sinusoids and portal areas. The possibility has to be borne in mind that these resulted from a

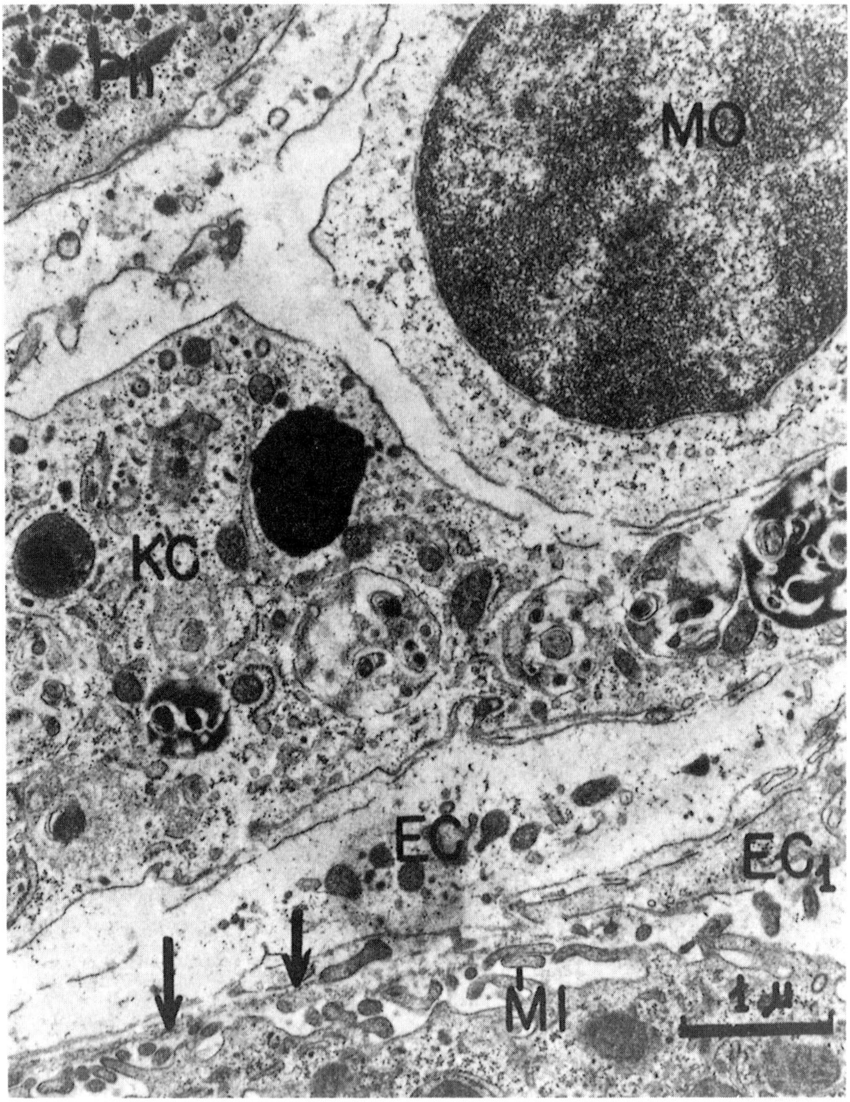

(a)

Figure 2 Electron micrographs from human *P. falciparum* infection[75]. (**a**) Enlarged Kupffer cell (KC) with dense and laminated bodies, surrounded by a single membrane, interpreted as malarial pigment. A mononuclear cell (MO) is also seen inside the sinusoid. Swollen endothelial cells (EC and EC_1) are seen partially overlapping and presenting beneath them a faint linear deposit interpreted as a basement membrane-like material (arrows). Microvilli (MI) are preserved. (**b**) Overlap of swollen endothelial cell (EC) cytoplasms. Part of a phagocyte, probably a granulocyte (Ph), is seen inside the sinusoidal lumen. Hepatocyte shows marked glycogen depletion, and scanty oedematous material (MI) (scale = μm)

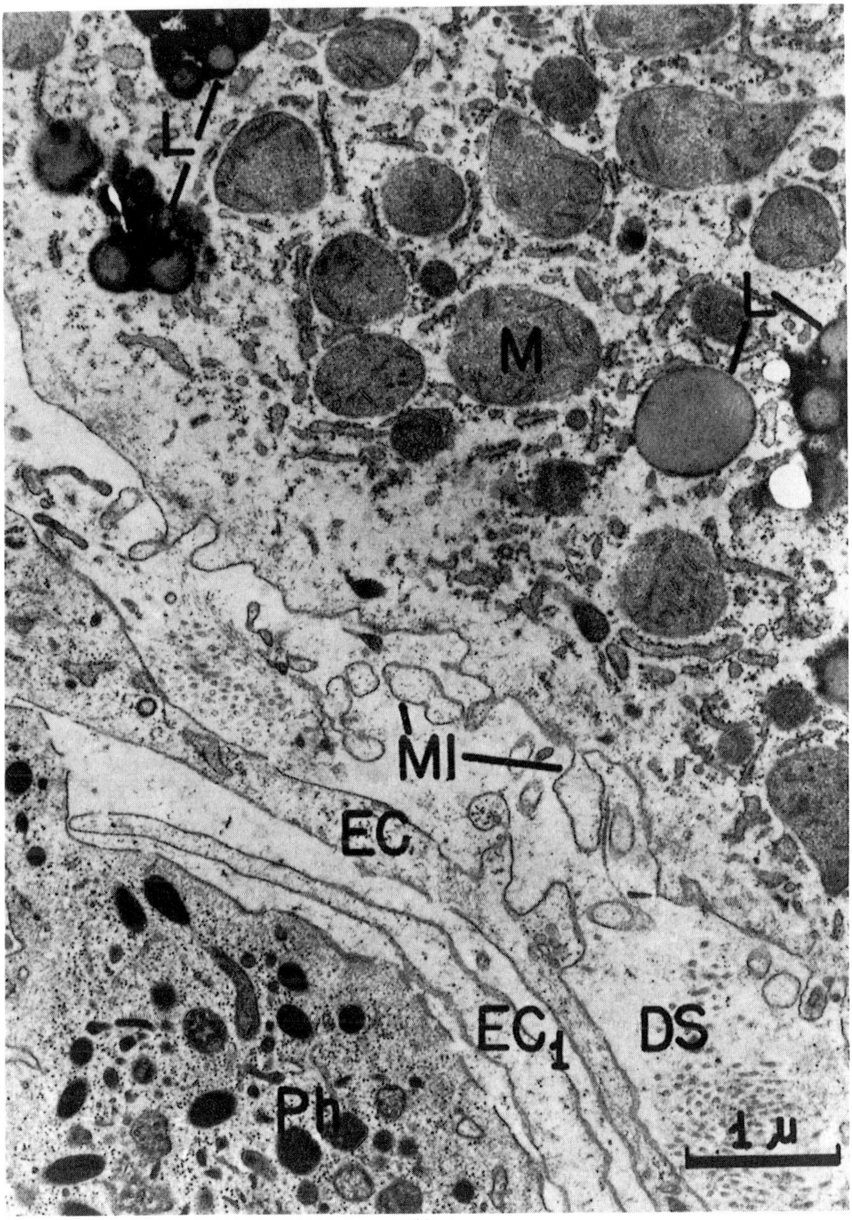

(b)

Figure 2 *continued*

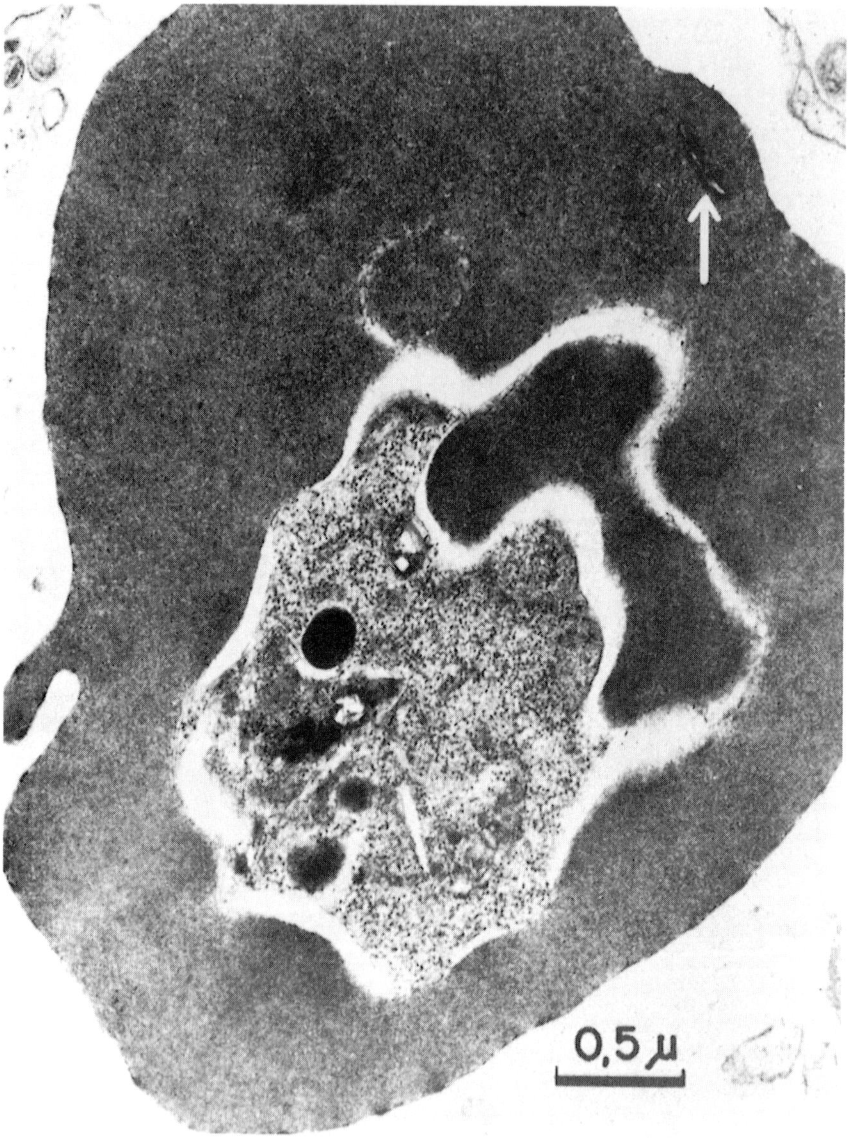

(a)

Figure 3 Parasitized intrasinusoidal erythrocytes[75]. (**a**) *P. falciparum* trophozoite within an erythrocyte, showing an irregular contour; the white arrow shows a cleft in the erythrocyte stroma. (**b**) Agglutinated erythrocytes, one of them parasitized with *P. vivax* and having a light stroma; arrows designate the clefts. (Scale = μm)

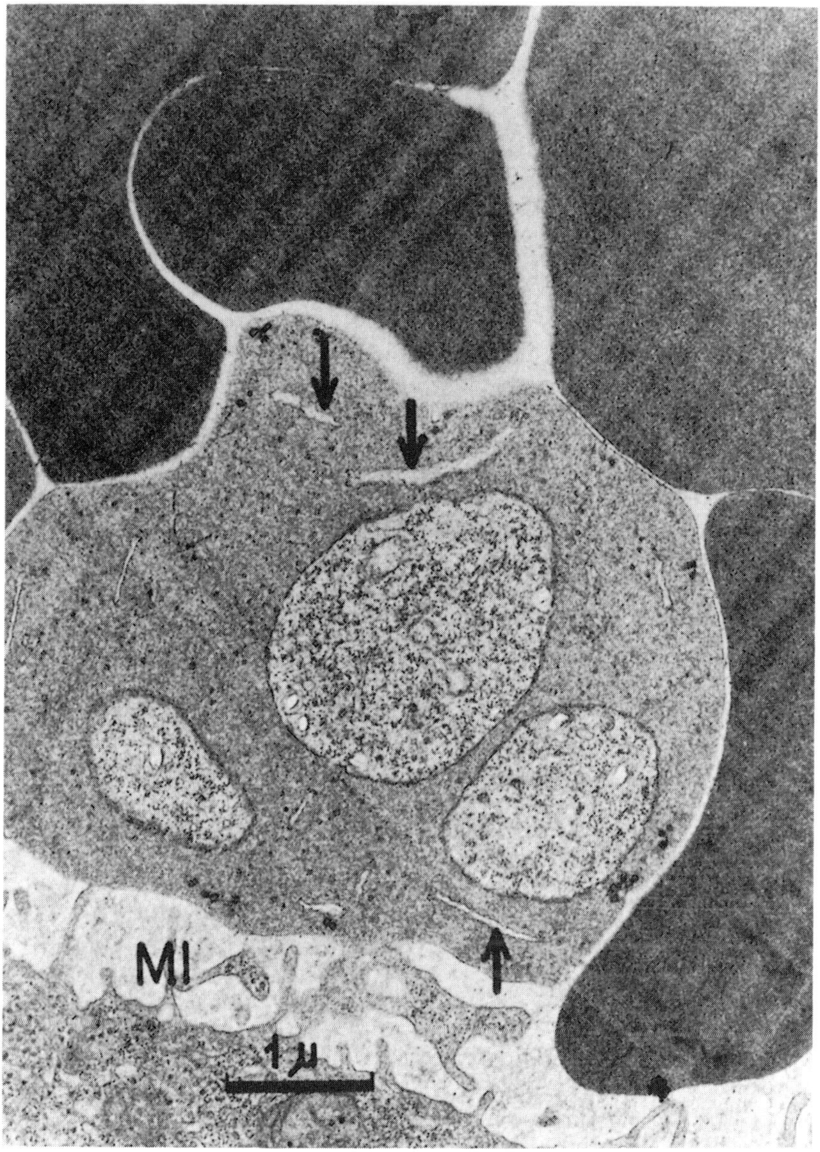

(b)

Figure 3 *continued*

coincident non-malarial infection and were not a direct result of *Plasmodium* sp. Overall, the morphological changes have been considered similar to those of *P. falciparum*, but less severe[56].

In the most chronic form of human malaria (i.e. that caused by *P. malariae*), the liver becomes enlarged and congested to only a moderate degree[56];

macroscopically the parenchyma shows diffuse pigmentation. Histologically the Kupffer cells and perilobular connective tissue contain pigment. An associated lymphadenopathy has been described by one group of investigators[77].

Warrell[60] has concluded that when coexistent viral hepatitis is excluded and post-mortem phenomena (e.g. centrizonal necrosis) have been taken into account, the histopathological changes are unimpressive. This is probably an accurate assessment of the situation in uncomplicated disease. However, in severe complicated disease there seems little doubt that centrizonal necrosis can be present during life, and that this probably contributes to some of the clinical manifestations of a severe *P. falciparum* infection (see below).

Whatever the infecting species, there seems no doubt that resolution of these changes after successful treatment and recovery is the rule[56]; residual changes are of minimal degree and Manson certainly seems to have been incorrect in concluding that chronic sequelae may follow[13]. However, in chronic malaria (caused by the non-*P. falciparum* parasites), the organ remains enlarged and hyperaemic, while the lobular structure is clearly delineated, and even more pronounced than in the normal organ – as a result of pigment deposition which is most marked in the periphery of the nodules. While there are very few recent studies of histopathology of the liver in malaria, it seems therefore extremely unlikely that long-term sequelae (e.g. cirrhosis) ever result from this group of infections[53].

HUMAN MALARIA: FUNCTIONAL HEPATIC ABNORMALITIES

The major problems in interpretation of the available data result from the fact that (1) most reported studies (as with those in experimental malaria) used techniques which did not measure hepatocellular function specifically, and (2) very little work on this subject has been carried out during the past two or three decades.

It seems probable that clinical signs, e.g. presence of jaundice and hepatomegaly, correlate approximately with the degree of disturbance of hepatocellular function[79]. Furthermore, the overall consensus is that the extent of these abnormalities is greatest in *P. falciparum* infection[80], despite the fact that an older study showed a lack of relationship between the degree of dysfunction, and either species or level of parasitaemia[58]. The jaundice associated with malaria usually contains a hepatocellular component, although haemolysis may be dominant[80,81–88]; most of these early studies used indices which are non-specific tests of hepatocellular function and have in the most part been relegated to the chemical pathology archives or museum. However, later investigators have measured serum transaminase concentrations[89–91], and these have largely confirmed earlier results in both *P. falciparum* and *P. vivax* infections. Approximately 60% of 38 American soldiers studied in Vietnam who were infected with *P. falciparum* had an elevated serum transaminase concentration[66]; this correlated well with biopsy–histology which was abnormal in most of them. In a single case report of *P. falciparum* malaria in a non-immune individual (which proved fatal), the liver was enlarged and tender, and although the serum transaminase concentrations were markedly elevated, the alkaline phosphatase was normal[92]. In West Africa, children with a fatal *P. falciparum* infection apparently show only minor evidence of parenchymal hepatic necrosis[93]; it is therefore probable that the immune status of the individual is of importance in determining the extent of hepatocellular dysfunction[80].

Several reports refer to liver function tests in *P. vivax* infection; however, the majority of these come from the Second World War period, or were carried out when this infection was used as a 'therapeutic' technique. The consensus of opinion was that changes were relatively mild and of a transitory nature, having resolved by 3–6 weeks after successful treatment[83]. In one investigation, abnormalities in hepatocellular function were demonstrated in the absence of overt damage to the liver parenchyma[71].

A correlation between the degree of elevation of transaminase concentration(s) and the presence (or absence) of tender hepatomegaly has been reported in Indian children infected with *P. vivax*[94]; alkaline phosphatase concentration was raised in nearly half of them (which perhaps reflected an obstructive component), and when investigated 6 weeks after successful treatment both clinical signs and enzyme concentrations had returned to normal. This latter study suggests that the extent of hepatocyte involvement in *P. vivax* infection is greater than was considered likely in some of the earlier reports[87]; these latter authors documented only transient dysfunction in 317 soldiers with chronic relapsing *P. vivax* infection, and no evidence of permanent impairment.

CLINICAL ASPECTS OF HEPATIC INVOLVEMENT IN *PLASMODIUM* SP. INFECTION

There are no clinical manifestations associated with hepatocyte involvement in the life cycle of *Plasmodium* sp. The sporozoite load which is injected by the mosquito is small, and although those hepatocytes which are infected are ultimately destroyed (see above) the overall impact of this on the human host is, at most, trivial[14].

Mild hepatomegaly, which is often tender, is common in geographical areas where malaria is endemic[66,93,95,96]. In a survey of over 1200 instances of acute malaria in British troops in West Africa during 1941–2, Hughes and Bomford[97] recorded hepatomegaly in 32 cases, and tenderness in 61; the most severe was 3 inches below the right costal margin. Fifteen per cent of 65 patients with a primary attack of *P. vivax* or *P. falciparum* infection studied in Sri Lanka had evidence of both hepatomegaly and jaundice[57]; these changes rapidly resolved after treatment. The nature of the jaundice is complex (see above), and while haemolytic and hepatocellular elements usually predominate, a cholestatic one may also play a part. Anaemia associated with malaria also has a multifactorial origin[98].

The differential diagnostic list includes several entities[51,57]: viral hepatitis, hepatic amoebiasis, typhoid 'hepatitis', EBV and CMV hepatitis, Q-fever, and the 'jaundice of acute bacterial infection', which in the tropics and subtropics is usually associated with pneumococcal lobar pneumonia or pyomyositis[51].

In order to study hepatic blood flow in severe acute *P. falciparum* malaria, Molyneux *et al.*[99] have recently carried out a clinical investigation using the peripheral disappearance curve for indocyanine green; this was performed in Thai adults and the data were interpreted using computer analysis. Figure 4 summarizes the result; a significant reduction in mean blood flow was demonstrated, and this returned to normal during convalescence ($p < 0.002$). In uncomplicated infection, however, the changes during acute infection compared with those in convalescence were not significant. These observations are entirely consistent with the histological results which were produced by Maegraith and his co-workers[36,41] (see above).

Whilst the Maegraith school initially favoured a venous outflow block to account for their results[69], a reduction in portal venous flow was later considered important[39]. The latter view coincides with that of Molyneux *et*

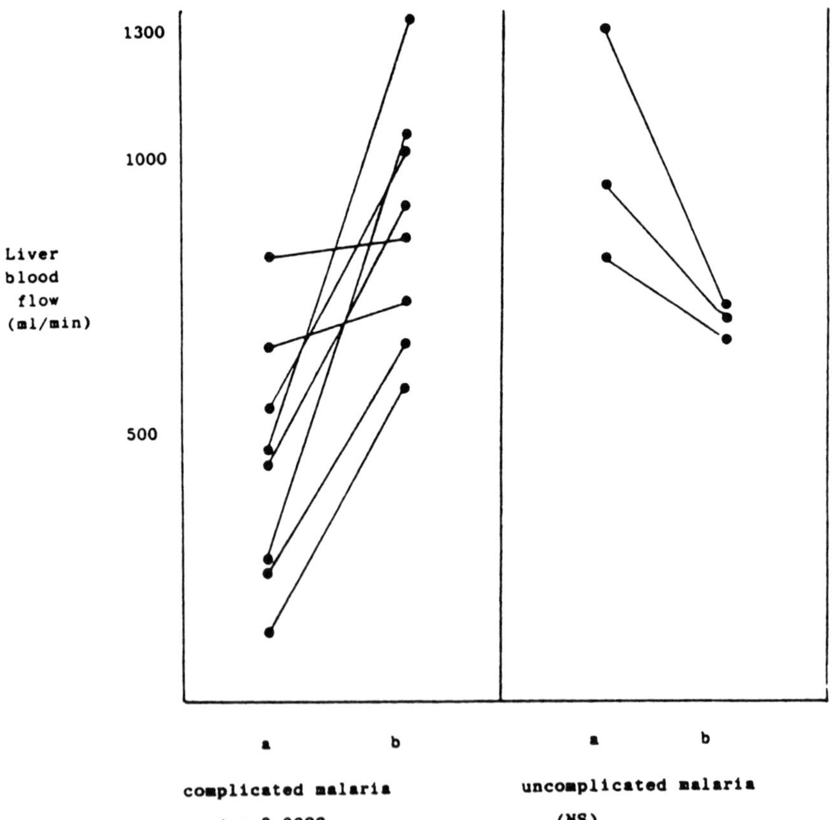

Figure 4 Liver blood flow measurements during acute *P. falciparum* malaria in Thai adults[99]: (*a*) during the acute infection, and (**b**) in convalescence. Severe complicated cases (left) are compared with uncomplicated cases (right).

al.; they demonstrated a concurrent reduction in small-intestinal absorption in their cases, and both events were accounted for by a generalized reduction in perfusion within the splanchnic bed.

Molyneux *et al.* consider, probably correctly, that these results might explain some of the clinical features of a complicated *P. falciparum* infection: (1) hypoglycaemia could result from a defect in hepatic gluconeogenesis; (2) lactic acidaemia and endotoxaemia may be exacerbated by a reduction in hepatic clearance of these compounds, and (3) metabolism of certain chemotherapeutic agents could be affected by reduced blood flow, even though serum transaminase concentrations are not necessarily elevated; quinine, for example, is largely metabolized by the hepatocyte.

In the light of their studies of hepatocellular function made in 1924, Sinton and Hughes[81] concluded that:

> the ingestion of glucose or laevulose is indicated in all cases of malaria, more especially in severe cases, to protect the liver cells and prevent further damage to the other functions of the liver, which are protected by the glycogen reserve of this organ.

With regard to the prognosis of liver involvement in malaria, few would now disagree that the changes are completely reversible, except the very long-standing reticuloendothelial changes in individuals who have spent a lifetime in an area endemic for malaria. Manson[13] considered:

> certain clinical facts about malarial hepatic congestion and malarial hepatitis are of importance: (i) such conditions do not tend to terminate in suppuration; (ii) they are almost always associated with splenic enlargement. These are important facts to recollect when it becomes a question of the diagnosis of malarial hepatitis from abscess of the liver. Another important fact to remember is that recent malarial enlargement of the liver is usually curable, depending as a rule on simple congestion; whereas old-standing malarial hepatic enlargement is usually incurable, depending as it always does, on hypertrophy of the connective tissue and a cirrhotic condition of the organ.

Apart from his comments on chronic disease, most present-day physicians would not be in major disagreement with these comments by the father of clinical tropical medicine.

Fredricks and Hoffbauer[86] commenting upon their results, published in 1945, concluded: 'malarial *therapy* (i.e. the introduction of a *P. vivax* infection by the physician) is ... contraindicated in the presence of clinically manifest disease (or for example, cirrhosis)'.

EFFECT OF CHEMOPROPHYLACTIC AND CHEMOTHERAPEUTIC AGENTS ON HEPATIC STRUCTURE AND FUNCTION

Some early reports raised the possibility that hepatic changes could result from the use of chemotherapeutic agents; however, most dismissed this association[73]. While the mechanism is not always clear, there is no doubt that some antimalarial compounds do possess hepatotoxic properties. Amodiaquine, which is no longer widely used for chemoprophylaxis, certainly possesses hepatotoxic properties (hepatocellular and cholestatic features are both involved)[7,100,101]. Hepatotoxicity has also been recently reported during mefloquine chemoprophylaxis[102]. Hepatitis and hepatic granulomas have been reported to be associated with 'Fansidar' (sulfadoxine + pyrimethamine) chemoprophylaxis[7]; it is likely that the sulphonamide component is responsible. Also, a granulomatous hepatitis has been reported in association with quinine administration[7,8]. The 4-aminoquinoline compound primaquine is used to eradicate the exoerythrocytic stage of *P. vivax* and *P. ovale* infection. Experimental evidence using the isolated perfused rat liver indicates that a *P. brugei* infection interferes with its metabolism and subsequent elimination[103]; although the degree of impairment increases with the severity of infection, this is not likely to have a great practical importance because primaquine is never indicated in the management of a *P. falciparum* infection.

The use of chemoprophylaxis by individuals with chronic liver disease (including cirrhosis) has not been adequately evaluated; this applies especially to long-term usage. The potential hepatotoxicity of mefloquine warrants special attention in this context.

MANAGEMENT OF HEPATOCELLULAR DYSFUNCTION IN *P. FALCIPARUM* MALARIA

Management consists basically in caring for a severely ill (sometimes unconscious) patient[7–9]. The major therapeutic measures should be directed at reducing the *P. falciparum* parasitaemia, correcting hypoglycaemia and pulmonary oedema, and monitoring renal function. Although the liver is often involved, it is unlikely that hepatocellular failure is ever the sole or indeed the predominant cause of death; this is usually a result of multi-organ failure. It is most unlikely that persisting hepatocellular dysfunction ever continues after recovery of a severe, complicated acute *P. falciparum* infection.

CONCLUSIONS

The hepatocyte plays an extremely important part in the human component of the life cycle of *Plasmodium* sp.; however, changes are restricted to the ultrastructural level, and have no significant effect *per se* on the health of the infected individual.

Compared with other major organs, e.g. the brain and kidneys, the liver comes off remarkably lightly in an acute malarial infection – even one resulting in complicated *P. falciparum* disease. Major changes focus on the reticuloendothelial components – the Kupffer cells and sinusoidal macrophages – both of which contain significant amounts of malarial pigment; the sinusoids also contain parasitized erythrocytes. These changes are present to some extent or other in all inhabitants of a region which possesses endemic malaria; an extreme instance consists of gross sinusoidal lymphocytosis which is one component of the syndrome – hyperreactive malarious splenomegaly.

Minor hepatocyte changes are present in all four human malarias; only in severe complicated *P. falciparum* infection do they assume clinical significance. Necrotic hepatocytes are usually confined to the centrilobular region. In experimental studies damage seems to be caused by anoxia resulting from reduced hepatic blood flow; a recent human study using an indirect method for blood-flow measurement has produced a result which is entirely consistent with these animal observations. Using a subhuman primate model, the mechanism for the blood-flow changes, which resemble a 'shock' syndrome, have been shown to be mediated via sympathetic activity. Whether tumour necrosis factor (TNF), which is markedly elevated in complicated *P. falciparum* infection, contributes to these changes is unknown. It seems most unlikely that in man the changes are ever sufficiently severe to produce isolated hepatocellular failure; when they do occur they usually coexist with evidence of multi-organ failure. Therefore, specific measures to counteract liver failure are not required, and reduction of the parasitaemia, care of the unconscious patient and monitoring of other system functions are all important. Certain chemoprophylactic and chemotherapeutic agents occasionally exert significant toxic effects on hepatocellular function.

References

1. Stringer, C. B. and Andrews, P. (1988). Genetic and fossil evidence for the origin of modern humans. *Science, NY*, **239**, 1263–8
2. Bruce-Chwatt, L. J. (1988). History of malaria from prehistory to eradication. In Wernsdorfer, W. H. and McGregor, I. (eds), *Malaria: principles and practice of malariology*, pp. 1–59. (Edinburgh, London: Churchill Livingstone)
3. Laveran, A. (1880). Note sur un nouveau parasite trouvé dans le sang de plusieurs malades atteints de fievre palustre. *Bull. Acad. Méd.*, 2nd series, **9**, 1235–6
4. Ross, R. (1897). On some peculiar pigmented cells found in two mosquitos fed on malarial blood. *Br. Med. J.*, **2**, 1786–8
5. Ross, R. (1898). Report on the cultivation of proteosoma, Labbé, in grey mosquitos. *Indian Med Gaz.*, **33**, 448–51
6. Manson, P. (1900). Experimental proof of the mosquito–malaria theory. *Br. Med. J.*, **2**, 949–51
7. Cook, G. C. (1986). *Plasmodium falciparum* infection: problems in prophylaxis and treatment in 1986. *Quart. J. Med.*, **61**, 1091–1115
8. Cook, G. C. (1988). Prevention and treatment of malaria. *Lancet*, **1**, 32–7
9. Cook, G. C. (1989). The great malaria problem: where is the light at the end of the tunnel? *J. Infect.*, **18**, 1–10
10. Strickland, G. T. (ed.) (1984). *Hunter's Tropical Diseases*, 6th edn, p. 530. (Philadelphia, London: W. B. Saunders)
11. Manson-Bahr, P. E. C. and Bell, D. R. (eds) (1987). *Manson's Tropical Diseases*, 19th edn, pp. 9–10. (London. Philadelphia: Baillière Tindall)
12. Goldsmith, R. and Heyneman, D. (eds) (1989). *Tropical Medicine and Parasitology*, p. 308 (Norwalk, Connecticut: Appleton & Lange)
13. Manson, P. (1898). *Tropical Diseases: a manual of the diseases of warm climates*, pp. 92–3. (London, Paris, New York, Melbourne: Cassell & Co.)
14. Hollingdale, M. R. (1985). Malaria and the liver. *Hepatology*, **5**, 327–35
15. Fairley, N. H. (1947). Sidelights on malaria in man obtained by subinoculation experiments. *Trans. R. Soc. Trop. Med. Hyg.*, **40**, 621–76

16. Shin, S. C. J., Vanderberg, J. P. and Terzakis, J. A. (1982). Direct infection of hepatocytes by sporozoites of *Plasmodium berghei*. *J. Protozool.*, **29**, 448–54
17. Sinden, R. E. and Smith, J. E. (1982). The role of the Kupffer cell in the infection of rodents by sporozoites of *Plasmodium*: uptake of sporozoites by perfused liver and the establishment of infection *in vivo*. *Acta Trop.*, **39**, 11–27
18. Meis, J. F. G. M., Verhave, J. P., Jap, P. H. K., Sinden, R. E. and Meuwissen, J. H. E. T. (1983). Malaria parasites – discovery of the early liver form. *Nature* (*Lond.*), **302**, 424–6
19. Meis, J. F. G. M., Verhave, J. P., Jap, P. H. K. and Meuwissen, J. H. E. T. (1985). Fine structure of exoerythrocytic merozoite formation of *Plasmodium berghei* in rat liver. *J. Protozool.*, **32**, 694–9
20. Mazier, D., Collins, W. E., Mellouk, S., Procell, P. M., Berbiguier, N., Campbell, G. H., Miltgen, F., Bertolotti, R., Langlois, P. and Gentilini, M. (1987). *Plasmodium ovale*: *in vitro* development of hepatic stages. *Exp. Parasitol.*, **64**, 393–400
21. Krotoski, W. A., Collins, W. E., Bray, R. S., Garnham, P. C. C., Cogswell, F. B., Gwadz, R. W., Killick-Kendrick, R., Wolf, R., Sinden, R., Koontz, L. C. and Stanfill, P. S. (1982). Demonstration of hypnozoites in sporozoite-transmitted *Plasmodium vivax* infection. *Am. J. Trop. Med. Hyg.*, **31**, 1291–3
22. Terzakis, J. A., Vanderberg, J. P., Foley, D. and Shustak, S. (1979). Erythrocytic merozoites of *Plasmodium berghei* in rat hepatic Kupffer cells. *J. Protozool.*, **26**, 385–9
23. Meis, J. F. G. M., Verhave, J. P., Jap, P. H. K., Sinden, R. E. and Meuwissen, J. H. E. T. (1983). Ultrastructural observations on the infection of rat liver by *Plasmodium berghei* sporozoites *in vivo*. *J. Protozool.*, **30**, 361–6
24. Verhave, J. P. and Meis, J. F. G. M. (1984). The biology of tissue forms and other asexual stages in mammalian plasmodia. *Experientia*, **40**, 1317–29
25. Aikawa, M. (1988). Fine structure of malaria parasites in the various stages of development. In Wernsdorfer, W. H. and McGregor, I. (eds), *Malaria*: *principles and practice of malariology*, pp. 97–129. (Edinburgh, London: Churchill Livingstone)
26. Shortt, H. E. and Garnham, P. C. C. (1948). Demonstration of a persisting exo-erythrocytic cycle in *Plasmodium cynomolgi* and its bearing on the production of relapses. *Br. Med. J.*, **1**, 1225–8
27. Shortt, H. E., Garnham, P. C. C., Covell, G. and Shute, P. G. (1948). The pre-erythrocytic stage of human malaria, *Plasmodium vivax*. *Br. Med. J.*, **1**, 547
28. Garnham, P. C. C. (1977). The continuing mystery of relapses in malaria. *Protozool. Abstr.*, **1**, 1–12
29. Garnham, P. C. C. (1987). The liver in malaria with special reference to the exoerythrocytic phase. *Ann. Trop. Med. Parasitol.*, **81**, 531–7
30. Garnham, P. C. C. (1988). Malaria parasites of man: life-cycles and morphology (excluding ultrastructure). In Wernsdorfer, W. H. and McGregor, I. (eds), *Malaria*: *principles and practice of malariology*, pp. 61–96. (Edinburgh, London: Churchill Livingstone)
31. Meis, J. F G. M. and Verhave, J. P. (1988). Exoerythrocytic development of malarial parasites. *Adv. Parasitol.*, **27**, 1–61
32. Hollingdale, M. R., Collins, W. E., Campbell, C. C. and Schwartz, A. L. (1985). *In vitro* culture of two populations (dividing and non-dividing) of exoerythrocytic parasites of *Plasmodium vivax*. *Am. J. Trop. Med. Hyg.*, **34**, 216–22
33. Brown, W. H. (1913). The renal complications of hematin intoxication and their relation to malaria. *Arch. Intern. Med.*, **12**, 315–21
34. Anderson, W. A. D. and Morrison, D. B. (1942). Role of parasite pigment (ferrihemic acid) in the production of lesions in malaria. *Arch. Pathol.*, **33**, 677–86
35. Rigdon, R. H. (1945). Malarial pigment: a consideration of the mechanism of elimination from the duck. *Am. J. Clin. Pathol.*, **15**, 489–93
36. Maegraith, B. G. (1948). *Pathological Processes in Malaria and Blackwater Fever*, p. 430. (Oxford: Blackwell)
37. Theakstone, R. D. G., Fletcher, K. A., Maskrey, P. and Maegraith, B. G. (1971). Ultrastructural studies of the effects of malarial toxic factors on normal mouse tissues. *Trans. R. Soc. Trop. Med. Hyg.*, **65**, 3–4
38. Rigdon, R. H. and Thomas, W. K. S. (1942). A study of the pathological lesions in *P. knowlesi* infection in *M. rhesus* monkeys. *Am. J. Trop. Med. Hyg.*, **22**, 329–39
39. Skirrow, M. B., Chongsuphajaisiddhi, T. and Maegraith, B. G. (1964). The circulation in

malaria. II. Portal angiography in monkeys (*Macaca mulatta*) infected with *Plasmodium knowlesi* and in shock following manipulation of the gut. *Ann. Trop. Med. Parasitol.*, **58**, 502–10
40. Skirrow, M. B. and Maegraith, B. G. (1964). The circulation in malaria. I. Portal angiograpy in the normal rabbit and monkey (*Macaca mulatta*). *Ann. Trop. Med. Parasitol.*, **58**, 491–501
41. Maegraith, B. and Fletcher, A. (1972). The pathogenesis of mammalian malaria. *Adv. Parasitol.*, **10**, 49–75
42. Sadun, E. H., Williams, J. S., Meroney, F. C. and Hutt, G. (1965). Pathophysiology of *Plasmodium berghei* infection in mice. *Exp. Parasitol.*, **17**, 277–86
43. Einheber, A., Wren, R. E., Rosen, H. and Martin, L. K. (1967). Ornithine carbamoyl-transferase activity in plasma of mice with malaria as an index of liver damage. *Nature*, **215**, 1489–91
44. Lal, D. M. and Hussain, Q. Z. (1978). Changes in transaminase activity in plasma and liver of albino mice infected with *Plasmodium berghei*. *Indian J. Med. Res.*, **67**, 362–6
45. Schnell, J. V., Siddiqui, W. A. and Geiman, Q. M. (1969). Analyses on the blood of normal monkeys and owl monkeys infected with *Plasmodium falciparum*. *Military Med.*, **134**, 1068–73
46. Wellde, B. T., Johnson, A. J., Williams, J. S. and Sadun, E. H. (1972). Experimental infection with *Plasmodium falciparum* in *Aotus* monkeys. *Am. J. Trop. Med. Hyg.*, **21**, 260–71
47. Jervis, H. R., Sprinz, H., Johnson, A. J. and Wellde, B. T. (1972). Experimental infection with *Plasmodium falciparum* in *Aotus* monkeys. *Am. J. Trop. Med. Hyg.*, **21**, 272–81
48. Riley, M. V. and Maegraith, B. G. (1961). A factor in the serum of malaria-infected animals capable of inhibiting the *in-vitro* oxidative metabolism of normal liver mitochondria. *Ann. Trop. Med. Parasitol.*, **55**, 489–97
49. Riley, M. V. and Maegraith, B. G. (1962). Changes in the metabolism of liver mitochondria of mice infected with rapid acute *Plasmodium berghei* malaria. *Ann. Trop. Med. Parasitol.*, **56**, 473–82
50. Fletcher, A. and Maegraith, B. (1966). The metabolism of the malaria parasite and its host. In Dawes, B. (ed.), *Advances in Parasitology*, vol. 10, pp. 31–48. (London: Academic Press)
51. Cook, G. C. (1980). The tropical liver: effect of chronic intestinal and reticuloendothelial infections. In *Tropical Gastroenterology*, pp. 59–66. (Oxford, New York, Delhi: Oxford University Press)
52. Edington, G. M. (1954). Cerebral malaria in the Gold Coast African: four autopsy reports. *Ann. Trop. Med. Parasitol.*, **48**, 300–6
53. Hutt, M. S. R. (1971). Some aspects of liver disease in Ugandan Africans. *Trans. R. Soc. Trop. Med. Hyg.*, **65**, 273–81
54. Cook, G. C. (1980). The tropical splenomegaly syndrome (TSS) and other splenic diseases in the tropics. In *Tropical Gastroenterology*, pp. 205–21. (Oxford, New York, Delhi: Oxford University Press)
55. Crane, G. G. (1986). Hyperreactive malarious splenomegaly (tropical splenomegaly syndrome). *Parasitol. Today*, **2**, 4–9
56. Boonpucknavig, V. and Boonpucknavig, S. (1988). The histopathology of malaria. In Wernsdorfer, W. H. and McGregor, I. (eds), *Malaria: principles and practice of malariology*, pp. 673–708. (Edinburgh, London: Churchill Livingstone)
57. Ramachandran, S. and Perera, M. V. F. (1976). Jaundice and hepatomegaly in primary malaria. *J. Trop. Med. Hyg.*, **79**, 207–10
58. Srichaikul, T. (1959). A study of pigmentation and other changes in the liver in malaria. *Am. J. Trop. Med. Hyg.*, **8**, 110–18
59. Aikawa, M., Suzuki, M. and Gutierrez, Y. (1980). Pathology of malaria. In Kreier, J. P. (ed.), *Malaria*, vol. 2, pp. 47–102. (New York: Academic Press)
60. Warrell, D. A. (1987). Pathophysiology of severe falciparum malaria in man. *Parasitology*, **94**, S53–S76
61. Aikawa, M. (1988). Human cerebral malaria. *Am. J. Trop. Med. Hyg.*, **39**, 3–10
62. Miller, L. H. (1989). Binding of infected red cells. *Nature* (*Lond.*), **341**, 18
63. Cook, G. C. (1990). *Parasitic Disease in Clinical Practice*, pp. 3–6 and 141–147. (Berlin: Springer-Verlag)
64. Dudgeon, L. S. and Clarke, C. (1917). A contribution to the microscopical histology of

malaria as occurring in the Salonika force in 1916, and a comparison of these findings with certain clinical phenomena. *Lancet*, **1**, 153–6
65. Winslow, D. J., Connar, D. H. and Sprinz, H. (1971). Malaria. In Marcial-Rojas, R. A. (ed.), *Pathology of Protozoal and Helminthic Diseases*, pp. 195–224. (Baltimore: Williams & Wilkins)
66. Deller, J. J., Cifarelli, P. S., Berque, S. and Buchanan, R. (1967). Malaria hepatitis. *Military Med.*, **132**, 614–20
67. Spitz, S. (1946). The pathology of acute falciparum malaria. *Military Surg.*, **99**, 555–72
68. Brito de, T., Meira, J. A. and Bassoi, O. N. (1962). Contribuicão ao estudo da malária. II. Patologia do fígado na malária aguda. *Rev. Inst. Med. Trop. São Paulo*, **4**, 105–11
69. Andrews, W. H. H. (1948). The liver lesions in malaria. *Trans. R. Soc. Trop. Med. Hyg. 1948*; **41**, 699–704
70. Klotz, O. (1929). Necrosis of the liver in malaria. *Am. J. Trop. Med.*, **9**, 241–8
71. White, L. G. and Doerner, A. A. (1954). Functional and needle biopsy study of the liver in malaria. *J. Am. Med. Assoc.*, **155**, 637–9
72. Corcoran, T. E., Hegstrom, G. J., Zoeckler, S. J. and Keil, P. G. (1953). Liver structure in nonfatal malaria. *Gastroenterology*, **24**, 53–62
73. McMahon, A. E., Kelsey, J. E. and Derauf, D. E. (1954). Hepatitis of malarial origin: clinical and pathologic study of fifty-four Korean veterans. *Arch. Intern. Med.*, **93**, 379–86
74. Aikawa, M. (1971). Parasitological review. *Plasmodium*: the fine structure of malarial parasites. *Exp. Pathol.*, **30**, 284–320
75. Brito de, T., Barone, A. A. and Faria, R. M. (1969). Human liver biopsy in *P. falciparum* and *P. vivax* malaria: a light and electron microscopy study. *Virch. Arch. Abt A, Path. Anat.*, **348**, 220–9
76. Rosen, S., Rycroft, D. W., Hano, J. E. and Barry, K. G. (1967). The liver in malaria; electron microscopic observations on a hepatic biopsy obtained 15 minutes post mortem. *Arch. Pathol.*, **83**, 271–7
77. Clark, H. C. and Tomlinson, W. J. (1949). The pathologic anatomy of malaria. In Boyd, M. F. (ed.), *Malariology*, vol. 2, pp. 874–903. (Philadelphia: W. B. Saunders)
78. Maegraith, B. (1948). Pathological processes in malaria. *Trans. R. Soc. Trop. Med. Hyg.*, **41**, 687–99
79. Kleeberg, J. and Birnhaum, D. (1948). Studies on liver damage in acute malaria. *Trans. R. Soc. Trop. Med. Hyg.*, **41**, 555–66
80. Fletcher, K. A. and Gilles, H. M. (1988). The chemical pathology of malaria. In Wernsdorfer, W. H. and McGregor, I. (eds), *Malaria: principles and practice of malariology*, pp. 647–71. (Edinburgh, London: Churchill Livingstone)
81. Sinton, J. A. and Hughes, T. A. (1924). The functional capacity of the liver in malaria with special reference to the levulose tolerance test. *Indian J. Med. Res.*, **12**, 409–22
82. Williams, R. G. (1927). The functions of the liver as affected by malaria induced by general paralytics. *Lancet*, **2**, 1071–3
83. Kopp, I. and Solomon, H. C. (1943). Liver function in therapeutic malaria. *Am. J. Med. Sci.*, **205**, 90–7
84. Kern, R. A. and Norris, R. F. (1944). Liver involvement in malaria. *US Naval Med. Bull., Washington*, **43**, 847–58
85. Mirsky, I. A., Brecht, R. von and Williams, L. D. (1944). Hepatic dysfunction in malaria. *Science*, **99**, 20–1
86. Fredricks, M. G. and Hoffbauer, F. W. (1945). A study of hepatic function in therapeutic malaria. *J. Am. Med. Assoc.*, **128**, 495–9
87. Lipincott, S. W., Ellerbrook, L. D., Hesselbrock, W. B., Gordon, H. H., Gottleib, L. and Marble, A. (1945). Liver function tests in chronic relapsing vivax malaria. *J. Clin. Invest.*, **24**, 616–22
88. Carter, A. B. and MacLagan, N. F. (1946). Some observations in liver function tests in diseases not primarily hepatic. *Br. Med. J.*, **2**, 80–2
89. von Fuhrmann, G. and Peltzer, F. (1959). Messung von enzym-activität bei einem fall von cerebraler malaria tropica. *Zeit. Tropenmed. Parasitol.*, **10**, 375–8
90. von Fuhrmann, G. (1962). Serumproteine und serumenzyme bei einigen tropischen erkrankungen. *Zeit. Tropenmed. Parasitol.*, **13**, 53–67

91. Sadun, E. H., Williams, J. S. and Martin, L. K. (1966). Serum biochemical changes in malarial infections in men, chimpanzees and mice. *Military Med.*, **131**, 1094–1106
92. Kapila, M., Lee, S. H., Gray, W. and Robson, A. (1982). Fatal falciparum malaria and the availability of parenteral antimalarial drugs in hospitals. *Br. Med. J.*, **284**, 1547–8
93. Edington, G. M. and Gilles, H. M. (1976). *Pathology in the Tropics*, 2nd edn, pp. 27–28 and 556. (London: Arnold)
94. Patwari, A., Aneja, S., Berry, A. M. and Ghosh, S. (1979). Hepatic dysfunction in childhood malaria. *Arch. Dis. Child.*, **54**, 139–41
95. Black, R. H. (1954). Enlargement of the liver due to malaria in natives of the south-west Pacific area. *Trans. R. Soc. Trop. Med. Hyg.*, **48**, 226–33
96. Walters, J. H. and Waterlow, J. C. (1954). Fibrosis of the liver in West African children. *Spec. Rep. Ser. Med. Res. Coun., London*, no. 285, p. 71
97. Hughes, S. B. and Bomford, R. R. (1944). Clinical features and treatment of malaria in British troops in west Africa. *Br. Med. J.*, **1**, 69–73
98. Phillips, R. E., Looareesuwan, S., Warrell, D. A., Lee, S. H., Karbwang, J., Warrell, M. J., White, N. J., Swasdichai, C. and Weatherall, D. J. (1986). The importance of anaemia in cerebral and uncomplicated falciparum malaria: role of complications, dyserythropoiesis and iron sequestration. *Quart. J. Med.*, **58**, 305–23
99. Molyneux, M. E., Looareesuwan, S., Menzies, I. S., Grainger, S. L., Phillips, R. E., Wattanagoon, Y., Thompson, R. P. H. and Warrell, D. A. (1989). Reduced hepatic blood flow and intestinal malabsorption in severe falciparum malaria. *Am. J. Trop. Med. Hyg.*, **40**, 470–6
100. Larrey, D., Castot, A., Pessayre, D., Merigot, P., Machayekhy, J.-P., Feldmann, G., Lenoir, A., Rueff, B. and Benhamou, J.-P. (1986). Amodiaquine-induced hepatitis: a report of seven cases. *Ann. Intern. Med.*, **104**, 801–3
101. Neftel, K. A., Woodtly, W., Schmid, M., Frick, P. G. and Fehr, J. (1986). Amodiaquine induced agranulocytosis and liver damage. *Br. Med. J.*, **292**, 721–3
102. Reisinger, E. C., Horstmann, R. D. and Dietrich, M. (1989). Tolerance of mefloquine alone and in combination with sulfadoxine-pyrimethamine in the prophylaxis of malaria. *Trans. R. Soc. Trop. Med. Hyg.*, **83**, 474–7
103. Mihaly, G. W., Date, N. M., Ireton, H. J. C. and Smallwood, R. A. (1987). The effect of malaria infection on primaquine elimination in the isolated perfused rat liver. *Biochem. Pharmacol.*, **36**, 225–8

15
The liver in leishmaniasis

A. D. M. BRYCESON

Leishmania donovani, and the closely related parasites of the complex that causes visceral leishmaniais (VL) may infect the liver. The parasite is transmitted by sandflies, from canine, rodent or human reservoirs, in four main zoogeographical zones which cover a large part of the tropics and subtropics in Europe, the Middle East, Asia and the Americas.

Most infections with *L. donovani* are subclinical. Epidemiological studies have suggested that for every clinical case of visceral leishmaniasis there may be 10 subclinical cases in Italy[1], and 30 in Kenya[2].

During an epidemic of VL in Italy, Pampiglione *et al.*[3] identified six individuals with a mild fleeting febrile illness that was associated with transient seropositivity and conversion to leishmanin positivity. In all six, liver biopsy revealed epithelioid cell granulomas, in one of which leishmania were identified (Figure 1). Thus in these patients the liver was the site of infection that healed spontaneously as a result of efficient cell-mediated immunity (CMI). In one patient persisting seropositivity over a 21-month period suggested persistent infection that might later produce clinical disease. More recently, in Brazil, it has been shown that malnutrition is important in determining whether disease will develop in subclinical seropositive children[4].

Not all infections with *L. infantum*, the Mediterranean parasite, reach the liver. In adults especially many infections produce typical self-healing sores of cutaneous leishmaniasis[5].

In those individuals who develop the syndrome of VL, however, the liver is more extensively infected, as part of the widespread parasitization of the reticuloendothelial system (RES), which reflects the failure or suppression of specific CMI. Interestingly, this failure is usually temporary, and over 70% of patients acquire CMI, as shown by lymphocyte transformation studies and leishmanin skin testing, within a few weeks of recovery from the disease[6]. In patients with established VL, liver biopsy classically shows marked hyperplasia and hypertrophy of Kupffer cells, which push out into the sinusoids (Figure 2). Many of the Kupffer cells are parasitized, with up to 10 amastigotes per cell. In early cases this endothelial proliferation is focal, but

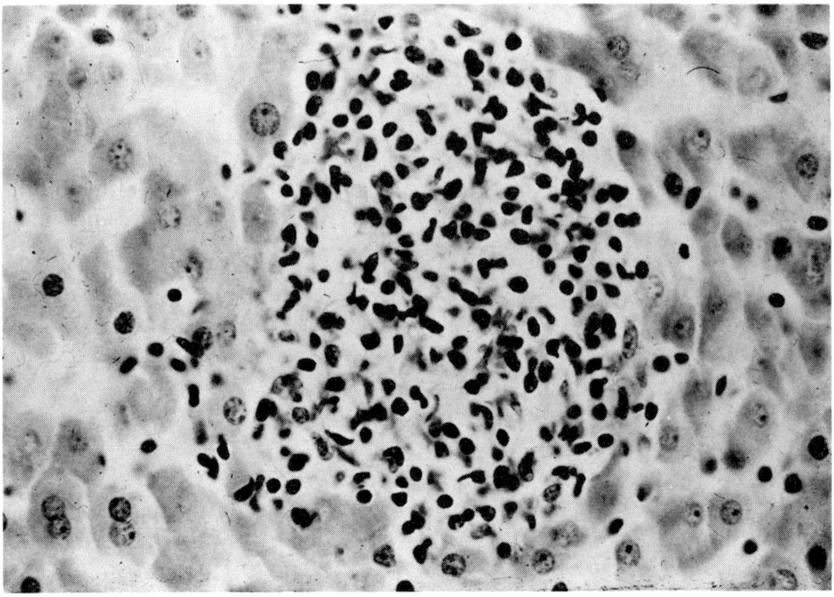

Figure 1 Granuloma in the liver of a case of self-healing, 'subclinical' leishmaniasis from Italy, comprising lymphocytes, histiocytes and a few epithelioid cells. (H&E ×600; courtesy of Professor Pampiglione)

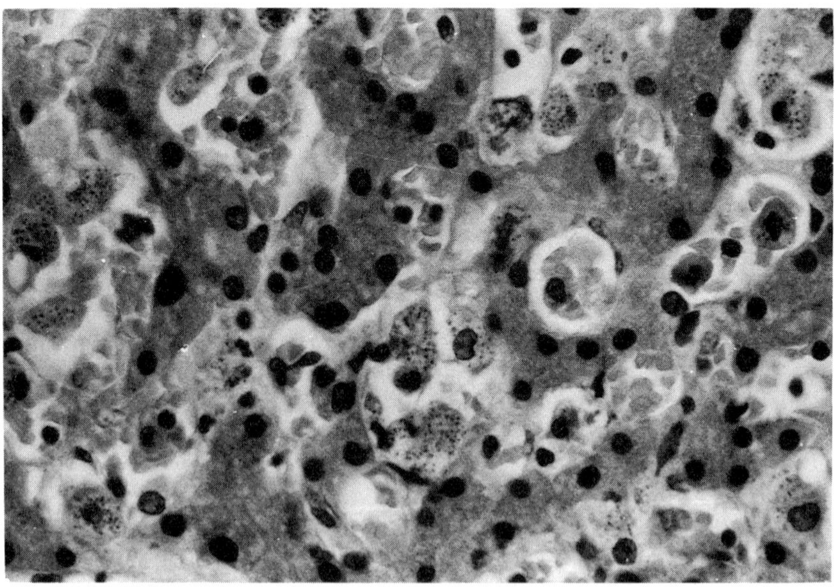

Figure 2 Classical pattern of liver in visceral leishmaniasis. Hypertrophy and hyperplasia of Kupffer cells, most of them parasitized, and which push out into the sinusoids. (H&E ×525; courtesy of Professor C. E. P. Corbett)

later extends throughout the sinusoids and sometimes to the centrilobular veins. In experimentally infected hamsters and monkeys (*Pithecus irus*) this proliferation may also extend to the portal veins, and the hyperplasia may be so intense that the sinusoids seem to be occluded and the cords of liver cells compressed into thin strands[7]. At this stage, in the hamster, hepatocytes are parasitized and show fatty degeneration; but in man hepatocytes are seldom seen to contain parasites. Usually hepatocytes appear healthy; but if venous congestion is severe there may be some atrophy, fatty change and occasional necrosis of groups or individual cells[8]. Parasitized histiocytes are also seen in the portal tracts. This classical pattern is also seen in patients with AIDS who develop VL[9] (Figure 3).

When parasites are numerous they are readily seen in sections stained routinely with haematoxylin and eosin. When scanty, immunoperoxidase is useful. Almost as common as the classical pattern, at least in Brazil, is a nodular pattern in which discrete granulomas are found in the lobules and the portal tracts, containing macrophages, lymphocytes and plasma cells, but without epitheloid cell differentiation[10] (Figure 4). Parasites are scanty and hepatocytes normal. Most common in Duarte and Corbett's series were cases showing a fibrogenic pattern characterized by intralobular proliferation of reticulin fibres and deposition of collagen bands, which in about half the cases led to multifocal perisinusoidal fibrosis. Lobular architecture, however was preserved. Only a few Kupffer cells and histiocytes are parasitised (Figure 5). Cases have been reported in which parasites could not be found, until the spleen was examined[8]. Presumably these variations reflect differing

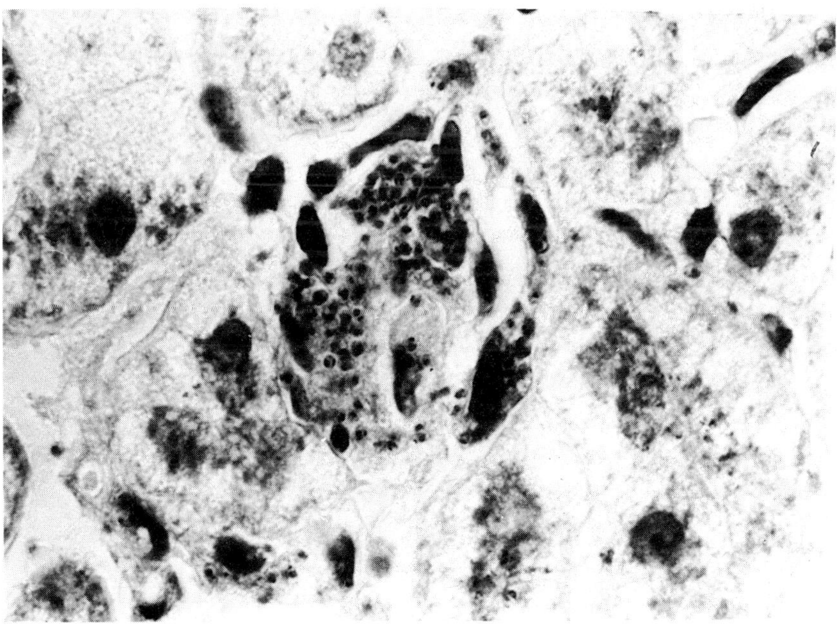

Figure 3 Kupffer cells, heavily parasitized with *Leishmania*, in the liver biopsy of a patient with AIDS. (Giemsa ×800; courtesy of Dr S. Falk)

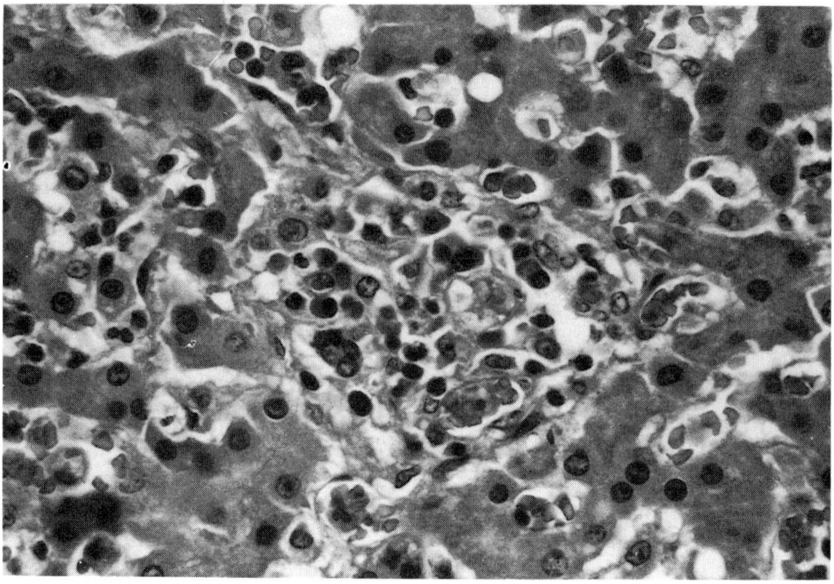

Figure 4 Nodular pattern in liver in visceral leishmaniasis. Collections of lymphocytes and plasma cells and macrophages without epithelial cell differentiation. Parasites are scanty (H&E × 520; courtesy of Profesor C. E. P.Corbett)

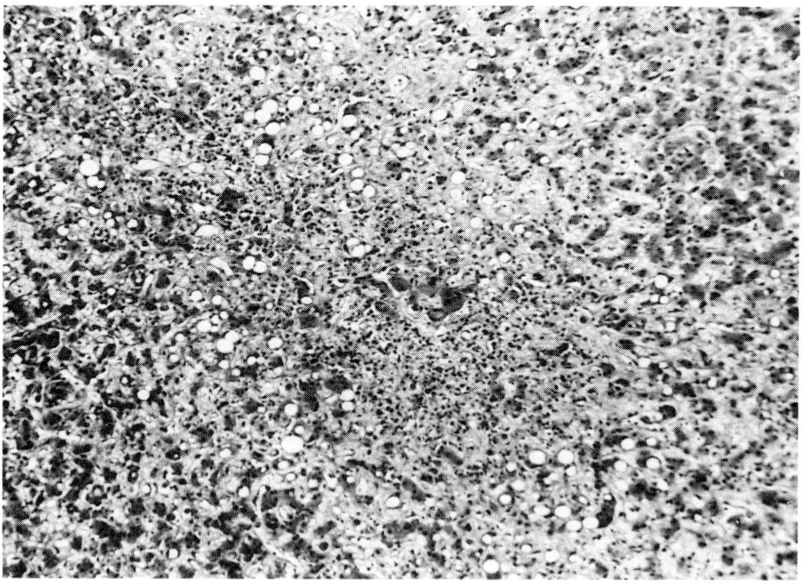

Figure 5 Diffuse introlobular fibrosis of the liver, showing bands of collagen tissue isolating small groups of liver cells. (H&E × 105; courtesy of Professor C. E. P. Corbett)

degrees of immune response, but no formal comparative study has been undertaken. In strains of inbred mice, however, liver histology clearly reflects a genetically determined immune response. Mice with no CMI show the classical pattern, while mice with CMI mount a necrotic response that destroys parasitized Kupffer cells and hepatocytes alike[12]. Moreno *et al.*[11] reported the appearance of fibrin ring granulomas in three patients of VL (Figure 6). The rings resembled those seen in Q fever and allopurinol hepatitis.

Finally, for the histopathologist, does VL cause any permanent liver damage? In 1908 Leonard Rogers, then Professor of Pathology at the Calcutta School of Tropical Medicine, described a 'peculiar intralobular cirrhosis of the liver produced by the protozoal parasite of kala azar'. He noted that it occurred only in very chronic cases, that had suffered from the disease for several years. The liver was smooth, unlike the usual hobnail cirrhosis. The fibrous tissue ran throughout the lobule parallel to and separating the columns of liver cells. The arrangement of the lobules themselves was unaltered, and there was very little proliferation of bile ducts. In the fibrous bands were seen lymphocytes and some epithelioid cells that might contain parasites. Ultimately liver cells atrophied and the patient developed ascites. In later series from India[21] this complication was seen less often, possibly because such chronic cases were less common and treatment had become available. But it has been described also by Duarte and Corbett from Brazil[10] and Daneshbod from Iran[22], and is probably a genuine, if nowadays rare, complication.

Certainly histopathologists need to understand the pathological processes

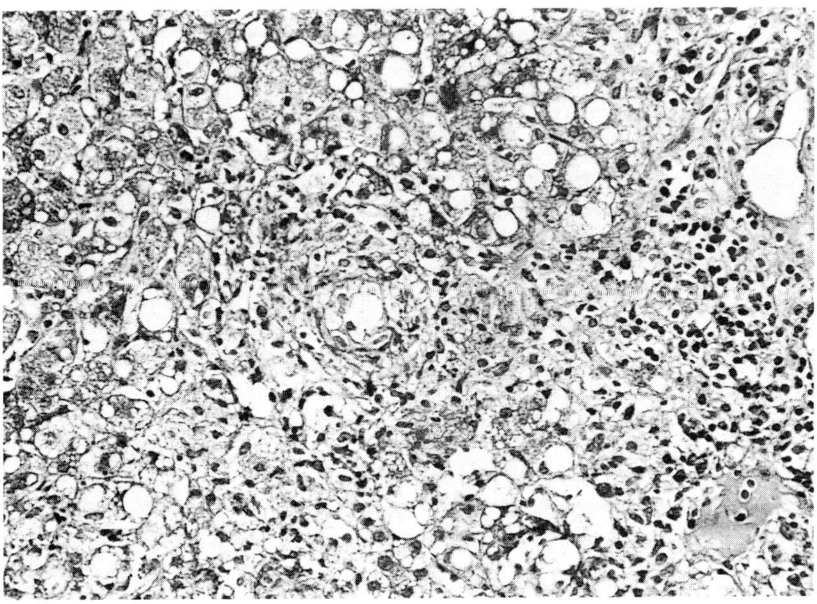

Figure 6 Hepatic granuloma with central vacuole and fibrinoid ring in a patient with visceral leishmaniasis. (H&E ×250; courtesy of Dr A. Moreno)

of the disease if they are to diagnose the disease correctly from biopsy specimens. These processes, as they affect the liver, may be summarized.

1. parasitization of the reticuloendothelial cells;
2. variable control of parasitization by ? CMI;
3. interstitial inflammation that may lead to fibrosis.

The clinical syndrome of VL comprises fever, hepatosplenomegaly, pancytopenia, hyperglobulinaemia (especially polyclonal IgG) and the production of a wide range of autoantibodies and immune complexes[13]. Nevertheless, and despite the massive parasitization of the reticuloendothelial system, most organs of the body continue to work well. The bone marrow is hyperplastic, but there may be maturation arrest and a negligible reticulocytosis. Renal biopsy has been performed in a few cases and shows mesangial thickening and proliferation of glomerular epithelial cells, and occasionally thickening of Bowman's membrane, with deposition of globulin and complement, but renal function is seldom impaired and albuminuria is rare. The submucosa of the small bowel, especially jejunum, is thickened and infiltrated with parasitized histiocytes, and in a few cases malabsorption of xylose and vitamin A has been demonstrated[14]. Pulmonary function has never been measured, but cough is common and histology shows an interstitial alveolitis[15] which is further evidence for Duarte and Corbett's concept of visceral leishmaniasis as an interstitial disease[10].

With regard to liver function, in a biochemical sense, the literature is confusing. Many series report abnormal tests, but not all have been controlled and the role of local endemic diseases such as hepatitis, malaria and schistosomiasis has not been considered. In Assam, however, Goswami[16] could find no additional cause for the modest elevation of serum bilirubin and alkaline phosphatase in half his adult patients with chronic kala-azar, with median duration of illness of 2–3 years. In a recent prospective study in Kenyan children, however, liver function was remarkably well preserved (Table 1). AST levels did not differ from those of 267 controls, and ALT levels were only minimally elevated. Prothrombin time was normal. Serum albumin levels were consistently low, but it is not known whether this results from defective synthesis or leakage from the gut lesion. Albumin levels return to normal within 2–3 weeks of starting treatment. Certainly globulin synthesis is increased. Bleeding is listed as a complication of VL, but on the rare occasions when prothrombin time has been measured and found to be prolonged, it has not been established whether the deficiency is nutritional, or due to malabsorption or to liver dysfunction. Jaundice is reported in 5–24% in different series, but its aetiology has not been investigated. In a

Table 1 Liver function in Kenyan visceral leishmaniasis

Laboratory test	*30 patients*	*267 controls*
Albumin (g/dl)	24 ± 4	42 ± 5
Globulin (g/dl)	35 ± 6	28 ± 4
Prothrombin (s)	13.5 (10–15)	13 (12–14)
Alanine transferase	35 (30–50)	24 (10–30)
Aspartate transferase	16 (10–30)	14 (5–25)

personal series of 95 patients with VL in Kenya, two became jaundiced and in each case it was due to intercurrent hepatitis B infection.

The diagnosis of VL rests on demonstrating the parasite. Most commonly this is achieved through aspiration of bone marrow, although splenic aspiration is more efficient, especially in early cases. Aspiration of the liver reveals parasites in 75–85% of cases[17]. The technique is simple and safe[18] and the specimen is examined by direct microscopy. If possible it should also be cultured. Aspiration is probably more efficient at detecting parasites than is biopsy or histology. If liver biopsy is performed a small part of the unfixed specimen should be set aside for parasitological examination.

Pentavalent antimonials remain the treatment of choice for VL. In the conventional dose of 10–20 mg Sb/kg body weight daily there is little or no toxicity. In some patients there is a modest induction of liver enzymes, which resolves spontaneously during or after treatment. When the drug is used at a higher dosage because of partial antimonial resistance, AST and ALT may rise to four or five times the normal value, but it is rarely necessary to withhold treatment[19]. Occasionally the physician becomes anxious and withholds treatment for a day or two (Figure 7). The most efficient treatment for antimony resistance is probably a pentavalent antimonial plus allopurinol. In Kenya, in children, no hepatotoxicity was noticed in five patients treated with this regimen[20] but I have noted rapidly rising enzymes in two out of

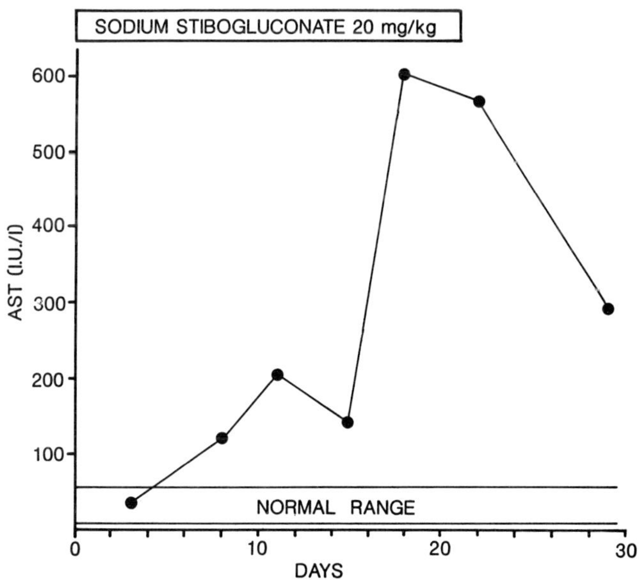

Figure 7 Serum levels of aspartate transaminase in treatment with sodium stibgluconate 20 mg Sb/kg body weight daily.

four European adults so treated. Patients with AIDS and VL may well need this regimen, and physicians should be alert to the possibility of hepatotoxicity.

VL is emerging as an AIDS disease[23], especially in southern Europe, but cases are being discovered with increasing frequency in non-endemic countries. Clinicians and pathologists need to be aware of its manifestations.

Acknowledgements

Professor C. E. P. Corbett, Dr A. Moreno, Professor S. Pampiglione and Dr S. Falk kindly provided illustrations. Permission to publish was granted by the editors of *Transactions of the Royal Society of Tropical Medicine and Hygiene* (Figure 1), *Revista do Instituto de Medicine Tropical de S. Paulo* (Figures 2, 4, 5, 6) and *Pathology Research and Practice* (Figure 3).

References

1. Pampiglione, S., Manson-Bahr, P. E. C., La Placa, M., Borgatti, M. A. and Musumeci, S. (1975). Studies in Mediterranean leishmaniasis. 3. The leishmanin test in kala-azar. *Trans. R. Soc. Trop. Med. Hyg.*, **69**, 60–8
2. Ho, M., Siongok, T. K., Lyerly, W. H. and Smith, D. H. (1982). Prevalence and disease spectrum in a new focus of visceral leishmaniasis in Kenya. *Trans. R. Soc. Trop. Med. Hyg.*, **76**, 741–5
3. Pampiglione, S., Manson-Bahr, P. E. C., Giungi, G., Giunti, A., Parenti, A. and Canestri Trotti, G. (1974). Studies in Mediterranean leishmaniasis 2. Asymptomatic cases of visceral leishmaniasis. *Trans. R. Soc. Trop. Med. Hyg.*, **68**, 447–53
4. Cerf, B. J., Jones, T. C., Badero, R., Sampaio, D., Teixcera, R. and Johnson, W. D. Jr (1987). Malnutrition a risk factor for severe visceral leishmaniasis. *J. Infect. Dis.*, **156**, 1030–3
5. Rioux, J. A., Lanotte, G., Maazoun, R. and Perello Pratlong, F. (1980). *Leishmania infantum* Nicolle, 1908, agent du bouton d'Orient antochtone. A propos l'identification biochemique de 2 souches isolees dans les Pyrenees-Orientales. *C.R. Acad. Sci., Paris*, **291**, 701–3
6. Ho, M., Koech, Iha, D. W. and Bryceson, A. D. M. (1983). Immuno-suppression in Kenyan visceral leishmaniasis. *Clin. Exp. Immunol.*, **51**, 207–14
7. Meleney, H. E. (1925). The histopathology of kala-azar in the hamster, monkey and man. *Am. J. Pathol.*, **1**, 147–68
8. Veress, B., Malik, M. O. A., Satir, A. A., and El Hassan, M. M. (1974). Morphological observations on visceral leishmaniasis in the Sudan. *Trop. Geogr. Med.*, **26**, 198–203
9. Falk, S., Helm, E. B., Hubner, K. and Stutte, H. J. (1988). Disseminated visceral leishmaniasis (kala azar) in acquired immunodeficiency syndrome (AIDS). *Pathol. Res. Pract.*, **183**, 253–5
10. Duarte, M. I. S. and Corbett, C. E. P. (1987). Histopathological patterns of the liver involvement in visceral leishmaniasis. *Rev. Inst. Med. Trop. Sao Paulo*, **29**, 131–6
11. Moreno, A., Marazuela, M., Yerba, M., Hernandez, M. J., Hellin, C. and Vargas, J. A. (1988). Hepatic fibrin ring granulomas in visceral leishmaniasis. *Gastroenterology*, **95**, 1123–6
12. Bradley, D. J. and Kirkley, J. (1977). Regulation of *Leishmania* populations with the host. 1. The variable course of *Leishmania donovani* infections in mice. *Clin. Exp. Immunol.*, **30**, 119–29
13. Pearson, R. D., de Alencar, J. E., Romito, R., Naidu, T. G., Young, A. C. and Davis IV, J. S. (1983). Circulating immune complexes and rheumatoid factors in visceral leishmaniasis. *J. Infect. Dis.*, **147**, 1102
14. Muigai, R., Gatei, D. G., Shaunak, S., Wozniak, A. and Bryceson, A. D. M. (1983). Jejunal

function and pathology in visceral leishmaniasis. *Lancet*, **2**, 476–9
15. Duarte, M. I. S., da Matta, V. L. R., Corbett, C. E. P., Laurenti, M. D., Chebabo, R. and Goto, H. (1989). Interstitial pneumonitis in human visceral leishmaniasis. *Trans. R. Soc. Trop. Med. Hyg.*, **83**, 73–6
16. Goswami, B. M. (1970). A study of cirrhosis of the liver due to chronic kala-azar. *J. Indian Med. Assoc.*, **54**, 315–20
17. Ho, E. A., Suong, T.-H. and Li, Y. (1948). Comparative merits of sternum, spleen and liver puncture in the study of human visceral leishmaniasis. *Trans. R. Soc. Trop. Med. Hyg.*, **41**, 629–36
18. Chulay, J. D. and Bryceson, A. D. M. (1983). Quantitation of amastigotes of *Leishmania donovani* in smears of splenic aspirates from patients with visceral leishmaniasis. *Am. J. Trop. Med. Hyg.*, **32**, 475–9
19. Chulay, J. D., Anzeze, E. M., Koech, D. K. and Bryceson, A. D. M. (1983). High-dose sodium stibogluconate treatment of cutaneous leishmaniasis in Kenya. *Trans. R. Soc. Trop. Med. Hyg.*, **77**, 717–21
20. Chunge, C. N., Gachini, G., Muigai, R., Wasunna, K., Rashid, J. R., Chulay, J. D., Anabwani, G., Oster, C. N. and Bryceson, A. D. M. (1985). Visceral leishmaniasis unresponsive to antimonial drugs. III. Successful treatment using a combination of sodium stibogluconate plus allopurinol. *Trans. R. Soc. Trop. Med. Hyg.*, **79**, 715–18
21. Sen Gupta, P. C., Chakravaty, N. K., Ray, H. N. and Das Gupta, B. (1956). The liver in kala-azar. *Ann. Trop. Med. Parasitol.*, **50**, 252–9
22. Daneshbod, K. (1972). Visceral leishmaniasis (kala-azar) in Iran: a pathologic and electron microscopic study. *Am. J. Clin. Pathol.*, **57**, 157–66
23. Smith, D., Gazzard, B., Lindley, R. P., Darwish, A., Reed, C., Bryceson, A. D. M. and Evans, D. A. (1989). Visceral leishmaniasis (kala azar) in a patient with AIDS. *AIDS*, **3**, 41–3

16
The liver in schistosomiasis

K. S. WARREN

INTRODUCTION

Schistosomiasis mansoni and japonica are part of the small group of infectious diseases that specifically involve the liver. It includes the liver flukes, hydatid cysts, amoebic liver abscess and the viral hepatitides. Yellow fever and leptospirosis, while often associated with jaundice, are multisystem diseases. A study of schistosomiasis requires a multidisciplinary approach focusing on hepatology and infectious disease; it also includes a major involvement with immunology and epidemiology.

An editorial entitled 'Schistomosiasis' in *Hepatology*, in 1984[1] bemoaned the fact that hepatologists have tended to neglect this often mispronounced disease – in the above case the miscreant being the redoubtable Henry Kissinger. The major thrust of the article was not that schistosomiasis is an infection of 100 million people, and a major national health problem in China, Egypt and Brazil, but that it provides a unique model for the understanding of several crucial aspects of liver disease including portal hypertension, portal-systemic encephalopathy, immunopathogenesis and fibrosis. In the area of infectious diseases, schistosomiasis has been the principal model in modern times for infectious agents which do not multiply within their hosts, for the study of the mechanisms of immunity and for the elucidation of the role of that 'enigmatic cell', the eosinophil.

Let me begin with the nuts and bolts of schistosomiasis as an infectious disease and a liver disease. This will be followed by a more detailed discussion of schistosomiasis as a model.

GEOGRAPHICAL DISTRIBUTION AND EPIDEMIOLOGY

Globally, 200 million people are infected with schistosomes. Of these about two-thirds carry the flukes, *Schistosoma mansoni* and *S. japonicum*, which reside in the portal and mesenteric venous systems of the gut. Two of the most populous countries in Africa, Egypt and Nigeria, and the largest country in Latin America, Brazil, consider schistosomiasis mansoni to be one of their principal health problems, as does China for schistosomiasis japonica. *S. mansoni* is endemic in parts of the Middle East and in most countries of Africa south of the Sahara. In the New World the infection is of significance in the Caribbean islands of Puerto Rico, Dominican Republic, Guadeloupe, Martinique and St Lucia; in South America it is endemic in Venezuela, Surinam and Brazil. *S. japonicum* is prevalent in China, the Philippines and Sulawesi in Indonesia; it has virtually died out in Japan. Other relatively rare schistosomes which involve the liver are *S. intercalatum* which occurs in parts of West Africa and *S. mekongi* (a *japonicum*-like organism) which is found sporadically in parts of Southeast Asia[2].

Schistosomiasis mansoni occurs almost exclusively in man, while schistosomiasis japonica is a zoonosis which involves many domestic and wild animals, the principal reservoirs being cattle and rats. The freshwater snail intermediate hosts of *S. mansoni* (*Biomphalaria* species) are aquatic while those of *S. japonicum* (*Oncomelania*) are amphibious. It is worthy of note that the schistosomes induce a highly fatal form of liver disease in their snail hosts. The larval form contained in the schistosome eggs excreted in human faeces hatches in fresh water and seeks and penetrates into its snail host where its final habitat is the 'hepatopancreas'. The organism then undergoes multiplication into thousands of cercariae which essentially destroy that vital organ, leading to high mortality.

Transmission is often seasonal and varies with the ecology. Infection is largely confined to certain times of the day; the infective forms of *S. mansoni* (cercariae) are shed by snails in large numbers between noon and 2 p.m.; *S. japonicum* cercariae are shed in small numbers in the evening; both survive under natural conditions for only a few hours.

In contrast to the snail, the stages of the human schistosomes in the human definitive host do not replicate. The adult male and female worms, each developing from a single invasive cercaria, have a mean lifespan of approximately 5 years. Worm burdens build up if there is repeated exposure to water containing the infected larvae. With respect to intensity of infection (the number of worms carried by the host) a peak is reached in the teens, from which it falls drastically thereafter. This change appears to be related largely to a decrease in exposure to infected water, but also may be associated with some degree of immunity occurring after prolonged infection. The distribution of schistosomes within the definitive hosts is overdispersed with only a small percentage – often less than 10% – of infected individuals carrying heavy worm burdens. Disease, as manifested by hepatomegaly and splenomegaly, is largely seen in those with heavy infections[3].

LIFE CYCLE

The schistosomes are called digenetic trematodes because their life cycle includes an asexual phase in freshwater snail 'intermediate hosts' and a sexual phase in mammalian 'definitive hosts', including man.

Parasite eggs passed in the faeces of the definitive host hatch in fresh water into ciliated miracidia which penetrate into specific species of snails. Within the snail they undergo several developmental stages multiplying asexually into thousands of tailed, free-swimming cercariae which escape the snail into water. Schistosome cercariae penetrate the skin of the definitive host directly, those of *S. mansoni* doing so in 5–10 min and those of *S. japonicum* as rapidly as 1 min.

Within the definitive host the schistosomes migrate from the skin to the lungs and thence to the portal venules where they develop into adult male and female worms, 10–30 mm in length. The paired worms then migrate to the mesenteric venules where they produce between 300 and 3000 eggs daily. Approximately half of these eggs pass through the intestinal mucosa and are excreted in the faeces.

CLINICAL FEATURES

Chronic schistosomiasis mansoni[4,5] and japonica[6] have been associated with a variety of systemic symptoms including weakness, abdominal pain and diarrhoea. Extensive field studies have revealed that these symptoms tend to be seen only in the small proportion of individuals with heavy infections. This was corroborated by investigations of a large number of patients seen over a period of years at a hospital for tropical diseases in the United Kingdom.

Hepatomegaly, and particularly splenomegaly, is also seen largely in those with heavy infections. Both organs are firm to hard in texture and non-tender. Many cases are detected incidentally on physical examination, or following an episode of haematemesis. Since the liver parenchyma is not involved in the pathogenic process, jaundice and the stigmata of chronic liver disease are not seen. Liver function tests are usually within or close to normal limits. Schistosomiasis occurs in many parts of the world where hepatitis is rife. Thus, patients with this parasitic infection and evidence of liver parenchymal dysfunction are often seen, but a synergistic interaction between the two infections has been demonstrated only in experimentally infected mice.

Patients with splenomegaly may show anaemia, leukopenia and thrombocytopenia. Eosinophilia is often observed in schistosome infections as in other helminth infections. Oesophageal varices are frequently found in those with splenomegaly. Haematemesis may occur erratically or fairly frequently. In those with pure hepatosplenic schistosomiasis portal-systemic encephalopathy is not observed during bleeding episodes.

Clinical manifestations of schistosomiasis may occur in the acute stages of infection and are useful for later diagnostic purposes. These include swimmer's itch, a maculopapular, pruritic rash following penetration of the skin by cercariae. It appears to be a sensitization phenomenon and occurs most frequently following infection by avian schistosomes. When there is a heavy primary infection, acute schistosomiasis or Katayama fever may be seen several weeks following exposure. This appears to be a serum sickness-like reaction with fever, hepatosplenomegaly, lymphadenopathy and eosinophilia.

Complications of hepatosplenic schistosomiasis include chronic salmonellosis, pulmonary schistosomiasis and cor pulmonale, glomerular involvement and nephrosis, and central nervous system disease. Susceptibility to *Salmonella* appears to occur in infection with all species of human schistosome. Clinical pulmonary disease is seen only after hepatosplenic schistosomiasis results in collateral circulation carrying schistosome eggs to the pulmonary arterioles. This results in granuloma formation and fibrosis which block blood flow and lead to cor pulmonale. Central nervous system involvement is rare. In the case of schistosomiasis mansoni the lower spinal cord is the site of granulomatous lesions leading to the development of paraplegia. In *S. japonicum* infection the cerebrum is the site of the lesions, resulting in focal seizures or generalized encephalopathy.

PATHOLOGY

The human liver in advanced hepatosplenic schistosomiasis has been described as follows:

> Pipestem fibrosis is the only human liver disease directly attributable to schistosome infection. Its precursor stages, observed incidentally at autopsy and in experimental infections of chimpanzees, begin with diffuse inflammatory infiltration around portal radicles proximal to pre-sinusoidal vessels containing egg granulomas. Next, the effected triads become fibrotic and enlarged. First, smaller, then larger portal vein branches become blocked by granulomas and disrupted by inflammation and fibrosis, or by organizing thrombi. Eggs and egg granulomas accumulate around these blockage sites, further contributing to portal enlargement. Simultaneously, the hepatic arteries enlarge and send out neovascular branches. Some portal vessels become dilated to angiomatoid proportions. Kupffer cells become prominent and pigment-laden but the liver parenchyma preserves its lobular and trabecular architecture showing only scattered and mild hepatocytic damage. In full blown schistosomal liver fibrosis the enlarged, whitish, fibrous triads surrounding portal vein lumina resemble the cross-sections of clay pipestems. The parenchyma between portal fields lacks the nodularity seen in Laennec's cirrhosis[7].

The spleen may become grossly enlarged and is firm in consistency, fibrotic and congested. It may be associated with hypersplenism accompanied by anaemia and pancytopenia.

DIAGNOSIS

Diagnosis of schistosomiasis must be done in terms of both the infection and the disease. Most cases of the infection do not manifest overt disease because of the overdispersed distribution of the parasite in the host, with the great majority of individuals having low-intensity infections. Conversely, it is possible to have the disease without the infection. This is because hepatosplenic disease usually takes one to two decades to develop while the mean lifespan of the worms is less than 5 years.

In endemic areas the prevalence of schistosomiasis can vary from a low to a very high percentage of the population. Intensity usually varies with prevalence. In non-endemic areas a key factor in the diagnosis is the physician's suspicion based on travel to or immigration from an endemic area. Other grounds for suspicion are eosinophilia suggesting a helminth infection, hepatomegaly, splenomegaly or, in the most extreme case, haematemesis. A geographical history is of great importance, not only in terms of which country but where in the country. Exposure to fresh water is essential; schistosomiasis is not transmitted in salt water or in chlorinated swimming pools. If both the geographical history and significant water contact are positive, a definitive diagnosis can be made by demonstration of eggs in the patient's faeces.

The best technique for doing this is the Kato thick smear, which is itself a form of concentrating faeces. A 500 mg sample of faeces that has been pressed through 105-mesh stainless steel bolting cloth is placed on a glass slide and covered with a cellophane coverslip impregnated with 50% glycerine. The slides are inverted and pressed onto a bed of filter paper, turned face up and left for a period of 24 h, during which time the faecal matter clears. For more rapid diagnosis it should be noted that a 20 mg faecal sample will clear in 15 min[8]. Although the embryo within the egg clears, the characteristic shape of the egg shell can easily be seen, and the eggs in the sample can be counted. Multiplication of the 50 mg sample by 20 gives the number of eggs per gram of faeces. Patients with less than 100 eggs/gram are considered to have light infections, those with counts between 100 and 400, moderate infections, and those with counts greater than 400, heavy infections.

A wide variety of immunological tests, both serological and intradermal, have been used. While many of them are highly sensitive they are not quantitative and suffer from frequent false-positive reactions. If eggs cannot be detected in the faeces, the intensity of infection is so low that it is unlikely to contribute to disease, the one exception being schistosomiasis of the central nervous system.

With respect to disease, liver enlargement may be observed in acute schistosomiasis 3–6 weeks after primary exposure, along with fever, lymphadenopathy and splenomegaly. This is essentially a transient syndrome, although occasionally it is fatal. Eggs may not be found in the faeces until 2 or 3 weeks after onset. In chronic schistosomal disease the liver is enlarged, smooth, firm and non-tender. As the disease progresses the spleen enlarges, in some cases extending well below the umbilicus, and is very firm in texture. It may be associated with a dragging sensation. Jaundice, emaciation, and stigmata of liver parenchymal damage are not present. Liver function tests including bilirubin, enzymes, serum proteins and even sensitive procedures such as bromsulphalein retention tend to be within normal limits. Needle biopsies of the liver are rarely diagnostic because of the focal nature of the lesions. Recently, it has been found that ultrasonography provides a very sensitive and virtually specific means of diagnosing pipestem fibrosis, revealing thickened fibrosed portal tracts and narrowed portal blood vessels[9]. This method can also determine the patency of the portal, splenic and superior mesenteric vessels. Another means of studying these vessels is by splenoportography. The presence of oesophageal varices can be determined by barium swallow and oesophagoscopy.

Differential diagnosis of hepatosplenic schistosomiasis includes portal vein thrombosis and rare granulomatous diseases of the liver such as sarcoidosis. A syndrome known as decompensated hepatosplenic schistosomiasis has been seen in endemic areas. These patients, infected with schistosomes, demonstrate a picture similar to cirrhosis of the liver with jaundice, stigmata of liver parenchymal damage, and deranged liver function tests. Many of them are suffering primarily from other forms of liver disease while concurrently having schistosomiasis.

TREATMENT AND PROGNOSIS

Treatment has been greatly simplified by the development of an excellent non-toxic drug, praziquantel-125[10]. The recommended dose for *S. mansoni* infection is 20 mg/kg twice in 1 day, and for *S. japonicum* 20 mg/kg three times in 1 day. Cure rates are 66–97% for schistosomiasis mansoni and 71–99% for schistosomiasis japonica. In those in which cure is not achieved intensity of infection is almost invariably reduced by over 90%. There is a significant reversal of parasite-induced morbidity after treatment, enlarged livers and spleens tending to regress in size. Praziquantel therapy is well tolerated, the incidence of side-effects usually ranging from 10% to 15%. They include abdominal pain or discomfort, nausea, vomiting, anorexia, and diarrhoea. There may also be headache, vertigo and dizziness, plus fever, urticarial rash and lassitude. On the basis of praziquantel's effectiveness and lack of serious toxicity it is recommended that all patients with schistosomiasis, even those with light infections, be treated.

It may occasionally be necessary to resort to splenectomy to control hypersplenism, but this should not be done until after drug treatment to determine if there is amelioration of this syndrome. Bleeding oesophageal varices should be treated by standard means. It is important to realize that portal-systemic encephalopathy does not occur in patients with pure hepatosplenic schistosomiasis. Repeated bleeding episodes may require oesophagoscopal or surgical means of treating the varices. Portacaval shunting is associated with a high incidence of encephalopathy; splenorenal shunting procedures are preferable.

It is worthy of note that the development of schistosomal disease can be prevented by periodic chemotherapy aimed at keeping the intensity of infection low. There is even evidence, from one highly endemic area, that following a single treatment hepatosplenic disease does not occur. Furthermore, there is enormous activity going on in laboratories all over the world to develop vaccines for schistosomiasis. Many different protective antigens, including not only those on the surface of the parasites but structural proteins and a wide variety of enzymes, have been isolated and cloned.

PREVENTION AND CONTROL

Until recently the major method of control of schistosomiasis was the use of molluscicides to destroy the snail intermediate host. Another approach has been to provide water supplies and latrines as a means of reducing transmission. Use of the new highly effective, single-dose, non-toxic drug praziquantel is clearly the most cost-effective means of controlling infection; it is also highly effective in controlling disease by sharply reducing the intensity of infection. Treatment may be targeted to the most heavily infected segments of the population, thereby preventing the occurrence of hepatosplenic schistosomiasis at relatively low cost[11].

SCHISTOSOMIASIS AS A MODEL

Schistosomiasis has the great advantage of being amenable for study in both man and mouse, that most useful and versatile of all laboratory animals. Mice can serve as models for infection with both *S. mansoni* and *S. japonicum* and for their associated forms of liver disease. Large numbers of patients can be gathered with different levels of infection and different stages of the disease. Mice can be infected with known numbers of worms. They develop hepatomegaly, splenomegaly, portal hypertension and oesophageal varices. They develop typical granulomatous lesions and periportal fibrosis, both of which can be studied quantitatively. They can be examined with virtually all of the tools of pathology, physiology, biochemistry and immunology.

With respect to liver disease in general, schistosomiasis provides several models which elucidate pathogenesis. They include the relative role of portal-systemic collateral circulation and liver parenchymal damage, the crucial role of the host immunological response, and the mechanisms of inflammation and liver fibrosis. Schistosomiasis has also been a model for helminth infections. These infectious agents do not replicate within the human host, a fact which has profound implications for the occurrence of disease. It also has been a model for research on eosinophilia, and the role of the eosinophil in immunity and disease.

The major disease syndrome associated with schistosome infections, both mansoni and japonicum, is hepatosplenic schistosomiasis. Most of these patients come to attention because of bleeding oesophageal varices. In spite of hepatomegaly, splenomegaly, portal hypertension and oesophageal varices they are usually in good health with none of the stigmata of chronic liver disease and virtually normal liver function tests. In the presence of severe periportal fibrosis their liver parenchymal cells are essentially normal in appearance and function. It is of particular interest, therefore, that when there is a severe haematemesis the patients do not develop hepatic coma. As a measure of the absorption and metabolism of blood products from the intestines, their arterial ammonia levels are within normal limits. Following portacaval shunt to prevent further haematemesis liver function drastically declines and the patients become susceptible to portal-systemic encephalopathy[12].

Schistosomiasis is an immunological disease. Its pathogenesis is related to the production of large numbers of eggs by the worm pairs situated in the mesenteric venules. Approximately half of these eggs break loose in the blood vessels and become sieved out in the presinusoidal portal venules where they induce granulomatous inflammation. Investigations of the microcirculation of the liver in mice revealed that the eggs alone do not cause significant obstruction, but the granulomas completely block portal venous circulation. Total liver blood flow remains within normal limits as there is marked neovascular formation of arterial vessels in the areas of inflammation and fibrosis[13].

Since the granulomas and subsequent fibrosis are essential factors in the pathogenesis of schistosomal disease the aetiology and dynamics of these lesions have been studied intensively. It has been demonstrated that the *S. mansoni* egg granuloma is an anamnestic reaction which is specific and can be transferred with cells and not with serum, thus constituting a cell-mediated immunological reaction. Inhibition of cell-mediated reactions by antilymphocyte serum and in nude athymic mice results in little or no granuloma formation. During the course of chronic schistosome infections modulation in granuloma formation occurs which may ameliorate or prevent the development of disease. This has been shown to be due to the presence of suppressor T cells and anti-idiotypic antibodies. These phenomena have been studied at the mediator (lymphokines and cytokines) and genetic levels[14].

Schistosomiasis has become the animal model of choice in the study of liver fibrosis. Examination of mice and humans infected with *S. mansoni* has revealed a high rate of collagen synthesis as determined by the formation of radiolabelled protein-bound hydroxyproline. There is also a marked increase in collagenase activity; thus the presence of fibrosis is related to an imbalance between collagen synthesis and degradation. A recent study has demonstrated that in chronic infection modulation of fibrotic events, as well as inflammation, occurs; inflammation was suppressed by cells and fibrosis both by cells and serum, suggesting independent mechanisms[15]. Furthermore, macrophages derived from granulomas elaborate factors which stimulate fibroblasts. In late chronic infections there is an increase in collagen degradation, and in post-treatment studies there has been a reversal of inflammation and fibrosis[13].

The relationship between infection and disease in helminth infections was first shown in the 1920s in clinical studies of hookworm[2]. It then became apparent that the anaemia induced by these bloodsucking parasites of the intestinal mucosa would occur only in those with heavy worm burdens, who constituted only a small percentage of hookworm infections. These observations were open to dispute at the time, and it was not until a half a century later that similar results were described in schistosomiasis, and in far greater detail[2]. It then became generally accepted that in virtually all helminth infections there is an overdispersed, negative binomial distribution of the parasites in their definitive hosts with only a very small proportion, usually less than 10%, bearing heavy worm burdens. Intensity of infection was correlated with the presence of hepatomegaly and splenomegaly. The practical outcomes of these observations are the use of quantitative egg-counting diagnostic procedures to aid in the assessment of the clinical status of the patient and to evaluate the necessity for treatment. The latter was particularly relevant in the past when only highly toxic drugs were available. Furthermore, this knowledge enables the development of control strategies in endemic areas targeted to treating only those with heavy worm burdens and calculated to maintain parasite levels below the disease-inducing threshold.

The eosinophil, which was discovered by Paul Ehrlich in 1879, has long been associated with helminth infections and allergies. Over the years it came to be called 'this enigmatic cell'. *In vitro* studies of the mechanism of immunity to schistosomiasis using cells from patients with schistosomiasis, and living schistosomula, demonstrated antibody-mediated cellular cytotoxicity with the eosinophil as one of the major killer cells. Scientists working on schistosomiasis then developed an antieosinophil serum which abrogated immunity not only in schistosome-challenged animals but in trichinosis as well. Thus for the first time a protective function for the eosinophil was demonstrated. More recently, using parasite models[16], including schistosomiasis (A. Sher, personal communication), the role of the cytokine IL 5 as a colony-stimulating factor for eosinophils has been defined, and an antibody against IL 5 has been shown to virtually eliminate eosinophilic reactions.

CONCLUSIONS

While schistosomiasis is a liver disease of importance, afflicting 5–10% of approximately 140 million people it has also served as a unique model for the understandng of the pathogenesis and pathophysiology of liver disease in general. By understanding the unique aspects of this helminth infection better diagnosis, treatment and control of this significant global health problem is facilitated.

References

1. Warren, K. S. (1984). Schistomosiasis. *Hepatology*, **4**, 979
2. Doumenge, J. P., Mott, K. E., Cheung, C., Villenave, D., Chapuis, Perrin, M. F. and Reaud-Thomas, G. (1987). *Atlas of the Global Distribution of Schistosomiasis.* (Geneva: Presses Universitaires de Bordeaux, World Health Organization)
3. Warren, K. S. (1981). The control of helminths: nonreplicating infectious agents of man. *Ann. Rev. Public Health*, **2**, 101–15 (annual reviews)
4. Prata, A. (1987). Schistosomiasis mansoni in Brazil. In Mahmoud, A. A. F. (ed.), *Schistosomiasis*, pp. 349–70. (London: Baillière Tindall)
5. Abdel-Wahab, M. F. and Mahmoud, S. S. (1987). Schistosomiasis mansoni in Egypt. In Mahmoud, A. A. F. (ed.), *Schistosomiasis*, pp. 371–96. (London: Baillière Tindall)
6. Olveda, R. M. and Domingo, E. O. (1987). Schistosomiasis japonica. In Mahmoud, A. A. F. (ed.) *Schistosomiasis*, pp. 397–418. (London: Baillière Tindall)
7. von Lichtenberg, F. (1987). Consequences of infections with schistosomes. In Rollinson, D.

and Simpson, A. J. G. (eds), *The Biology of Schistosomes: From Genes to Latrines*, p 185. (London: Academic Press)

8. Peters, P. A. S. and Kazura, J. W. (1987). Update on diagnostic methods for schistosomiasis. In Mahmoud, A. A. F. (ed.), *Schistosomiasis*, pp. 419–34. (London: Baillière Tindall)
9. Homeida, M., Abdel-Gadir, A. F., Cheever, A. W., Bennett, J. L., Arbab, B. M., Abdel-Salem, I. M., Defalla, A. A. and Nash, T. E. (1988). Diagnosis of pathologically confirmed Symmer's periportal fibrosis by ultrasonography: a prospective blinded study. *Am. J. Hyg. Trop. Med.*, **38**, 86–91.
10. King, C. H. and Mahmoud, A. A. F. (1989). Drugs five years later, praziquantel. *Ann. Intern. Med.*, **110**, 290–6
11. Mahmoud, A. A. F., Siongok, T. A., Ouma, J., Houser, H. B. and Warren, K. S. (1983). Effect of targetted mass treatment on intensity and morbidity in schistosomiasis mansoni: 3-year follow-up of a community in Machakos, Kenya. *Lancet*, **1**, 849–51
12. Warren, K. S., Reboucas, G. and Baptista, A. G. (1965). Ammonia metabolism and hepatic coma in hepatosplenic schistosomiasis: patients studied before and after portocaval shunt. *Ann. Intern. Med.*, **62**, 1113–33
13 Warren, K. S. (1987). Determinants of disease in human schistosomiasis. In Mahmoud, A. A. F. (ed.), *Schistosomiasis*, pp. 349–70 (London: Baillière Tindall)
14. Boros, D. L. (1989) Immunopathology of *Schistosoma mansoni* infection. *Clin. Microbiol. Rev.*, **2**, 250–69
15. Olds, G. R., El Meneza, S., Mahmoud, A. A. F. and Kresina, T. F. (1989). Differential immunoregulation of granulomatous inflammation, portal hypertension, and hepatic fibrosis in murine schistomosiasis mansoni. *J. Immunol.*, **142**, 3605–11
16. Coffman, R. L., Seymour, B. W. P., Hudak, S., Jackson, J. and Rennick, D. (1989). Antibody to interleukin-5 inhibits helminth-induced eosinophilia in mice. *Science*, **245**, 308–10

17
Pharmacotherapy of hepatic hydatid disease

J. REICHEN, J. COTTING and U. STEIGER

Hydatid disease is a tapeworm infestation essentially due to two parasites – *Echinococcus granulosus* and *E. alveolaris* – a third form, *E. vogeli*, occurs only in the Latin Americas and will not be considered further. The definitive hosts for *E. granulosus* include dogs, wolves, jackals and various felines; the intermediate hosts are ungulates such as sheep and cattle. *E. granulosus* is found mostly in sheep- and cattle-raising areas; tapeworm control in dogs has been used successfully to decrease human infestation. The definitive host for *E. alveolaris* is the fox, the intermediate hosts being small rodents, in particular voles. Man is thought to get infected by eating berries contaminated by egg-containing faeces from infested foxes. Direct contact with infested foxes or – less commonly – cats and dogs, is also thought to lead to infection. For both parasites, man is a 'false' intermediate host since the life cycle of the parasite stops in man.

The two diseases differ not only in their life cycle but also in their natural history in man; in both, radical surgery where feasible is the preferred treatment. The results of surgical procedures have recently been reviewed[1-3] and will not be considered further. Radical surgery is not possible in every case, however. For this reason, pharmacotherapy is still an important modality for treatment of inoperable disease. Moreover, since intraoperative spillage of cyst contents is the major factor in recurrence of disease, preoperative sterilization of parasites is desirable. Indeed, preoperative treatment has recently been shown to sterilize hydatid cysts in the majority of cases[4] (see below). The mainstays of pharmacotherapy are the benzoimidazoles, which are thought to act by inhibiting the microtubular system of the parasites[5]. There is considerable experience with two drugs of this family, namely mebendazole and albendazole. Experience with praziquantel, the third drug shown to have *in vitro* activity[6], is very limited in man[7]; this drug holds much promise, however, since it has quite a good safety record[8].

CLINICAL PHARMACOLOGY OF THE BENZOIMIDAZOLES

Mebendazole was originally designed as an intestinal parasitocidal agent and selected for its low absorption and – thereby – lack of systemic effects. With heroic doses ranging up to 20 g/d it is possible, however, to achieve therapeautic mebendazole concentrations in plasma and cysts[9,10]. Absorption can be increased by administering the drug together with a fatty meal[11]; another measure to increase mebendazole plasma concentrations is to inhibit its metabolism by cimetidine[12]; the results of this combination therapy are controversial, however[13]. Plasma levels of $>250\,\mu$mol/l are aimed at[14]; because of the poor absorption there is virtually no relationship between dose and plasma levels[9,15]; frequent monitoring is therefore advisable. Mebendazole is usually well tolerated, the major side-effects being hepatotoxicity and neutropenia, necessitating drug withdrawal in up to 10% of cases. A compilation of the major side-effects from various sources[2,15–17] is given in Table 1.

Albendazole, a congener of mebendazole, is much better absorbed than mebendazole. Its absorption can be further improved by giving it together with a fatty meal[18,19]. Albendazole is a prodrug since it is rapidly and virtually quantitatively metabolized to albendazole sulphoxide[19,20]; the sulphoxide has parasitostatic properties of its own[21], while the further metabolites, in particular albendazole sulphone, are inactive.

Similar to mebendazole, effective cyst levels which depend on the plasma levels are achieved with albendazole[22]. Albendazole appears to have a higher incidence of adverse reactions, in particular of hepatotoxicity and of neutropenia. Side-effects, compiled from various sources[16,23], including our own unpublished experience, are listed in Table 1. In our experience transaminase elevation is an almost universal phenomenon, while overt hepatitis requiring discontinuation of the drug occurs in less than 5%. We have observed two cases of neutropenia (10%) necessitating withdrawal of the drug in one patient. Albendazole is embryotoxic[21] and appropriate precautions are necessary when using this drug in women of child-bearing age.

E. GRANULOSUS

E. granulosus is usually acquired from infested dogs. The histology of the cyst wall is represented schematically in Figure 1; the germinal layer

Table 1 Side-effects of benzoimidazole parasitostatic drugs: the incidence was extracted from the various series quoted in the text (percentages)

	Mebendazole	*Albendazole*
Transaminase elevation	5–30	30–100
Overt hepatitis	<5	5–7
Cholestasis	rare	rare
Neutropenia	13–26	3–25
Mild anaemia	5	<5
Hair loss	2–9	2–20
Allergic phenomena	2–5	?

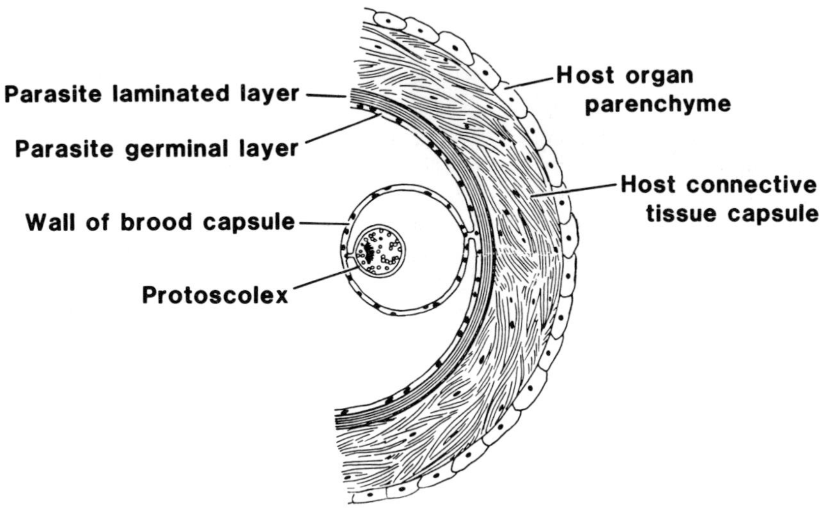

Figure 1 Schematic representation of a hydatid cyst due to *E. granulosus*

containing live parasites is surrounded by a parasite-derived laminated layer. The parasite evokes an immune response leading to formation of a collagenous capsule by the host which may calcify. Radiologically, *E. granulosus* presents as cysts; differentiation from simple or congenital liver cysts can often be made by the presence of daughter cysts or hydatid sand in the cyst lumen. Daughter cysts occur in up to 65% of hydatid cysts[24–25]; the presence of 'sand' is not pathognomonic since debris can be found in up to 50% of simple cysts[24]. Rim calcification favours the diagnosis of a hydatid cyst. Diagnosis – and differentiation against *E. multilocularis* – can be made by a highly sensitive ELISA[26].

Hydatid cysts grow slowly, increasing in size by 1–5 cm per year[27]. An interesting study on the natural history of hydatid cysts has been reported from Turkana, Kenya[25]; the results of this study are summarized in Figure 2; it is important to realize that spontaneous growth arrest, and even disappearance, perhaps due to evacuation into the biliary tree[28], occurs in a sizeable percentage of patients. This finding has to be taken into account when evaluating studies on pharmacotherapy of *E. granulosus*.

The rather slow growth of hydatid cysts provides the explanation for the finding that symptoms usually occur only after many years of infestation. The symptoms are mostly due to mass effects: a feeling of fullness, palpable mass, gastric outlet obstruction or biliary obstruction often associated with rupture of the cyst into the biliary tree[28]. In rare cases the primary manifestation can be due to superinfection of the cyst; the cysts can burst, thereby liberating highly antigenic substances. Up to 10% of cases therefore present initially with allergic symptoms or outright anaphylactic shock[29]. Due to this possibility diagnostic puncture is strongly discouraged in spite of recent advocacy of this procedure[30]. Other complications in a large surgical series included rupture into the biliary tree in 16.3%, superinfection

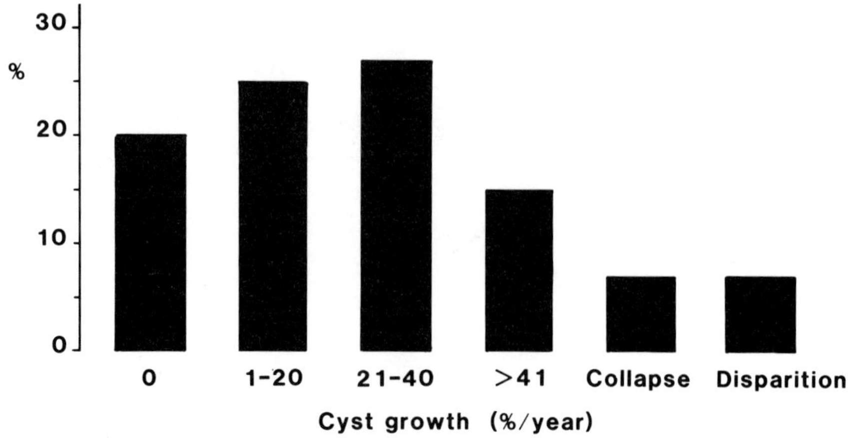

Figure 2 Growth of hydatid cysts due to *E. granulosus*. ($n = 44$). This is a longitudinal sonographic follow-up in Turkana, Kenya. Of note is that some of the cysts can collapse or disappear spontaneously. Drawn from the data of Romig *et al.*[25]

in 11%, rupture into the peritoneal space in 4.3% and bronchobiliary and cutaneous fistulae in 1.3%[31].

Wherever feasible, radical surgery is the treatment of choice; however, even in supposedly radically operated patients, recurrence rates of up to 22% have been described[1,32]. Cyst rupture before or during surgery is the main determinant of recurrence[32]; prophylactic treatment with one of the benzimidazoles has therefore been advocated[4]; in this study only 1/14 patients treated with albendazole preoperatively for more than 1 month had viable protoscolices, while 2/2 patients treated for shorter time intervals had live parasites. Mebendazole seems to be parasitostatic at best, since even with prolonged treatment with this drug 50% unequivocally viable parasites were detected and none had been definitively killed[9].

There are no controlled trials of any of the benzomidazoles available. Several studies have reported a beneficial effect of mebendazole on inoperable or recurrent hydatid disease[13,16,33–35]. A summary of the results of mebendazole in 231 patients is given in Figure 3. While it is obvious that 'cures', usually defined as cyst collapse and complete calcification, occur in between 40% and 80% of cases, treatment failures are frequent. The drug is currently considered parasitostatic at best; this contention is supported by the finding of over 50% viable protoscolices even after prolonged mebendazole treatment[9].

For this reason much hope has been put into the better-absorbable drug, albendazole. While the experience with this drug in hepatic hydatid disease due to *E. granulosus* is still limited[16,23,35,36], much higher response rates have been achieved (see Figure 3). Of major interest in this context is the cooperative WHO trial comparing mebendazole and albendazole[16]. This trial is analysed for *E. granulosus* in Table 2; the response rates given in the table refer to all forms of *E. granulosus*. Unfortunately, hepatic lesions were

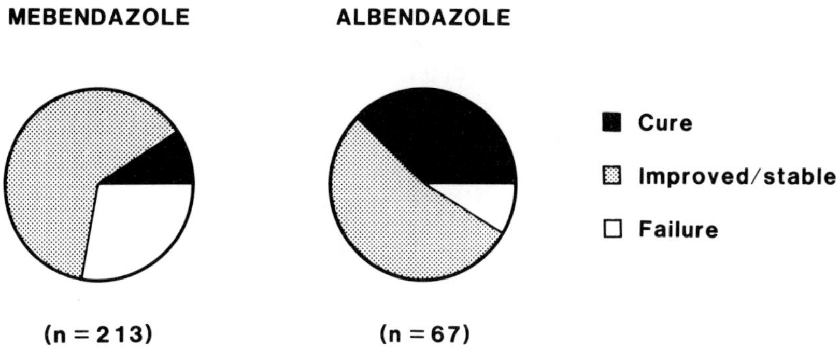

Figure 3 Comparison of the efficacy of mebendazole and albendazole on *E. granulosus* hepatic cysts. The data are summarized from various trials quoted in the text

not analysed separately. Experience in other trials shows that hepatic and pulmonary lesions have much better response rates than lesions in other locations. Therefore, the percentages given in Table 2 probably represent minimal estimates of response rates. Follow-up data on the WHO trial are not yet published, but confirm the trend in favour of albendazole (J. Horton, personal communication).

E. ALVEOLARIS

The scolices of *E. alveolaris* grow invasively and have the capacity to metastasize spontaneously to distant organs; biologically, this parasite behaves very much like a slowly growing malignant tumour. This is due to the fact that, in contrast to *E. granulosus*, *E. alveolaris* does not induce the formation of a fibrous capsule. *E. alveolaris* can also produce hepatic necrosis, which is not seen with *E. granulosus*. The liver is the primary site in over 90% of cases. Radiologically, *E. alveolaris* also often presents as a malignant tumour; typical on CT are areas of mixed densities[37], often with calcifications, and a cuneiform peripheral location. The advent of highly sensitive and

Table 2 Collaborative trial (Besançon, Sofia, Zurich) comparing mebendazole and albendazole in *E. granulosus*.

	Mebendazole	*Albendazole*
All cysts (*n*)	85	30
Hepatic cysts (*n*)	32	14
Success	9.4%	16.7%
Partial resolution	4.7%	13.3%
Improvement	47.1%	46.7%
Failure	38.8%	23.3%

The data were extracted from Davis *et al.*[16]. The percentages given refer to all cysts, since the data for hepatic cysts were not given individually. This represents minimal estimates since most authors found that hepatic and peritoneal cysts had better response rates than cysts in other locations parasite-specific ELISAs has helped diagnosis considerably[26].

Time from infection to onset of symptoms is thought to range from 5 to 15 years[2,38]. Before the advent of non-invasive screening techniques such as serology and ultrasound, up to 50% of patients presented initially with obstructive jaundice[38], often associated with cholangitis. In heavily infested areas, such as the Jura mountains of France, presentation with jaundice has decreased to 30% since screening programmes for populations at risk, have been installed[38].

In contrast to *E. granulosus*, radical surgery is rarely feasible; resectability rates of 26–58% have been reported[33], but none of these authors gave late recurrences. Cure is rare, and recurrences up to 25 years after supposedly radical surgery have been described[39]. Orthotopic liver transplantation has been used as treatment modality in this disease; early results are encouraging[40]. Ten-year survival in inoperable patients is only 10–30%[33,41]. The course of the disease is almost invariably complicated by biliary symptoms such as obstruction and cholangitis, and by the complications of portal hypertension[2,17,38,41].

The growth rate of *E. alveolaris* is slower than that of *E. granulosus*. Thus, Luder *et al.* found an average growth rate of 10 ml/year in patients with recurrent alveolar disease after supposedly radical surgery[42]; there was a wide range, however, growth rate ranging from 3.8 to 221 ml/year (see Figure 4).

Mebendazole has clearly been shown to lead to an arrest of growth, and even regression in some instances[16–17,33,42,43]. The literature is difficult to evaluate since patients are reported repeatedly as part of different trials. A compilation of the results is given in Figure 5. The trials of Wilson *et al.*[44], as well as that of Amman and collaborators[17], reported an increase in life expectancy in treated patients as compared to historical controls; 10-year survival in the latter study was 84%. Mebendazole is probably parasitostatic

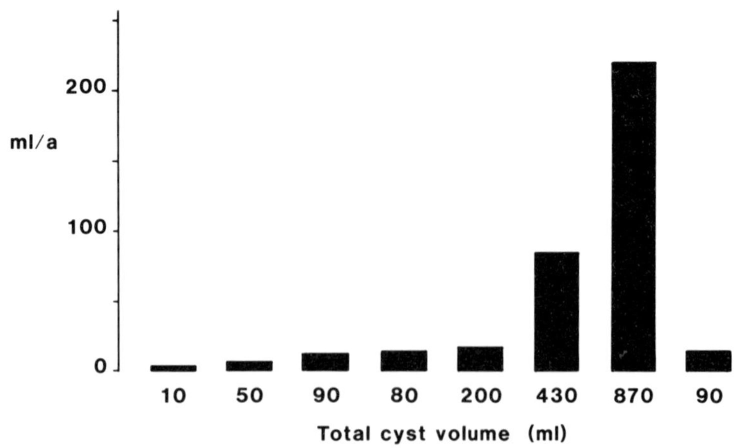

Figure 4 Growth rate of *E. alveolaris*, redrawn from Luder *et al.*[42]. The growth rate was determined by stereological methods from consecutive CT scans and is expressed as ml/year. Growth rate is given as a function of total cyst volume determined by stereology

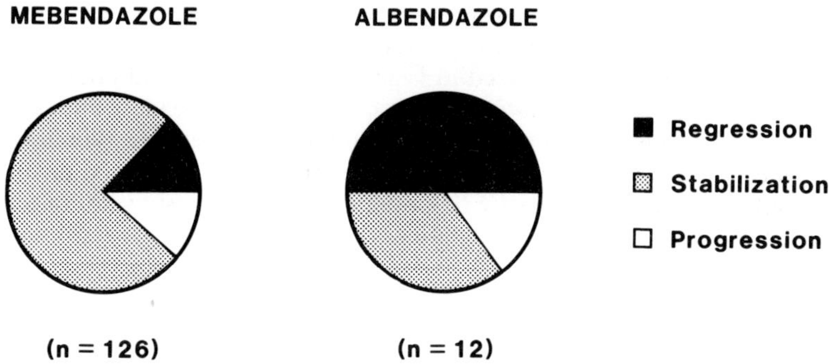

Figure 5 Comparison of the efficacy of mebendazole and albendazole in *E. alveolaris*. The data are compiled from various sources quoted in the text

and not truly parasitocidal; thus Rausch *et al.*[43] found 27% viable parasites remaining in surgically resected specimens (as opposed to 73% in untreated controls).

Virtually no data are available on the effects of albendazole in *E. alveolaris*. Wilson *et al.* treated seven patients, two of whom were operated upon after 58 and 84 days of albendazole treatment; the parasite had been killed in both instances[44]. In our series viable parasites were found in two patients after a treatment period of 26 and 96 days, respectively; whether this represents inadequate time of treatment, or whether albendazole is parasitostatic only, remains unsettled at present. A multicentre trial of the WHO has started 20 patients on albendazole[16].

We have treated 12 patients with either inoperable *E. alveolaris* or patients who showed progression during mebendazole therapy (Table 3). Two of these patients had presumably radical surgery, and evaluation would be premature. In the remaining 10 patients we observed regression of the lesion in two,

Table 3 Experience in Berne with albendazole in 12 patients with *E. alveolaris*.

Patient	*Pre-Rx**	*Operation*	*Follow-up (months)*	*Radiology*	*Remarks*
AV	+	+	8	Stable	—
BA	–	+	6	Stable	—
BC	–	+	11	Regression	Desobstruction
DM	–	+	13	NED†	Radical surgery
EA	+	+	20	Progressive	—
LK	–	+	5	Stable	—
MA	–	–	24	Stable	Desobstruction
PH	+	+	18	Stable	—
RM	+	+	22	Regression	—
SV	–	–	12	Progressive	Desobstruction
TR	–	–	22	Stable	—
VU	–	–	10	NED†	Radical surgery

Albendazole was administered in 4-week cycles at 200 mg p.o. t.i.d., interrupted by a 2-week drug-free interval

* Pretreated with mebendazole for >1 year; the switch to albendazole was made because of progressive disease in spite of adequate serum levels

† No evidence of disease

stabilization in six and frank progression in two patients after a mean follow-up period of 15 months. The results of these two, as well as of the patients of Wilson *et al.*, are demonstrated in Figure 5. Three of our 12 patients were completely obstructed at initiation of therapy; two were considered inoperable and transplantation was considered. Awaiting transplantation, albendazole was started, and in both desobstruction occurred; the evolution in one of these patients is shown in Figure 6. Under albendazole, resolution of biliary obstruction occurred in all three patients. While spontaneous resolution of biliary obstruction is known to occur – presumably to passage of debris and/or evacuation of parasite material into the biliary tree, this seems too much of a coincidence, and we are inclined to ascribe the favourable evolution to the drug. Of note is that the parasite in one of the desobstructed patients showed evidence of progression in spite of the desobstruction.

CONCLUSIONS

The benzimidazole parasitostatic drugs are active against both *E. granulosus* and *E. alveolaris*. In *E. granulosus* albendazole may be parasitocidal; it will presumably replace mebendazole because of its better bioavailability. Mebendazole leads to true growth arrest in *E. alveolaris* but is clearly only parasitostatic. Early results with albendazole in this devastating disease are encouraging, but more active compounds are clearly needed to achieve cyst sterilization in all cases.

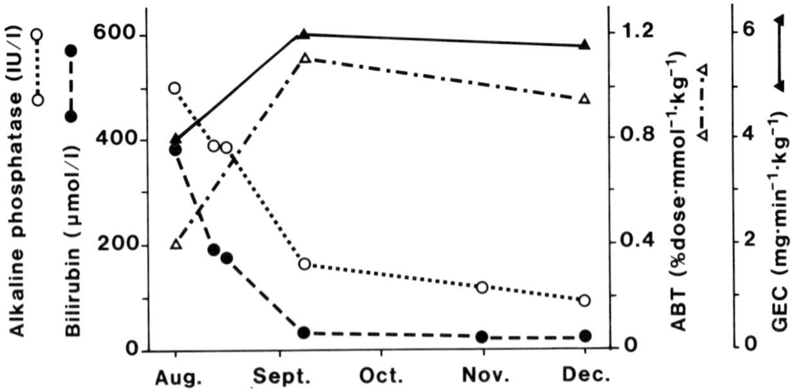

Figure 6 Desobstruction presumably induced by albendazole in patient A.M. (see also Table 3). The patient was completely obstructed and awaiting transplantation. Albendazole was started at the beginning of August 1986; prompt desobstruction occurred, as documented by the rapid and sustained fall in serum bilirubin and alkaline phosphatase. Liver function recovered, as evidenced by the sustained increase in galactose elimination capacity (GEC) and aminopyrine *N*-demethylation (ABT). The patient has remained well; the parasite is stable radiologically

Acknowledgements

J.R. is the recipient of a Research Career Development Award from the Swiss National Foundation for Scientific Research (No. 3.731), supported by SNF grant No. 32.9365. We wish to thank Dr J. Horton from Smith-Kline-French, Welwyn Garden City, for supplying the albendazole to our patients.

References

1. Langer, B. (1987). Surgical treatment of hydatid disease of the liver. *Br. J. Surg.*, **74**, 237–8
2. Miguet, J. P. and Bresson-Hadni, S. (1989). Alveolar echinococcosis of the liver. *J. Hepatol.*, **8**, 373–9
3. Chipponi, J. and Huguier, M. (1986). Les kystes hydatiques du foie operes en France. Epidemiologie, attitudes diagnostiques et therapeutiques. Etude de 306 cas. *Gastroenterol. Clin. Biol.*, **10**, 419–23
4. Morris, D. L. (1987). Pre-operative albendazole therapy for hydatid cyst. *Br. J. Surg.*, **74**, 805–6
5. Laclette, J. P., Guerra, G. and Zetina, C. (1980). Inhibition of tubulin polymerization by mebendazole. *Biochem. Biophys. Res. Commun.*, **92**, 417–23
6. Taylor, D. H., Morris, D. L., Richards, S. K. and Reffin, D. (1988). Echinococcus multilocularis: In vivo results with albendazole and praziquantel. *Trans. R. Soc. Trop. Med. Hyg.*, **82**, 611–15
7. Henriksen, T. H., Klungsoyr, P. and Zerihun, D. (1989). Treatment of disseminated peritoneal hydatid disease with praziquantel. *Lancet*, **1**, 272
8. King, C. H. and Mahmoud, A. F. (1989). Drugs five years later: praziquantel. *Ann. Intern. Med.*, **110**, 290–6
9. Luder, P. J., Witassek, F., Weigand, K., Eckert, J. and Bircher, J. (1985). Treatment of cystic echinococcosis (*Echinococcus granulosus*) with mebendazole: assessment of bound and free drug levels in cyst fluid and of parasite vitality in operative specimens. *Eur. J. Clin. Pharmacol.*, **28**, 279–85
10. Braithwaite, P. A., Roberts, M. S., Allan, R. J. and Watson, T. R. (1982). Clinical pharmacokinetics of high dose mebendazole in patients treated for cystic hydatid disease. *Eur. J. Clin. Pharmacol.*, **22**, 161–9
11. Muenst, G. J., Karlaganis, G. and Bircher, J. (1980). Plasmaconcentrations of mebendazole during treatment of echinococcosis. Preliminary results. *Eur. J. Clin. Pharmacol.*, **17**, 375–8
12. Bekhti, A. and Pirotte, J. (1987). Cimetidine increases serum mebendazole concentrations. Implications for treatment of hepatic hydatid cysts. *Br. J. Clin. Pharmacol.*, **24**, 390–2
13. Luder, P. J., Siffert, B., Witassek, F., Meister, F. and Bircher, J. (1986). Treatment of hydatid disease with high oral doses of mebendazole. Long-term follow-up of plasma mebendazole levels and drug interactions. *Eur. J. Clin. Pharmacol.*, **31**, 443–8
14. Witassek, F., Burkhardt, B., Eckert, J. and Bircher, J. (1981). Chemotherapy of alveolar echinococcosis – comparison of plasma mebendazole concentrations in animals and man. *Eur. J. Clin. Pharmacol.*, **20**, 427–33
15. Woodtli, W., Bircher, J., Witassek, F., Eckert, J., Wuethrich, B. and Ammann, R. W. (1985). Effect of plasma mebendazole concentrations in the treatment of human echinococcosis. *Am. J. Trop. Med. Hyg.*, **34**, 754–60
16. Davis, A., Pawlowski, Z. S. and Dixon, H. (1986). Multicentre clinical trials of benzimidazole-carbamates in human echinococcosis. *Bull. WHO*, **64**, 383–8
17. Ammann, R., Tschudi, K., von Ziegler, M., Meister, F., Cotting, J., Eckert, J., Witassek, F. and Freiburghaus, A. (1988). Langzeitverlauf bei 60 Patienten mit alveolaerer Echinokokkose unter Dauertherapie mit Mebendazol (1976–1985). *Klin. Wochenschr.*, **66**, 1060–73
18. Marriner, S. E., Morris, D. L., Dickson, B. and Bogan, J. A. (1986). Pharmacokinetics of albendazole in man. *Eur. J. Clin. Pharmacol.*, **30**, 705–8
19. Lange, H., Eggers, R. and Bircher, J. (1988). Increased systemic availability of albendazole when taken with a fatty meal. *Eur. J. Clin. Pharmacol.*, **34**, 315–17

20. Rolin, S., Souhaili-El Amri, H., Batt, A. M., Levy, M., Bagrel, D. and Siest, G. (1989). Study of the in vitro bioactivation of albendazole in human liver microsomes and hepatoma cell lines. *Cell Biol. Toxicol.*, **5**, 1–14
21. Delatour, P. R. and Gyurik, R. J. (1981). Albendazole: a comparison of relay embryotoxicity with embryotoxicity of individual metabolites. *Am. Res. Vet.*, **12**, 159–67
22. Morris, D. L., Chinnery, J. B., Georgiou, G., Stamatakis, G. and Golematis, B. (1987). Penetration of albendazole sulphoxide into hydatid cysts. *Gut*, **28**, 75–80
23. Morris, D. L., Dykes, P. W., Marriner, S., Bogan, J., Burrows, F., Skeene-Smitz, H. and Clarkson, M. J. (1985). Albendazole – objective evidence of response in human hydatid disease. *J. Am. Med. Assoc.*, **253**, 2053–7.
24. Harris, K. M., Morrisl, D. L., Tudor, R., Toghill, P. and Hardcastle, J. D. (1986). Clinical and radiographic features of simple and hydatid cysts of the liver. *Br. J. Surg.*, **73**, 835–8
25. Romig, T., Zeyhle, E., Macpherson, C. N. L., Rees, P. H. and Were, J. B. O. (1986). Cyst growth and spontaneous cure in hydatid disease. *Lancet*, **1**, 861
26. Gottstein, B., Schantz, P. M., Todorov, T., Saimot, A. G. and Jacquier, P. (1986). An international study on the serological differential diagnosis of human cystic and alveolar echinococcosis. *Bull. WHO*, **64**, 101–5
27. Sierra, J., Oviedo, J., Berthier, M. and Leiguarda, R. (1985). Growth rate of secondary hydatid cysts of the brain. *J. Neurosurg.*, **62**, 781–2
28. Van Steenbergen, W., Fevery, J., Broeckaert, L., Ponette, E., Marchal, G., Baert, A., Penninckx, F., Kerremans, R. and De Groote, J. (1987). Hepatic echinococcosis ruptured into the biliary tract. *J. Hepatol.*, **4**, 133–9
29. Werczberger, A., Colhman, J., Wertheim, G., Gunders, A. E. and Chowers, I. (1979). Disseminated echinococcosis with repeated anaphylactic shock. *Chest*, **74**, 482–4
30. Hira, P. R., Lindberg, L. G., Francis, I., Shweiki, H., Shaheen, Y., Leven, H. and Behbehani, K. (1988). Diagnosis of cystic hydatid disease: role of aspiration cytology. *Lancet*, **2**, 655–7
31. Akinoglu, A., Bilgin, I. and Erkocac, E. U. (1985). Surgical management of hydatid disease of the liver. *Can. J. Surg.*, **28**, 171–4
32. Little, J. M., Hollands, M. J. and Ekberg, H. (1988). Recurrence of hydatid disease. *World J. Surg.*, **12**, 700–4
33. Schantz, P. M., Van den Bossche, H. and Eckert, J. (1982). Chemotherapy for larval echinococcosis in animals and humans: Report of a workshop. *Z. Parasitenkd.*, **67**, 5–26
34. Kammerer, W. S. and Schantz, P. M. (1984). Long term follow-up of human hydatid disease (*Echinococcus granulosus*) treated with a high-dose mebendazole regimen. *Am. J. Trop. Med. Hyg.*, **33**, 132–7
35. Okelo, G. B. A. (1986). Hydatid disease: Research and control in Turkana. III. Albendazole in the treatment of inoperable hydatid disease in Kenya – a report on 12 cases. *Trans. R. Soc. Trop. Med. Hyg.*, **80**, 193–5
36. Saimot, A. G., Cremieux, A. C., Hay, J. M., Meulemans, A., Giovanangeli, M. D., Delaitre, B. and Coulaud, J. P. (1983). Albendazole as a potential treatment for human hydatidosis. *Lancet*, **2**, 652–6
37. Didier, D., Weiler, S., Rohmer, P., Lasseque, A., Deschamps, J. P., Vuitton, D., Miguet, J. P. and Weill, F. (1985). Hepatic alveolarechinococcosis: Correlative US and CT study. *Radiology*, **154**, 179–86
38. Bresson-Hadni, S., Miguet, J. P., Vuitton, D., Meyer, J. P., Becker, M. C., Didier, D., Coche, G., Weill, F., Carbillet, J. P., Landecy, G., Mantion, G. and Gillet, M. (1988). L'echinococcose alveolaire hepatique humaine. *Sem. Hôp. Paris*, **64**, 2692–701
39. Mosimann, F. (1980). Is alveolar hydatid disease of the liver incurable? *Ann. Surg.*, **192**, 118–23
40. Gillet, M., Miguet, J. P. and Mantion, G. (1988). Orthotopic liver transplantation in alveolar echinococcosis of the liver: analysis of a series of 6 patients. *Transplant. Proc.*, **20**, 573–6
41. Wilson, J. F. and Rausch, R. L. (1980). Alveolar hydatid disease: A review of clinical features of 33 indigenous cases of *E. multilocularis* infection in Alaskan eskimoes. *Am. J. Trop. Med. Hyg.*, **29**, 1340–55
42. Luder, P. J., Robotti, G., Meister, F. P. and Bircher, J. (1985). High oral doses of mebendazole interfere with growth of larval echinococcus multilocularis lesions. *J. Hepatol.*, **1**, 369–77
43. Rausch, R. L., Wilson, J. F., McMahon, B. J. and O'Gorman, M. A. (1986). Consequences

of continuous mebendazole therapy in alveolar hydatid disease – with a summary of a ten-year clinical trial. *Ann. Trop. Med. Parasitol.*, **80**, 403–19

44. Wilson, J. F., Rausch, R. L., McMahon, B. J., Schantz, P. M., Trujillo, D. E. and O'Gorman, M. (1987). Albendazole therapy in alveolar hydatid disease: a report of favorable results in two patients after short-term therapy. *Am. J. Trop. Med. Hyg.*, **37**, 162–8

Section IV: Viral Infections of the Liver

18
The hepadnaviruses: a review of replication and persistence

J. SUMMERS

In this paper I will attempt briefly to review the group of viruses known as hepadnaviruses, and to describe in general terms their biology, what we know about the way in which they replicate themselves in liver cells, and how this knowledge impacts on our ability to devise theoretically successful schemes of antiviral therapy. Hepadnaviruses are represented by the prototype virus, human hepatitis B virus, which is the aetiological agent of chronic liver disease in many millions of infected individuals. Hepadnaviruses, however, are also found is several animal species, some of which have provided valuable experimental models for laboratory studies of replication and pathogenesis. For example, a virus found in marmots in the eastern United States, known as the woodchuck hepatitis virus (WHV)[1], is closely related structurally and biologically to the human hepatitis B virus, yet is restricted in its host range to woodchucks and closely related species[2]. WHV was shown shortly after its discovery to cause chronic infections in wild animals which result in chronic active hepatitis and in hepatocellular carcinoma when the animals are kept in captivity[1,3,4]. A similar oncogenic virus has been described in Beechey ground squirrels[5,6] and has been extensively studied as a model for hepadnavirus replication. Finally, an avian virus, the duck hepatitis B virus (DHBV)[7] is commonly found in domestic flocks of Pekin ducks, and has been particularly valuable as a model for laboratory studies of virus replication. Early in these studies, W. S. Robinson proposed the name 'hepadnavirus'[8] to describe this family of viruses related to the human hepatitis B virus. The name was derived from their two salient characteristics; that is, *hepa*totrophic *DNA* viruses. Hepadnaviridae is the family name adopted by the International Committee on Virus Nomenclature.

Extensive epidemiological studies over the past 20 years since the discovery of hepatitis B virus have been, and continue to be, the primary source of general information about the most important reservoirs of hepadnavirus infection, modes of transmission and pathogenic risks of infection. Although the mode of existence of this virus and its interaction with the human population is extremely complicated, at the risk of oversimplification I would like to summarize those points which are related in important or useful ways to the intracellular viral replication cycle.

First, although horizontal transmission among adult humans can be a significant source of acute, or less often chronic, hepatitis, vertical transmission – that is, transmission from one generation to the next – appears most important in establishing the virus in populations in areas of high endemicity[9,10]. Vertical transmission results in patterns of distribution that resemble the distribution of genetic traits within populations. The mechanisms of vertical transmission are not entirely understood, but most often involve perinatal transmission from mother to infant[11]. In addition there is a significant risk of sexual transmission, providing an additional indirect paternal route[12]. The distribution of other known hepadnaviruses of animals suggests the same dependence on vertical transmission, although this has not been as extensively studied. The clearest case of vertical transmission among animal hepadnaviruses occurs in transmission of the duck hepatitis B virus from infected laying hens to the developing embryo *in ovo*[7,13–15].

The predominance of vertical transmission of HBV shows that first, HBV infections must be capable of chronicity that spans early infancy through the ages of reproduction, and second that, in general, pathogenic progression of the infections during this period is not sufficient to prevent host reproduction and consequent virus transmission. In fact, both predictions are well documented: chronic viral infection is most often sub-clinical, and the onset of severe aspects of chronic liver disease is often delayed for several decades. This long period of latent pathogenesis provides us with a window during which treatment or cure of HBV infections can result in the prevention of disease. It is therefore the purpose of our work to understand the molecular strategies that are used by HBV to maintain an infection of such extreme persistence over decades.

Hepadnaviruses are small DNA-containing viruses that consist of an inner nucleocapsid, containing DNA, and an outer envelope (Figure 1). Serological assays for antibodies to the nucleocapsid or core antigen, and for the envelope or surface antigen, are important tools in diagnosis of HBV infections. Virus particles and empty envelope particles are secreted into the blood by infected hepatocytes by an active process that does not involve death of the cell. Thus, large numbers of hepatocytes, perhaps all hepatocytes, in an infected host are capable of being infected by hepadnaviruses with no deleterious effect on the host. Rather than persisting in infected individuals by 'hiding' in a protected compartment, or by becoming inactive and latent, HBV is maximally expressed at all times. It is remarkable that the host immune response is so ineffectual in resolving these overt chronic infections, and the mechanism by which the virus evades the immune system is not understood (a discussion of this phenomenon is beyond the scope of this article). In fact the absence of liver disease in many patients who are chronically infected with HBV, and particularly the absence of hepatocellular injury in animals infected with hepadnaviruses, strongly suggests that the nature of the hepadnavirus replication cycle is totally consistent with normal hepatocyte function. It is of interest then, from both a theoretical and a practical standpoint, to understand how virus production and assembly occurs in

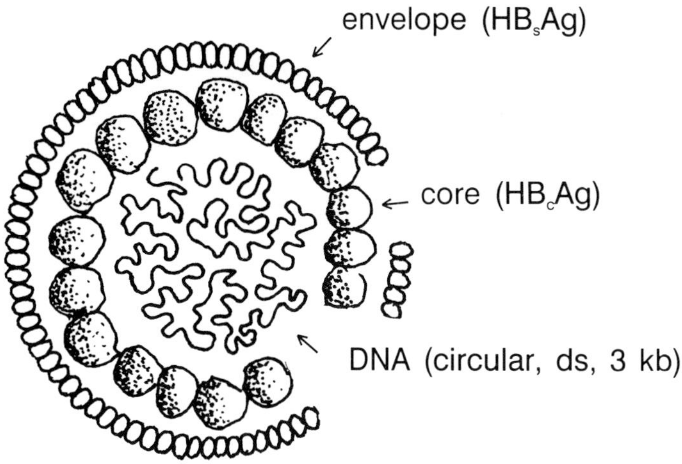

Figure 1 Structure of hepadnaviruses. The structure of the virion is shown schematically. The diameter of the complete virion is 42 nm and that of the nucleocapsid core is 27 nm

hepatocytes in the absence of cell injury.

Several years ago, W. S. Mason and I, studying the replication cycle of the duck hepatitis B virus, found that this virus possessed an unexpected but familiar lifestyle inside the infected cell[16,17]. Although the virus particle contained a DNA genome it replicated its genome by transcribing copies of RNA continuously in the infected cell and then using these RNA genomes, or pregenomes, as templates to produce DNA genomes by reverse transcription, much as retroviruses use their RNA genomes to produce the DNA provirus. An outline of the replication cycle as it was then understood is shown in Figure 2.

Infecting viral DNA first appears in the nucleus as a free circular double-stranded DNA whose two strands are covalently closed[18] (a). This covalently closed circular DNA is then transcribed by cellular enzymes to generate messenger RNAs that encode the three groups of viral structural proteins, core, envelope and DNA polymerase (b). In addition, transcription generates RNA copies of the entire DNA, which we named the 'pre-genomes' (c), and in the presence of the viral proteins the pregenomes are assembled into nucleocapsid particles (d), which are capable of enzymatically reverse transcribing the RNA molecules within them into double-stranded DNA. Such DNA synthesis takes place in the cytoplasm of the infected cell (e), and capsids that contain mature viral DNA are assembled into envelopes and secreted from the infected cell by exocytosis (f).

In this model it can be seen that the initial product of virus infection, the covalently closed circular viral DNA, plays a crucial role in the maintenance of virus production. Without the presence of this molecule in the nucleus to serve as a template for the production of mRNA and pregenomes, virus production would cease. We have therefore focused our work in recent years on understanding the formation and fate of closed circular DNA in infected

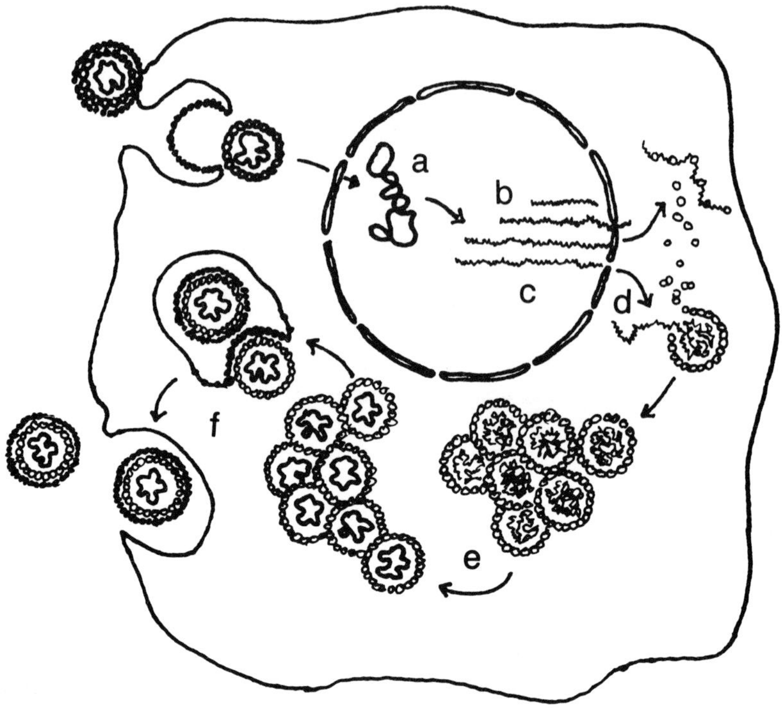

Figure 2 The replication cycle of hepadnaviruses. The replication cycle of the duck hepatitis B virus in duck hepatocytes is shown schematically. Letters a–f refer to the discussion in the text.

cells. As a result of the work of Jan Tuttleman and Christine Pourcel in my laboratory we subsequently refined this model to include an early phase of infection and a late phase of infection, based on the metabolism of closed circular DNA.

This refinement was necessitated by the fact that the model accounts for the presence of only one molecule of closed circular DNA in the nucleus, derived directly from the infecting virus, but in fact there are multiple copies of closed circular viral DNA in chronically infected cells. This observation raised the possibility that closed circular viral DNA might possess an independent mechanism of replication, different from that used to produce virion DNA, that would account for this amplification. We were able to study this problem using a cell culture system developed for the growth of the duck hepatitis B virus *in vitro*[19]. Using this system we were able to determine that replication, or amplification, of the number of copies of infecting viral closed circular DNA occurred early in infection, by 4 days, at a time when no detectable virus was being released into the medium. This early amplification appeared to be necessary for the production of significant amounts of virus, probably through a gene dosage effect.

With the knowledge that initial viral closed circular DNA is capable of amplification, we postulated that copy number control is exerted over the viral closed circular DNA, otherwise unregulated DNA replication would produce an escalating production of viral gene products, and rapid cell death. Examples of such unregulated viral replication resulting in cell death are common among both RNA and DNA viruses. In initial attempts to understand the regulation of closed circular DNA synthesis, Tuttleman *et al.* investigated the mechanism of synthesis of this DNA in cultured hepatocytes[20].

The results clearly demonstrated that closed circular DNA amplification occurred through the reverse transcription pathway and was probably accomplished by transport of a fraction of the newly synthesized cytoplasmic viral DNA into the nuclear compartment (Figure 3). Thus, closed circular DNA amplification appeared to be an alternative pathway of viral DNA transport, occurring as a shunt to the pathway of viral secretion. One hypothesis to account for the nuclear transport of newly synthesized viral DNA would be that the nucleocapsid possesses an intrinsic ability to deliver DNA to the nucleus, as required during the initial virus infection, and that early amplification is an expression of that property of the nucleocapsid. Regulation of amplification would then consist of modifying that property of the capsid and redirecting capsid transport to the secretory pathway, mediated by acquisition of the viral envelope. This model would assign a pivotal role to the envelope proteins in regulating amplification of closed circular DNA.

We tested this notion using a genetic approach and new methods of *in vitro* cultivation of the duck hepatitis B virus, worked out in my laboratory over the past two years. We also borrowed heavily from the results of

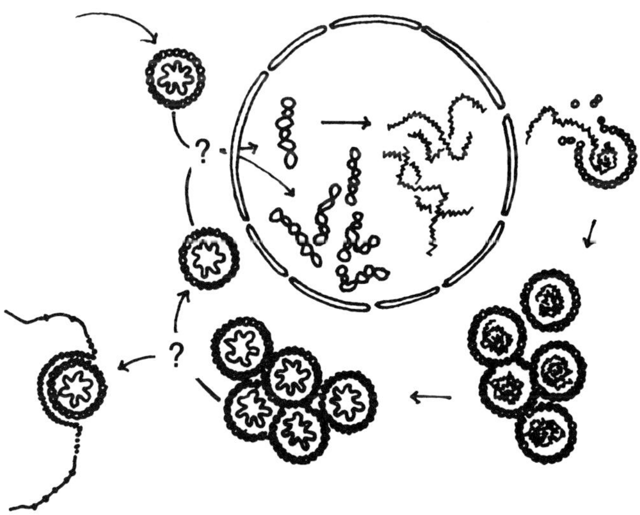

Figure 3 Intracellular amplification of cccDNA. The mechanism for amplification of cccDNA described by Tuttleman *et al.*[20] is shown schematically. Infecting virus and virus secretion is not shown.

others[21–25] who have reported the production of HBV after transfection of a variety of human hepatoma cell lines with cloned viral DNA. The experiments were carried out in my laboratory with John Pugh, and in collaboration with Arthur Horwich, at Yale Medical School[26].

The cell line Huh-7 was found to be capable of producing infectious duck hepatitis B virus particles after transfection with cloned viral DNA-containing plasmids[27]. These cells, however, are not susceptible to infection with DHBV, nor do they produce viral closed circular DNA, whose metabolism we wish to study. However, viral particles infectious for duck hepatocytes can be produced in Huh-7 cells, and *in vitro* mutagenesis of the infectious plasmid DNA can be used to generate genomes with mutations in predetermined locations. These mutated genomes can be packaged into particles infectious for duck hepatocytes by complementation with a second mutant genome after cotransfection of Huh-7 cells with both plasmid DNAs.

In order to construct a plasmid that would provide the viral proteins for packaging, we deleted both copies of a 12 base pair sequence in the viral genome insert, direct repeat 1 (DR1) (Figure 4). DR1 is required for correct initiation of synthesis of both the minus and plus strand DNA[28–30]. When

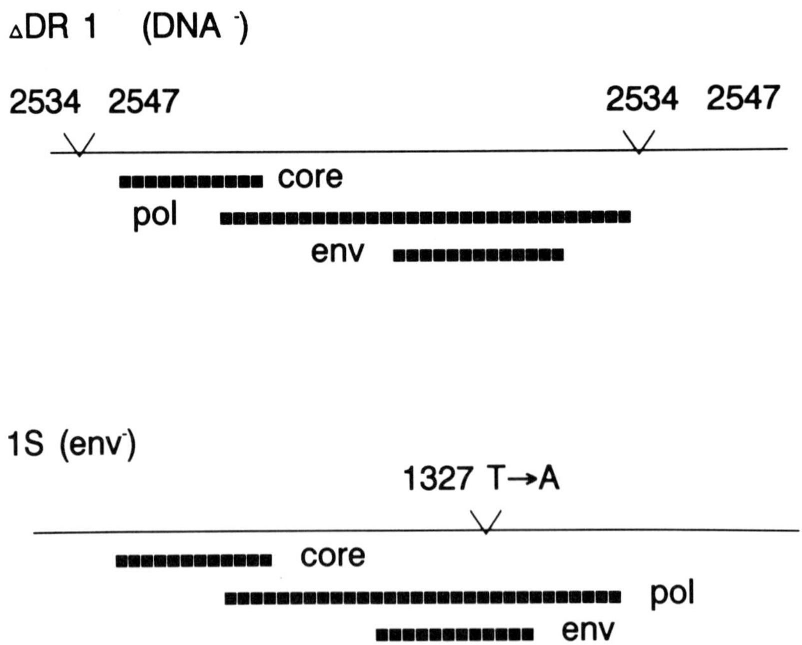

Figure 4 Structures of ΔDR 1 (top) and 1s (env-) (lower) mutants. The nucleotides joined by deletion or altered by base substitution are indicated above the site of the mutation (v). The approximate locations of the three major open reading frames encoding core (core), polymerase (pol), and envelope (env) proteins are indicated by broken lines. The pregenome coding region is indicated by the solid line. Nucleotides are numbered from the Eco RI site

this plasmid containing the mutated viral genome was transfected into Huh-7 cells it was able to direct the synthesis of DNA polymerase, envelope and capsid (core) proteins, but was unable to produce viral DNA or infectious virus particles. Other mutant genomes defective in the core, polymerase and envelope genes, but containing DR1, were constructed in the same way to test the ability of ΔDR1 plasmid to provide each viral function for packaging *in trans* in cotransfection experiments. Since ΔDR1 was able to provide these functions and consequently to rescue the individual mutant genomes into viral particles, yet was unable to produce viral DNA copies of itself, cotransfection of mutant plasmids with ΔDR1 produced helper-free mutant virus stocks that could be used to infect hepatocytes *in vitro*.

We used this system to test the properties of an envelope-deficient mutant genome when packaged and introduced into primary hepatocytes. The mutation that resulted in envelope deficiency consisted of single base changes which result in translational termination of all envelope proteins in the 'S' region, but do not alter the coding sequence of the overlapping polymerase gene (Figure 4). This mutant plasmid is capable of viral DNA synthesis, but cannot produce enveloped particles or infectious virus. We asked whether such a defect in virus envelope production would have an effect on the synthesis or accumulation of closed circular DNA.

An example of the growth of this mutant in primary hepatocytes compared with the growth and spread of wild-type virus is shown in Figure 5. With similar numbers of infected cells the mutant shows a rapid accumulation of viral replicative intermediates, surpassing that seen in the wild-type infection at early times, followed by the disappearance of viral DNA at later times. Closed circular DNA is synthesized by the mutant-infected cells, indicating that envelope production is not required for closed circular DNA amplification. The striking difference in the amounts of closed circular DNA accumulated in the mutant as compared to the wild-type infected cells suggests that closed circular DNA accumulation is not controlled, and therefore that envelope production is necessary for control of closed circular DNA accumulation. The reduction in the amount of mutant virus replication in the cultures, seen at later time points, is paralleled by a reduction in the number of cells that stain for viral core antigen between 6 and 20 days after infection, while cultures infected with wild-type virus show clear evidence of virus spread during this period (Figure 6). This disappearance of infected cells in the cultures suggests that lack of such control of intracellular virus replication results in cellular death, and that a critical mechanism for maintenance of a persistent non-cytopathic infection is the control of closed circular DNA accumulation. The phenotype of the mutant, and related envelope mutants, are currently under further study.

We tentatively conclude that hepadnaviral replication is regulated inside the infected cell by a process that is related to virus secretion. This regulation would ensure that virus replication does not escalate to a level harmful to the cell and the host. The selective pressure for such a regulatory mechanism is the ability of the infected host to transmit viral infection vertically to the next generation.

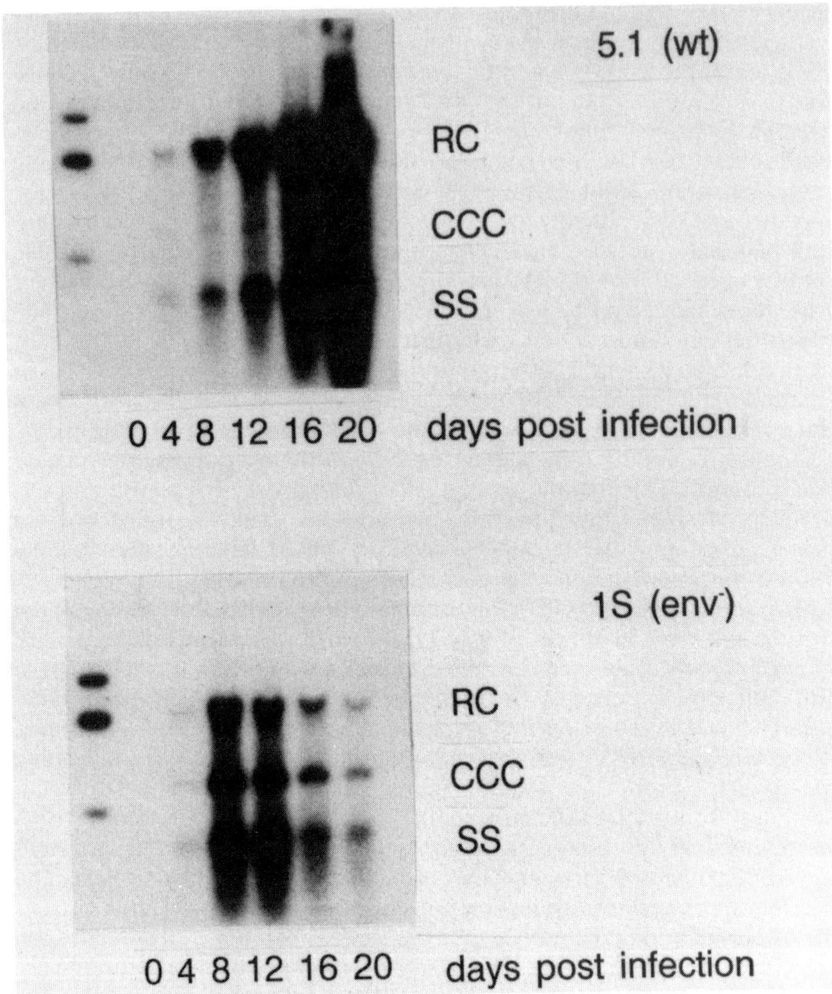

Figure 5 Growth of wild-type and envelope mutant viruses in primary duck hepatocytes. Virus particles containing wild-type or mutant genomes were used to infect primary duck hepatocytes at a multiplicity of 0.01. Infected dishes were harvested at the times indicated and total DNA was extracted from the dishes. Viral DNA was assayed by agarose gel electrophoresis and blot hybridization. Relaxed circular (RC), covalently closed circular (CCC), and single-stranded (SS) DNA positions are indicated

DISCUSSION

What does knowledge of the mechanisms of hepadnaviral persistence tell us useful about antiviral therapy? First, we can say that in order to cure infected cells and return them to their preinfected state, closed circular viral DNA must be eliminated from the cell, and the ability of the cell to regenerate new closed circular DNA must be inhibited. Closed circular DNA synthesis is dependent on reverse transcription of RNA to DNA, and therefore can

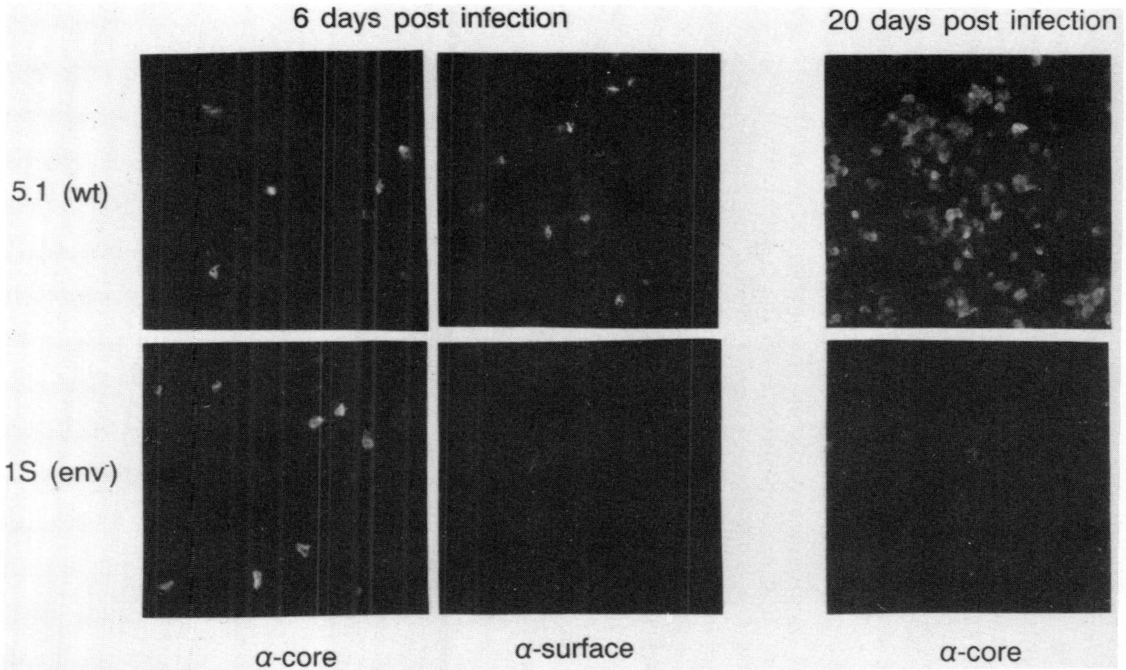

Figure 6 Immunofluorescent staining of infected hepatocytes. Cells infected in the experiment in Figure 6 were fixed at 6 days and 20 days p.i. and stained for DHBV envelope or core antigens. At day 6 no cells could be seen staining for envelope proteins in cultures infected with the envelope mutant, although core antigen staining cells were evident. At 20 days p.i., wild-type virus infection has spread throughout the culture, but in cultures infected with the envelope mutant staining cells were rare. The results suggest that the mutant-infected cells died between 6 and 20 days p.i.

be expected to be inhibited by inhibitors of virion DNA production.

Pre-existing closed circular DNA, however, is not itself sensitive to inactivation by inhibitors of viral DNA synthesis, since it does not replicate itself directly. The stability of closed circular DNA in infected cells is unknown at present, and experiments are under way to measure how long this species, and therefore the potential for virus production, remains in the cell in the absence of new viral DNA synthesis. This potential might be recognized in individuals undergoing antiviral therapy with drugs that merely inhibit viral DNA synthesis as a rebound of virus production following cessation of treatment.

Finally, the potential for inducing hepatocellular destruction by interference with the viral replication cycle is further illustrated by these studies. Chisari *et al.*[31] have previously shown that prevention of envelope particle (surface antigen) secretion in transgenic mice expressing hepatitis B surface antigen results in progressive chronic disease in the liver, due to slow accumulation of viral envelope proteins in the endoplasmic reticulum of hepatocytes with cytopathic consequences. Likewise, this study suggests that interference with assembly of enveloped virus in infected cells may cause cell death by allowing the escalation of intracellular virus replication to a cytopathic level. Such induced hepatocellular damage could be either beneficial to the objectives of antiviral therapy, in the case of patients with scattered virus-producing hepatocytes, or could lead to liver failure when a majority of hepatocytes are infected.

References

1. Summers, J., Smolec, J. M. and Snyder, R. (1978). A virus similar to human hepatitis B virus associated with hepatitis and hepatoma in woodchucks. *Proc. Natl. Acad. Sci., USA*, **75**, 4533–7
2. Seeger, C., Marion, P. L., Ganem, D. and Varmus, H. E. (1987). *In vitro* recombinants of ground squirrel and woodchuck hepatitis viral DNAs produce infectious virus in squirrels. *J. Virol.*, **61**, 3241–7
3. Popper, H., Shih, J.-W., Gerin, J. L., Wong, D.-C., Hoyer, B. H., London, W. T., Sly, D. L. and Purcell, R. H. (1981). Woodchuck hepatitis and hepatocellular carcinoma: correlation of histologic with virologic observations. *Hepatology*, **1**, 91–8
4. Popper, H., Roth, L., Purcell, R. H., Tennant, B. C. and Gerin, J. L. (1987). Hepatocarcinogenicity of the woodchuck hepatitis virus. *Proc. Natl. Acad. Sci.*, USA, **84**, 866–70
5. Marion, P. L., Oshiro, L. S., Regnery, D. C., Scullard, G. H. and Robinson, W. S. (1980). A virus in Beechey ground squirrels that is related to hepatitis B virus of humans. *Proc. Natl. Acad. Sci., USA*, **77**, 2941–5
6. Marion, P. L., Van-Davelaa, M. J., Knight, S. S., Salazar, F. H., Garcia, G., Popper, H. and Robinson, W. S. (1986). Hepatocellular carcinoma in ground squirrels persistently infected with ground squirrel hepatitis virus. *Proc. Natl. Acad. Sci., USA*, **83**, 4543–6
7. Mason, W. S., Aldrich, C., Summers, J. and Taylor, J. M. (1982). Asymmetric replication of duck hepatitis B virus DNA in liver cells: free minus-strand DNA. *Proc. Natl. Acad. Sci., USA*, **79**, 3997–4001
8. Robinson, W. S., Miller, R. H. and Marion, P. L. (1987). Hepadnaviruses and retroviruses share genome homology and features of replication. *Hepatology*, **7** (1 Suppl), 64S–73S
9. Stevens, C. E., Beasley, R. P., Tsui, J. and Lee, W. C. (1975). Vertical transmission of hepatitis B antigen in Taiwan. *N. Engl. J. Med.*, **292**, 771–4
10. Stevens, C. E., Neurath, R. A., Beasley, R. P. and Szmuness, W. (1979). HBeAg and anti-HBe detection by radioimmunoassay: correlation with vertical transmission of hepatitis B

virus in Taiwan. *J. Med. Virol.*, **3**, 237–41

11. Anderson, K. E., Stevens, C. E., Tsuei, J.-J., Lee, W.-C., Sun, S.-C. and Beasley, P. (1975). Hepatitis B antigen in infants born to mothers with chronic hepatitis B antigenemia in Taiwan. *Am. J. Dis. Child.*, **29**, 1389–92
12. Tassopoulos, N. C., Papaevangelou, G. J., Roumeliotou-Karayannis, A., Ticehurst, J. R., Feinstone, S. M. and Purcell, R. H. (1987). Detection of hepatitis B virus DNA in asymptomatic hepatitis B surface antigen carriers: relation to sexual transmission. *Am. J. Epidemiol.*, **126**, 587–91
13. Urban, M. K., O'Connell, A. P. and London, W. T. (1985). Sequence of events in natural infection of Pekin duck embryos with duck hepatitis B virus. *J. Virol.*, **55**, 16–22
14. O'Connell, A. P., Urban, M. K. and London, W. T. (1983). Naturally occurring infection of Pekin duck embryos by duck hepatitis B virus. *Proc. Natl. Acad. Sci., USA*, **80**, 1703–6
15. Tagawa, M., Robinson, W. S. and Marion, P. L. (1987). Duck hepatitis B virus replicates in the yolk sac of developing embryos. *J. Virol.*, **61**, 2273–9
16. Summers, J. and Mason, W. S. (1982). Replication of the genome of a hepatitis B-like virus by reverse transcription of an RNA intermediate. *Cell*, **29**, 403–15
17. Mason, W. S., Seal, G. and Summers, J. (1980). Virus of Pekin ducks with structural and biological relatedness to human hepatitis B virus. *J. Virol.*, **36**, 829–36
18. Mason, W. S., Halpern, M. S., England, J. M., Seal, G., Egan, J., Coates, L., Aldrich, C. and Summers, J. (1983). Experimental transmission of duck hepatitis B virus. *Virology*, **131**, 375–84
19. Tuttleman, J. S., Pugh, J. C. and Summers, J. W. (1986). In vitro experimental infection of primary duck hepatocyte cultures with duck hepatitis B virus. *J. Virol.*, **58**, 17–25
20. Tuttleman, J. S., Pourcel, C. and Summers, J. (1986). Formation of the pool of covalently closed circular viral DNA in hepadnavirus-infected cells. *Cell*, **47**, 451–60
21. Sureau, C., Romet-Lemonne, J. L., Mullins, J. I. and Essex, M. (1986). Production of hepatitis B virus by a differentiated human hepatoma cell line after transfection with cloned circular HBV DNA. *Cell*, **10**, 37–47
22. Tsurimoto, T., Fujiyama, A. and Matsubara, K. (1987). Stable expression and replication of hepatitis B virus genome in an integrated state in a human hepatoma cell line transfected with the cloned viral DNA. *Proc. Natl. Acad. Sci., USA*, **84**, 444–8
23. Yaginuma, K., Shirakata, Y., Kobayashi, M. and Koike, K. (1987). Hepatitis B virus (HBV) particles are produced in a cell culture system by transient expression of transfected HBV DNA. *Proc. Natl. Acad. Sci., USA*, **84**, 2678–82
24. Sells, M. A., Chen, M.-L. and Acs, G. (1987). Production of hepatitis B virus particles in Hep G2 cells transfected with cloned hepatitis B virus DNA. *Proc. Natl. Acad. Sci., USA*, **84**, 1005–9
25. Galle, P. R., Schlicht, H. J., Fischer, M. and Schaller, H. (1988). Production of infectious duck hepatitis B virus in a human hepatoma cell line. *J. Virol.*, **62**, 1736–40
26. Horwich, A. L., Furtak, K., Pugh, J. and Summers, J. (1989). Synthesis of hepadnavirus particles containing replication-defective DHBV genomes in cultured Huh-7 cells. *J. Virol.* (In press)
27. Pugh, J. C., Yaginuma, K., Koike, K. and Summers, J. (1988). Duck hepatitis B virus (DHBV) particles produced by transient expression of DHBV DNA in a human hepatoma cell line are infectious in vitro. *J. Virol.*, **62**, 3513–16
28. Lien, J. M., Aldrich, C. E. and Mason, W. S. (1986). Evidence that a capped oligoribonucleotide is the primer for duck hepatitis B virus plus-strand DNA synthesis. *J. Virol.*, **57**, 229–36
29. Molnar-Kimber, K. L., Summers, J. W. and Mason, W. S. (1984). Mapping of the cohesive overlap of duck hepatitis B virus DNA and of the site of initiation of reverse transcription. *J. Virol.*, **51**, 181–91
30. Lien, J. M., Petcu, D. J., Aldrich, C. E. and Mason, W. S. (1987). Initiation and termination of duck hepatitis B virus DNA synthesis during virus maturation. *J. Virol.*, **61**, 3832–40
31. Chisari, F. V., Filippi, P., Buras, J., McLachlan, A., Popper, H., Pinkert, C. A., Palmiter, R. D. and Brinster, R. L. (1987). Structural and pathological effects of synthesis of hepatitis B virus large envelope polypeptide in transgenic mice. *Proc. Natl. Acad. Sci., USA*, **84**, 6909–13

19
Hepatitis B virus carrier and hepatocellular carcinoma

H. E. BLUM, T. J. LIANG and J. R. WANDS

INTRODUCTION

Infection with hepatitis B virus (HBV) is endemic throughout much of the world, with an estimated 200 million people carrying persistent HBV infection. HBV infects only humans and certain non-human primates; it belongs to a group of hepatotropic DNA viruses (the hepadnaviruses) that includes HBV and the hepatitis viruses of the woodchuck (WHV)[1], ground squirrel (GSHV)[2], tree squirrel (TSHV)[3], Pekin duck (DHBV)[4] and heron (HHBV)[5]. In humans, HBV infection is associated with a wide spectrum of clinical presentations ranging from the healthy carrier state to acute or chronic hepatitis and liver cirrhosis. Further, chronic HBV infection is involved in the development of hepatocellular carcinomas (HCCs), a major cause of death from cancer throughout the world.

The geographical coincidence between a high prevalence of HBV infection and high incidence of HCCs, the fact that HBV carriers are more than 100-fold more likely than non-carriers to develop HCCs, the presence of integrated viral DNA in a large proportion of HCCs and the development of HCCs in hepadnavirus-infected woodchucks, ground squirrels and Pekin ducks all strongly suggest a relationship between viral infection and malignant transformation of hepatocytes. However, the molecular mechanisms leading to the malignant transformation of liver cells are still poorly defined.

In recent years, important advances have been made in the study of the biology of HBV and the virus-host cell interaction at the molecular level[6–9]. This paper will review the epidemiology of HBV infection and HCC development, the clinical and pathological characteristics of HCCs in HBV carriers and current concepts of molecular hepatocarcinogenesis.

EPIDEMIOLOGY OF HBV INFECTION AND HCC

Three lines of epidemiological evidence suggest that the majority of the HCCs throughout the world are associated with HBV infection: geography, case–control studies and prospective studies.

Geography

There is a striking geographical correlation between the prevalence of hepatitis B surface antigen (HBsAg) and the annual incidence of HCCs for most, if not all, areas of the world[10]. Very high rates of HCCs (>20 per 100 000 population and year) are observed in China, Southeast Asia and South African blacks; high rates (10–20 per 100 000 population and year) are documented in Japan, southern Europe and Bulgaria; intermediate rates (5–10 per 100 000 population and year) in Poland, Romania, Hungary, Yugoslavia, Austria, Germany, France and Belgium; and low rates (<5 per 100 000 population and year) in Canada, USA, Latin America, UK, Scandinavia, Israel, India and Australia. High incidence rates are also found in Chinese in Hawaii or California, and in Alaskan Eskimos. The geographical relationship between HBsAg prevalence and HCC incidence holds true for all countries and populations mentioned above. A possible exception at present is Greenland, where the HCC incidence appears lower than expected from the HBsAg carrier rate.

Case–control studies

In many areas of the world the prevalence of HBV markers in patients with HCC has been analysed. All studies, independent of the geographical region, demonstrate an excess frequency of HBsAg positivity in patients with HCC as compared to healthy controls or the general population (Table 1). In most areas of the world HBsAg prevalence is higher in HCC patients with cirrhosis than in patients without cirrhosis. Further, a significant number of patients with HCC is HBsAg-negative but positive for anti-HBc or anti-HBs. These findings suggest that serological recovery from HBV infection does not always indicate complete resolution of HBV-associated clinical disease. Similar data have recently been obtained in the woodchuck model of hepadnavirus infection[19] (see below).

Prospective studies

A prospective general population study in 22 707 Taiwanese men[11,20] demonstrated an HCC incidence of 528 per 100 000 men and year in HBsAg-

Table 1 HBV serology in patients with HCC

Country	*HBsAg (%)*	*Anti-HBc (only) (%)*	*Anti-HBs (%)*	*Reference*
Taiwan	97	1	2	11
Hong Kong	38/88*			12
South Africa	53/61†	16/17	8/12	13
Japan	34		24	14
Japan	7/27			15
Greece	37	16	39	16
Great Britain	14/37			17
Austria	9/19			18

* Patients without cirrhosis/patients with cirrhosis
† 8/17% HBeAg+; 64/48% anti-HBe+

positive individuals as compared to 3 per 100 000 and year in HBsAg-negative individuals (Table 2). No HCC developed in persons negative for all HBV markers. HBV carriers, therefore, have an approximately 200-fold higher risk of developing an HCC than non-infected individuals. HCC and cirrhosis accounted for more than 50% of the deaths among HBV carriers as compared to less than 2% of the deaths among non-carriers.

Taken together, the epidemiological data indicate that HBV infection plays a central role in the aetiology and pathogenesis of HCC development. While 85–90% of the annual incidence of HCCs worldwide (estimated to be about 250 000) are associated with chronic HBV infection, the independent oncogenic potential of other factors has been established[21]: viral infections other than HBV, toxins, hormones and various diseases leading to the development of cirrhosis (Table 3). Among these aetiological factors, alcohol is probably one of the leading causes of HCCs in the Western world, most frequently developing in the setting of macronodular cirrhosis. Further, the tumour-promoting contribution of some of these agents as cofactors to the development of HCCs in HBV carriers has been demonstrated or epidemiologically suspected[22,23] (e.g. alcohol, aflatoxins, androgens).

Table 2 Prospective study of HBV carriers in Taiwan, 1975–83[11]

HBVserology	*Subjects (n)*	*HCC (n)*	*HCC Risk (per 100 000 and year)*
HBsAg positive	3454	113	528
HBsAg negative	19 253	3	3
anti-HBc + only	2248	1	7
anti-HBs +	15 570	2	2
HBV –	1272	0	0
Total	22 707	116	82

Table 3 Factors associated with HCC development

Viral infections
- HBV
- HCV*

Toxins
- Alcohol
- Aflatoxins
- Thorotrast
- Vinyl chloride

Hormones
- Oral contraceptives
- Androgens

Various other conditions associated with development of liver cirrhosis
- Primary biliary cirrhosis
- Haemochromatosis
- Alpha-1-antitrypsin deficiency
- Tyrosinaemia

* Chronic infection with hepatitis C virus

CLINICAL AND PATHOLOGICAL CHARACTERISTICS OF HBV INFECTION AND HCC

Infection with HBV induces a wide spectrum of clinical presentations, ranging from the 'healthy' carrier state to acute or chronic hepatitis and liver cirrhosis. Further, chronic HBV infection is clearly associated with the development of HCCs (see above). Prospective studies have shown that in 60–70% of individuals HBV infection is clinically inapparent. The outcome of infection in a given individual is largely dependent on the age at infection: in adults only 5–10% of individuals develop chronic HBV infection, while in newborns and children more than 90% go on to a chronic HBV carrier state[24].

Natural course of chronic HBV infection

Clinically, chronic HBV infection can present either as a 'healthy' HBV carrier state or as chronic hepatitis B. The clinical characteristics of these two presentations and their potential to lead to HCCs (Table 4) are significant from both a clinical and scientific point of view. HBV carriers have been followed prospectively in a number of clinical studies. In clinically asymptomatic patients a single or follow-up liver biopsy both in children and adults most frequently shows mild abnormalities (e.g. non-specific alterations or CPH) which are stable for many years and rarely progress to a more serious form of liver disease[25–27]. Clinical and histological studies in children, however, indicate a high frequency of ALT elevation and histological alterations ranging from non-specific changes to CAH[28,29]. These data suggest that a true 'healthy' HBV carrier state, as defined above (Table 4), may be infrequent. Rather, the chronic HBV carrier state should be viewed as a continuum ranging from very mild/focal and clinically/histologically inapparent or only transiently identifiable disease with a low HCC potential to clinically symptomatic active/aggressive liver disease with a high risk of malignant transformation.

The factors determining the clinical course and eventual outcome in a given HBV carrier are poorly defined as yet. In a prospective study from Taiwan the factors contributing to the development of cirrhosis in HBV

Table 4 Clinical characteristics of chronic HBV carriers

		Chronic hepatitis B	
	'Healthy' HBV carrier	*Asymptomatic*	*Symptomatic*
Symptoms	–	–	+
Signs	–	–	+
ALT elevation	–	(+)	+++
Liver histology	NL*	NS–CPH†	NS–CAH–cirrhosis‡
Progression and HCC development	(±)	+	+++

* Normal except for ground glass hepatocytes
† NS-CPH represents spectrum from nonspecific to chronic persistent hepatitis
‡ NS-CAH-cirrhosis represents spectrum from nonspecific hepatic inflammation to chronic hepatitis with or without cirrhosis

Table 5 Prospective study of asymptomatic HBV carrier children in Taiwan[28]

13/18	*ALT elevations*
	moderate
	frequently transient
18/18	*Histological abnormalities*
	15/18 non-specific changes
	3/18 CPH

carriers were assessed[30]: patients who experienced hepatic decompensation, repeated exacerbation without HBeAg to anti-HBe seroconversion or with HBeAg reappearance were found to develop cirrhosis most frequently. In a study from Italy[31], by contrast, 54% of patients with CAH serologically positive for HBsAg and anti-HBe developed cirrhosis within 4–5 years. Whether this aggressive clinical course is related to a specific HBV mutation, resulting in a stop codon at the end of the pre-C gene, remains to be determined[32,33].

Pathological characteristics

From a pathological point of view, 60–90% of HBV-associated HCCs arise in the setting of liver cirrhosis, mostly of the macronodular type[25,26]. Further, in most HCC patients without cirrhosis, portal fibrosis and/or cellular infiltrates are found[15]. From these data one is led to believe that there is probably no HBV-induced HCC arising in a completely normal liver. Rather, some hepatocellular necrosis and inflammation followed by regeneration may be required in the malignant transformation process. Given the fact that hepatocyte necrosis, inflammation and regeneration are highly associated with hepatocarcinogenesis (see below), it is reasonable to assume that the risk of malignant transformation correlates with the duration and degree of the underlying liver disease. In this context, liver cirrhosis clearly presents the most significant precursor lesion with the highest risk of malignant transformation. At the same time, however, any form of chronic hepatitis B, even if clinically and/or histologically undetectable, carries a low but definite risk of progressing to HCC. Taken together, the data suggests that the duration and severity of HBV-induced liver disease are key determinants for the development.

Risk factors

The clinical and pathological characterization of HBV carriers has allowed us to define a number of factors indicating a high risk of developing an HCC (Table 6). The highest risks have males older than 40 years with liver cirrhosis. The significance of viral markers other than HBsAg (anti-HBc, HBeAg, anti-HBe) is less clear. The presence of anti-HBc IgM, however, may indicate an especially high risk for the development of HCC[34–37], possibly reflecting low-level HBV replication. From the case–control studies mentioned above

Table 6 Pathology in HBV carrier children in Taiwan[29]

	Asymptomatic (%) ($n = 37$)	*Symptomatic* (%) ($n = 29$)
Male	62	93
ALT > 300 U/l	5	34
Jaundice	0	34
Splenomegaly	0	21
Mother HBsAg+	39	69
Liver histology		
Normal*	11	0
Non-specific	49	3
CPH	35	24
CAH	5	38
Cirrhosis	0	35

* Except for ground-glass hepatocytes

(Table 1) it is clear, however, that even serological recovery from HBV infection with presence of anti-HBs does not always indicate complete resolution of HBV-induced clinical disease, and can be associated with the development of HCC.

MOLECULAR HEPATOCARCINOGENESIS

The molecular mechanisms leading from chronic HBV infection to the malignant transformation of liver cells are still poorly defined. Molecular studies of human HCCs and animal models, however, have begun to identify key steps in hepatocarcinogenesis. While all molecular concepts of HCC development would need to take into consideration the various epidemiological, clinical and pathological aspects mentioned above, it is important to emphasize that the malignant transformation of hepatocytes is probably a unicellular event sequentially followed by tumour growth and later metastasis, representing the clonal expansion of the transformed liver cell[38–43].

Human HCCs

In most HBV-related HCCs, HBV DNA has been found integrated into the host cellular genome[6–8]. HBV DNA integrations have also been identified in non-tumorous liver from patients with chronic HBV infection with or

Table 7 Risk factors for HCC development

Cirrhosis	60–90% of HCCs associated with macronodular cirrhosis (risk 5 × over non-cirrhotics)	
Male sex	HCC 3–5 × more frequent in males than in females	
Age	Annual HCC incidence increases with age:	
	Maximum in Asia:	50–60 years
	Maximum in Africa:	30–40 years
HBV marker	Anti-HBc IgM	
Cofactors	Alcohol, aflatoxins, androgens	

without HCC[44–48]. The structure of integrated viral DNAs and of their flanking host cellular sequences has been analysed in great detail: HBV DNA integrations are usually subgenomic in size, may be colinear with the genome or may be inverted and frequently contain multiple rearrangements, including deletions, direct and inverted duplications and translocations. Depending on the physical structure and the degree of methylation of the integrated viral DNA sequences, viral proteins (HBsAg, HBcAg, HBxAg or polymerase gene products) are expressed in HCC cells[49–52]. However, because of the rearrangements, pregenomic RNA as an intermediate of viral DNA replication is not transcribed from integrated viral DNA species.

The molecular mechanisms controlling viral DNA integration and possibly excision–reintegration are so far unknown. HBV integrations have been identified on many chromosomes (chromosomes 2, 3, 4, 5, 6, 7, 9, 11 and 17). The integration appears to be a non-directed random event. The only aspect of viral integration that seems to be non-random is the frequent use of sequences near the direct repeats DR1 and DR2 within the viral genome as integration sites[53]. Possibly, integration of viral DNA is favoured by intracellular accumulation of HBV DNA molecules during the natural course of infection[54]. No common structure of HBV DNA integrations has been found in the HCC tissues, and the pattern of HBV DNA integration in the HCC is frequently different from that in the non-tumorous part of the liver from the same patient[47].

Animal models

Animal models of hepadnavirus infection and studies with transgenic mice have begun to yield new insight into the relationship between chronic HBV infection and HCC development. HCCs have been observed in woodchucks[19,55,56], ground squirrels[57] and Pekin ducks[58,59]. In woodchucks the relative risk of developing an HCC is essentially 100% for animals with persistent antigenaemia, acquired either naturally or experimentally[55]. Similar to HBV-associated HCCs (Table 1), HCCs were also observed in woodchucks serologically recovered from acute WHV infection[19,60] indicating a significant risk of HCC development (approximately 5%) even after seroconversion to anti-WHs. The risk was found to be even higher for serologically recovered animals with persistence of WHV DNA in the liver[19]. Similar to HBV, WHV DNA integrations appear to be random and display multiple rearrangements.

In transgenic mice the overexpression of the large HBsAg (pre S1/pre S2/S protein) in hepatocytes induces a sequence of hepatocellular changes which closely resemble chronic viral hepatitis[61–63], leading from 'ground-glass' hepatocytes to liver cell necrosis, hyperplasia and eventually to neoplasia. In this system there is a direct correlation between the level of viral gene expression, the extent of liver cell injury and neoplasia development. Liver cell injury appears to be a direct consequence of viral gene expression. Interestingly, in transgenic mice adult males have higher HBsAg levels in serum than females[64]. It remains to be established, however, to what extent this process occurs during HBV infection in man.

Current concepts of molecular hepatocarcinogenesis

While activation of c-myc[64], a steroid thyroid hormone receptor[66] and a retinoic acid receptor[67,68] have been identified in some HCCs, and HBV DNA has been found integrated in a sequence homologous to v-erb-A and steroid receptor genes[69], in most tumours studied so far there is no clear evidence that viral integration contributes directly to tumorigenesis. In view of the genetic changes detected in HBV-associated HCCs, including deletions, translocations and rearrangements, the loss of tumour-suppressing genes may also contribute to tumour development, analogous to the observations made in retinoblastoma, colorectal cancer, breast cancer and other malignancies[70,71].

In our hypothesis of molecular hepatocarcinogenesis (Table 8) the key event is the rearrangement/disorganization of cellular DNA in a single hepatocyte. This event is dependent on increased liver cell regeneration/-mitoses and inflammation in response to hepatocyte necrosis. This liver disease-related aspect carries a definite but low oncogenic potential, probably similar to chronic hepatitis from other causes (Table 3). In the setting of chronic hepatitis B, however, HBV DNA makes a specific contribution to the malignant transformation by integration into the cellular genome, presumably during liver cell mitoses. The frequency of HBV DNA integrations is dependent, among other factors, on the duration and severity of the underlying liver disease. Critical DNA integrations can eventually induce the rearrangement of cellular DNA (structural changes) and/or the dysregulation of cellular or viral gene expression (functional changes). These changes in turn can result in the activation of cellular oncogenes or, more likely, in the inactivation or loss of tumour-suppressing genes, finally leading to the malignant phenotype.

This concept of hepatocarcinogenesis (Figure 1) accommodates many, if not all, of the molecular data available to date, as well as the epidemiological,

Table 8 Concepts of molecular hepatocarcinogenesis

Key event: Rearrangement/disorganization of cellular DNA in a single hepatocyte

1. *Liver disease-related aspects*
   Increased liver cell *regeneration-mitoses* and *inflammation* in response to hepatocyte necrosis (? promoted by humoral factors, e.g., lymphokines)
2. *HBV DNA-related aspects*
   Non-directed, random integration of HBV DNA into hepatocyte DNA resulting in *rearrangement* of cellular DNA (structural changes) or *dysregulation* of cellular or viral gene expression (functional changes):
   (a) activation of cellular oncogenes
   (b) inactivation of tumour-suppressing genes
3. *Contribution of cofactors*
   Cellular DNA rearrangement possibly promoted through exogenous factors (e.g. aflatoxins). Autonomous, clonal expansion of malignantly transformed hepatocyte possibly promoted through exogenous or host factors (e.g. androgens)

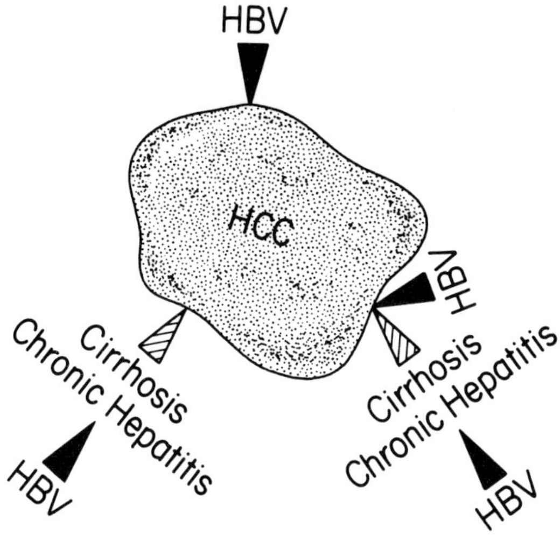

Figure 1 Possible mechanisms of HBV-induced hepatocarcinogenesis

clinical and pathological observations in patients with HCC, and allows for the contribution of other cofactors, such as alcohol, aflatoxins and androgens, as tumour-promoting agents.

SUMMARY AND PERSPECTIVES

Epidemiological, clinico-pathological and molecular data demonstrate a causal relationship between HBV infection and HCC development. Central to the malignant transformation of the hepatocyte is chronic hepatitis with liver cell necrosis–inflammation–regeneration, resulting in increased number of mitoses. In this setting, HBV DNA makes a specific contribution to malignant transformation by integration into the cellular genome. Critical integrations may eventually induce structural and/or functional changes in the biology of the hepatocyte with activation of cellular oncogenes or, more likely, inactivation of tumour-suppressing genes.

The scientific challenge of the future lies in the identification of the cellular and molecular events leading to or contributing to the malignant phenotype of HCC cells. Clinically, major efforts will be directed towards improving the efficiency of antiviral therapies in patients with chronic hepatitis B, as well as the early recognition of HCCs in a subclinical and potentially treatable/curable stage. Most important, however, will be the systematic implementation of HBV vaccination in high HBsAg prevalence areas. The preventive strategies hold the promise not only of reducing morbidity and mortality from chronic HBV infection and cirrhosis, but also of preventing the development of HCCs, one of the world's more frequent malignancies.

Acknowledgements

The support of H. E. Blum by a Hermann-and-Lilly-Schilling professorship from the Stifterverband fuer die Deutsche Wissenschaft is gratefully acknowledged. This work was supported in part by grants AA-02666, CA-35711, AA-08169 and HD-20469 from the National Institutes of Health. J. R. Wands is the recipient of a Research Scientist Award AA-00048. The authors gratefully acknowledge the assistance of Mrs Kristin Cambria-Shaw in the preparation of the manuscript.

References

1. Summers, J., Smolec, J. M. and Snyder, R. (1978). A virus similar to hepatitis B virus associated with hepatitis and hepatoma in woodchucks. *Proc. Natl. Acad. Sci., USA*, **75**, 4533–7
2. Marion, P. L., Oshiro, L. S., Regnery, D. C., Scullard, G. H. and Robinson, W. S. (1980). A virus in Beechey ground squirrels that is related to hepatitis B virus of humans. *Proc. Natl. Acad. Sci., USA*, **77**, 2941–4
3. Feitelson, M. A., Millman, I. and Blumberg, B. S. (1986). Tree squirrel hepatitis B virus: antigenic and structural characterization. *Proc. Natl. Acad. Sci., USA*, **83**, 2233–7
4. Mason, W. S., Seal, G. and Summers, J. (1980). Virus of Pekin ducks with structural and biological relatedness to human hepatitis B virus. *J. Virol.*, **36**, 829–36
5. Sprengel, R., Kaleta, E. F. and Will, H. (1988). Isolation and characterization of hepatitis B virus endemic in herons. *J. Virol.*, **62**, 3832–9
6. Tiollais, P., Pourcel, C. and Dejean, A. (1985). The hepatitis B virus. *Nature*, **317**, 489–95
7. Ganem, D. and Varmus, H. E. (1987). The molecular biology of the hepatitis B viruses. *Ann. Rev. Biochem.*, **56**, 651–93
8. Schoedel, F., Sprengel, R., Weimer, T., Fernholz, D., Schneider, R. and Will, H. (1989). Animal hepatitis B viruses. *Adv. Viral. Oncol.*, **8**, 73–102
9. Mason, W. S. and Taylor, J. M. (1989). Experimental systems for the study of hepadnavirus and hepatitis delta virus infections. *Hepatology*, **9**, 635–45
10. Okuda, K. and Beasley, R. P. (1982). Epidemiology of hepatocellular carcinoma. In Okuda, K. and MacKay, I. (eds), *Hepatocellular Carcinoma*, pp. 9–30. (Geneva: UICC Report 17)
11. Beasley, R. P. and Hwang, L.-Y. (1984). Hepatocellular carcinoma and the hepatitis B virus. *Sem. Liver Dis.*, **4**, 113–21
12. Gibson, J. B., Wu, P. C., Ho, J. C. I. and Lauder, J. J. (1980). HBsAg, hepatocellular carcinoma and cirrhosis in Hong Kong. A necropsy study. *Br. J. Cancer*, **42**, 370–7
13. Kew, M. C. (1989). Hepatocellular carcinoma with and without cirrhosis. A comparison in Southern African blacks. *Gastroenterology*, **97**, 136–9
14. The Liver Cancer Study Group of Japan (1984). Primary liver cancer in Japan. *Cancer*, **54**, 1747–55
15. Okuda, K., Nakashima, T., Kojiro, M., Kondo, Y. and Wada, K. (1989). Hepatocellular carcinoma without cirrhosis in Japanese patients. *Gastroenterology*, **97**, 140–6
16. Tassopoulos, N. C., Theodoropoulos, G., Sjogren, M. H., Engle, R. and Purcell, R. H. (1989). Serological markers of hepatitis B virus and infections in Greek adults with primary hepatocellular carcinoma. *Infection*, **17**, 23–5
17. Melia, W. M., Wilkinson, M. L., Portmann, B. C., Johnson, P. J. and Williams, R. (1984). Hepatocellular carcinoma in the noncirrhotic liver: a comparison with that complicating cirrhosis. *Q. J. Med.*, **33**, 391–400
18. Ferenci, P., Dragosics, B., Marosi, L. and Kiss, F. (1984). Relative incidence of primary liver cancer in cirrhosis in Austria. Etiological considerations. *Liver*, **4**, 7–14
19. Korba, B. E., Wells, F. V., Baldwin, B., Cole, P. J., Tennant, B. C., Popper, H. and Gerin, J. L. (1989). Hepatocellular carcinoma in woodchuck hepatitis virus-infected woodchucks: presence of viral DNA in tumor tissue from chronic carriers and animals serologically recovered from acute infections. *Hepatology*, **9**, 461–70

20. Beasley, R. P., Hwang, L.-Y., Lin, C.-C. and Chien, C.-S. (1981). Hepatocellular carcinoma and hepatitis B virus. *Lancet*, **2**, 1129–33
21. Lisker-Melman, M., Martin, P. and Hoofnagle, J. H. (1989). Conditions associated with hepatocellular carcinoma. *Med. Clin. N. Am.*, **73**, 999–1009
22. Itoh, S. and Shimoji, K. (1986). Effects of alcohol on the liver in HBsAg carriers. *Am. J. Gastroenterol.*, **81**, 779–82
23. Van Rensburg, S. J., Cook-Mozzafari, P., van Schalkwyk, D. J., van der Watt, J. J., Vincint, T. J. and Purchase, I. F. (1985). Hepatocellular carcinoma and dietary aflatoxin in Mazambique and Transkei. *Br. J. Cancer*, **51**, 713–26
24. Hoofnagle, J. H., Shafritz, D. A. and Popper, H. (1987). Chronic type B hepatitis and the 'healthy' HBsAg carrier state. *Hepatology*, **7**, 758–63
25. Popper, H. (1986). The relation between hepatitis B virus infection and hepatocellular carcinoma. *Hepato-gastroenterology*, **33**, 2–5
26. Popper, H., Shafritz, D. A. and Hoofnagle, J. H. (1987). Relation of the hepatitis B virus carrier state to hepatocellular carcinoma. *Hepatology*, **7**, 764–72
27. Lok, A. S. F. and Lai, C.-L. (1988). A longitudinal follow-up of asymptomatic hepatitis B surface antigen-positive Chinese children. *Hepatology*, **8**, 1130–3
28. Chang, M.-H., Hwang, L.-Y., Hsu, H.-C., Lee, C.-Y., and Beasley, R. P. (1988). Prospective study of asymptomatic HBsAg carrier children in the perinatal period: Clinical and liver histologic studies. *Hepatology*, **8**, 374–7
29. Hsu, H.-C., Lin, Y.-H., Chang, M.-H., Su, I.-J., and Chen, D.-S. (1988). Pathology of chronic hepatitis B virus infection in children with special reference to the intrahepatic expression of hepatitis B virus antigens. *Hepatology*, **8**, 378–82
30. Liaw, Y.-F., Tai, D.-I., Chu, C.-M. and Chen, T. J. (1988). The development of cirrhosis in patients with chronic B hepatitis: a prospective study. *Hepatology*, **8**, 493–6
31. Fattovich, G., Brollo, L., Alberti, A., Pontisso, P., Giustina, G. and Realdi, G. (1988). Long-term follow-up of anti-HBc positive chronic active hepatitis B. *Hepatology*, **8**, 1651–4
32. Brunetto, M. R., Stemler, M., Schoedel, F., Will, H., Ottobrelli, A., Rizzetto, M., Verme, G. and Bonino, F. (1989). Identification of HBV variants which cannot produce precore derived HBeAg and may be responsible for severe hepatitis. *Ital. J. Gastroenterol.*, **21**, 151–4
33. Carman, W. F., Jacyna, M. R., Hadziyannis, S., Karayiannis, P., McGarvey, M. J., Makvis, A. and Thomas, H. C. (1989). Mutation preventing formation of hepatitis B e antigen in patients with chronic hepatitis B infection. *Lancet*, **2**, 588–91
34. Sjogren, M. H., Lemon, S. M., Chung, W. K., Sun, H. S. and Hoofnagle, J. H. (1984). IgM antibody to hepatitis B core antigen in Korean patients with hepatocellular carcinoma. *Hepatology*, **4**, 615–18
35. Roggendorf, M., Hwang, L.-Y., Beasley, R. P., Chen, P. H., Chen, T.-C., Lo, K.-R. and Deinhardt, F. (1987). Anti-HBc IgM in cases of hepatocellular carcinoma and cirrhosis in Taiwan. *J. Hepatol.*, **5**, 268–73
36. Sjogren, M. H., Dusheiko, G. M., Kew, M. C. and Song, E. (1988). Hepatitis B virus infection and hepatocellular carcinoma: Correlation between IgM antibody to hepatitis B core antigen, hepatic Be antigen and hepatitis B DNA. *Am. J. Trop. Med. Hyg.*, **39**, 582–5
37. Lai, M. C., Tong, M. J., Nowicki, M. J. and Lee, S.-D. (1988). Is anti-HBc IgM a useful test in patients with HBsAg-positive chronic hepatitis or primary hepatocellular carcinoma? *Hepatology*, **8**, 514–17
38. Hino, O., Kitagawa, T., Koike, K., Kobayashi, M., Hara, M., Mori, W., Nakashima, T., Hattori, N. and Sugano, H. (1984). Detection of hepatitis B virus DNA in hepatocellular carcinoma in Japan. *Hepatology*, **4**, 90–5
39. Esumi, M., Aritaka, T., Arii, M., Suzuki, K., Tanikawa, K., Misuo, H., Mima, T. and Shikata, T. (1986). Clonal origin of human hepatoma determined by integration of hepatitis B virus DNA. *Cancer Res.*, **46**, 5767–71
40. Imazeki, F., Omata, M., Yokosuka, O. and Okuda, K. (1986). Integration of hepatitis B virus DNA in hepatocellular carcinoma. *Cancer*, **58**, 1055–60
41. Blum, H. E., Offensperger, W.-B., Walter, E., Offensperger, S., Wahl, A., Zeschnigk, C. and Gerok, W. (1987). Hepatocellular carcinoma and hepatitis virus infection: molecular evidence for monoclonal origin and expansion of malignantly transformed hepatocytes. *J. Cancer Res. Clin. Oncol.*, **113**, 466–72
42. Tsuda, H., Hirohashi, S., Shimosato, Y., Terada, M. and Hasegawa, H. (1988). Clonal origin

of atypical adenomatous hyperplasia and clonal identity with hepatocellular carcinoma. *Gastroenterology*, **95**, 1664–6

43. Chen, P.-J., Chen, D.-S., Lai, M.-Y., Chang, M.-H., Huang, G.-H., Yang, P.-M., Sheu, J.-C., Lee, S.-C., Hsu, H.-C. and Sung, J.-L. (1989). Clonal origin of recurrent hepatocellular carcinomas. *Gastroenterology*, **96**, 527–9
44. Hada, H., Arima, T., Togawa, K., Okada, Y., Morichika, S. and Nagashima, H. (1986). State of hepatitis B viral DNA in the liver of patients with hepatocellular carcinoma and chronic liver disease. *Liver*, **6**, 189–98
45. Yaginuma, K., Kobayashi, H., Kobayashi, M., Morishima, T., Matsuyama, K. and Koike, K. (1987). Multiple integration site of hepatitis B virus DNA in hepatocellular carcinoma and chronic active hepatitis tissues from children. *J. Virol.*, **61**, 1808–13
46. Lai, M.-Y., Chen, D.-S., Chen, P.-J., Lee, S.-C., Shen, J.-C., Huang, G.-T., Wei, T.-C., Lee, C.-S., Yu, S.-C., Hsu, H.-C. and Sung, J. L. (1988). Status of hepatitis B virus DNA in hepatocellular carcinoma. *J. Med. Virol.*, **25**, 249–58
47. Tanaka, Y., Esumi, M. and Shikata, T. (1988). Frequent integration of hepatitis B virus DNA in noncancerous liver tissue from hepatocellular carcinoma patients. *J. Med. Virol.*, **26**, 7–14
48. Tozuka, S., Uchida, T., Suzuki, K., Esumi, M. and Shikata, T. (1989). State of hepatitis B virus DNA in hepatocytes of patients with non-carcinomatous liver disease. *Arch. Pathol. Lab. Med.*, **113**, 20–5
49. Yokosuka, O., Omata, M., Imazeki, F., Ito, Y. and Okuda, K. (1986). Hepatitis virus RNA transcripts and DNA in chronic liver disease. *N. Engl. J. Med.*, **315**, 1187–92
50. Bowyer, S. M., Dusheiko, G. M., Schoub, B. D. and Kew, M. C. (1987). Expression of hepatitis B virus genome in chronic hepatitis B carriers and patients with hepatocellular carcinoma. *Proc. Natl. Acad. Sci., USA*, **84**, 847–50
51. Imazeki, F., Yaginuma, K., Omata, M., Okuda, K., Kobayashi, M. and Koike, K. (1987). RNA transcripts of hepatitis B virus in hepatocellular carcinoma. *Hepatology*, **7**, 753–7
52. Su, T.-S., Lui, W.-Y., Lin, L.-H., Hans, S.-H. and P'eng, F.-K. (1989). Analysis of hepatitis B virus transcripts in infected human livers. *Hepatology*, **9**, 180–5
53. Shih, C., Burk, K., Chou, J.-M., Yang, C.-Y., Lee, C.-S., Zeldis, J., Isselbacher, K. J., Wands, J. R. and Goodman, H. M. (1987). Imprecise site-specific recombination of hepatitis B virus in hepatoma. *J. Virol.*, **61**, 4391–8
54. Raimondo, G., Burk, R. D., Lieberman, H. M., Muschel, J., Hadziyannis, S. J., Will, H., Kew, M. C., Dusheiko, G. M. and Shafritz, D. A. (1988). Interrupted replication of hepatitis B virus in liver tissue of HBsAg carriers with hepatocellular carcinoma. *Virology*, **166**, 103–12
55. Popper, H., Roth, L., Purcell, R. H., Tennant, B. C. and Gerin, J. L. (1987). Hepatocarcinogenicity of the woodchuck hepatitis virus. *Proc. Natl. Acad. Sci., USA*, **84**, 866–70
56. Rogler, C. E., Hino, O. and Su, C.-Y. (1987). Molecular aspects of persistent woodchuck hepatitis virus and hepatitis B virus infection and hepatocellular carcinomas. *Hepatology*, **7**, 74S–78S
57. Marion, P. L., van Davelaar, M. J., Knight, S. S., Salazar, F. H., Garcia, G., Popper, H. and Robinson, W. S. (1986). Hepatocellular carcinoma in ground squirrels persistently infected with ground squirrel hepatitis virus. *Proc. Natl. Acad. Sci., USA*, **83**, 4543–6
58. Yokosuka, O., Omata, M., Zhou, Y.-Z., Imazeki, F. and Okuda, K. (1985). Duck hepatitis B virus DNA in liver and serum of Chinese ducks: integration of viral DNA in a hepatocellular carcinoma. *Proc. Natl. Acad. Sci., USA*, **82**, 5180–4
59. Imazeki, F., Yaginuma, K., Omata, M., Okuda, K., Kobayashi, M. and Koike, K. (1988). Integrated structure of duck hepatitis B virus DNA in hepatocellular carcinoma. *J. Virol.*, **62**, 861–5
60. Mitamura, K., Hoyer, B. H., Ponzetto, A., Nelson, J., Purcell, R. H. and Gerin, J. L. (1982). Woodchuck hepatitis virus DNA in woodchuck liver tissue. *Hepatology*, **2**, 47S–50S
61. Chisari, F. V., Pinkert, C. A., Milich, D. R., Filippi, P., McLachlan, A., Palmiter, R. D. and Brinster, R. L. (1985). A transgenic mouse model of the chronic hepatitis B surface antigen carrier state. *Science*, **230**, 1157–60
62. Chisari, F. V., Filippi, P., Buras, J., McLachlan, A., Popper, H., Pinkert, C. A., Palmiter, R. D. and Brinster, R. L. (1987). Structural and pathological effects of synthesis of hepatitis B virus large envelope polypeptide in transgenic mice. *Proc. Natl. Acad. Sci., USA*, **84**, 6909–13

63. Chisari, F. V. (1989). The hepatitis B virus large envelope polypeptide can cause liver cell injury and multifocal nodular hyperplasia in transgenic mice. In Bannasch, P., Keppler, D. and Weber, G. (eds), *Liver Cell Carcinoma*, pp. 165–168. (Lancaster: MTP Press)
64. DeLoia, J. A., Burk, R. D. and Gearhart, J. D. (1989). Developmental regulation of hepatitis B surface antigen expression in two lines of hepatitis B virus transgenic mice. *J. Virol.*, **63**, 4069–73
65. Hsu, T.-Y., Moeroey, T., Etiemble, J., Louise, A., Trepo, C., Tiollais, P. and Buendia, M.-A. (1988). Activation of c-myc by woodchuck hepatitis virus insertion in hepato-cellular carcinoma. *Cell*, **55**, 627–35
66. de The, H., Marchio, A., Tiollais, P. and Dejean, A. (1987). A novel steroid thyroid hormone receptor-related gene inappropriately expressed in human hepatocellular carcinoma. *Nature*, **330**, 667–70
67. Brand, N., Petkovich, M., Krust, A., Chambon, P., de The, H., Marchio, A., Tiollais, P. and Dejean, A. (1988). Identification of a second human retinoic acid receptor. *Nature*, **332**, 850–3
68. Benbrook, D., Lernhardt, E. and Pfahl, M. (1988). A new retinoic acid receptor identified from a hepatocellular carcinoma. *Nature*, **333**, 669–72
69. Dejean, A., Bougueleret, L., Grzeschik, K.-H. and Tiollais, P. (1986). Hepatitis B virus integration in a sequence homologous to v-erb-A and steroid receptor genes in a hepatocellular carcinoma. *Nature*, **332**, 70–2
70. Friend, S. H., Dryja, T. P. and Weinberg, R. A. (1988). Oncogenes and tumor-suppressing genes. *N. Engl. J. Med.*, **318**, 618–22
71. Green, M. R. (1989). When the products of oncogenes and anti-oncogenes meet. *Cell*, **56**, 1–3

20
Treatment of chronic hepatitis B

J. H. HOOFNAGLE

INTRODUCTION

Chronic hepatitis B is estimated to affect 200–300 million persons, or 5% of the world's population[1]. The condition is common in underdeveloped areas of the world and particularly China, Southeast Asia and Subsaharan Africa. In the United States and in Europe chronic hepatitis B is relatively uncommon. A population-based seroepidemiological study recently carried out in the United States[2] showed that 0.43% of the population have hepatitis B surface antigen (HBsAg) in serum, suggesting that there are at least 1 million Americans chronically infected with hepatitis B virus (HBV).

CHRONIC HEPATITIS B: NATURAL HISTORY

The natural history of chronic hepatitis B has been the subject of many studies throughout the world. In general, chronic infection with HBV can be separated into two phases: an early 'replicative' phase and a later 'non-replicative' phase (Figure 1).

The onset of chronic HBV infection is usually associated with a mild, subclinical hepatitis[1]. However, even before symptoms occur, or the serum aminotransferase levels become abnormal, serum HBV markers such as HBsAg, hepatitis B e antigen (HBeAg), HBV DNA and DNA polymerase activity become detectable and rise to high and sustained levels. Serum aminotransferase levels vary initially but then usually remain 2–10-fold elevated above the upper limit of the normal range. Symptoms are minimal, if present at all. This 'replicative' phase of illness is marked by variable degrees of hepatic inflammation and necrosis, the presence of detectable levels of HBV in serum and replicative forms of the virus in the liver.

The severity and clinical course of chronic hepatitis B during this replicative phase are quite variable. In some patients the disease is rapidly progressive, the virus remains detectable, and the patient develops cirrhosis and disability from liver disease within a few years of onset of infection. In other patients the disease waxes and wanes in severity, periods of mild disease activity are

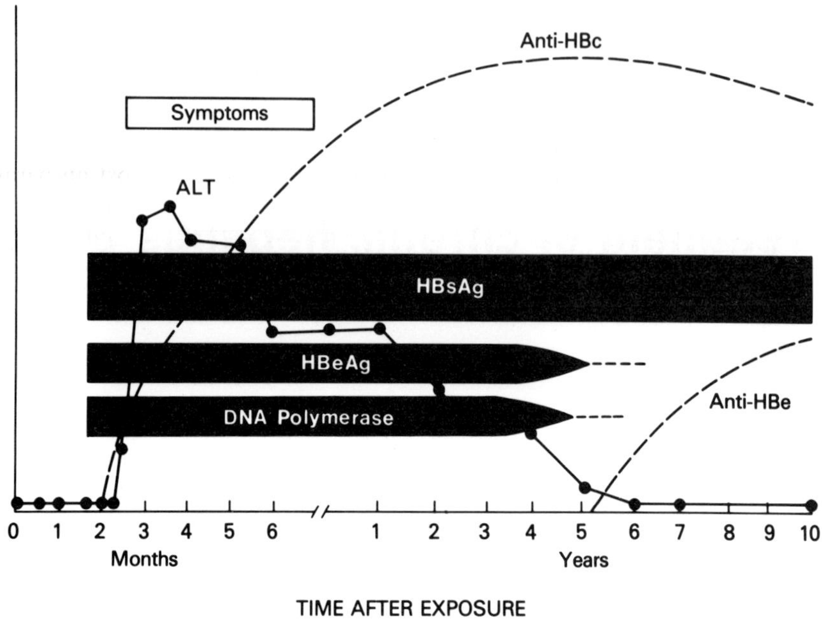

Figure 1 The clinical, serum biochemical and serological course of a typical case of chronic hepatitis B. After a 5-year period of chronic hepatitis there is a spontaneous improvement in disease with fall of serum aminotransferase activities into the normal range and loss of serum markers of hepatitis B virus replication despite continued presence of HBsAg. Abbreviations: HBsAg, hepatitis B surface antigen; HBeAg, hepatitis B e antigen; DNA-p, DNA polymerase activity; HBV, hepatitis B virus; ALT, alanine aminotransferase; anti-HBc, antibody to hepatitis B core antigen; anti-HBe, antibody to HBeAg

followed by exacerbations of disease, and the patient may develop cirrhosis after many years of infection. In other patients the disease is mild or moderate, but ultimately the patient enters a spontaneous remission.

Indeed, in 60–70% of patients spontaneous resolution of the active viral replication and chronic hepatitis eventually occurs, despite the fact that most patients remain HBsAg positive[3]. Serological studies show that the remission in disease is marked by an abrupt fall in serum levels and disappearance of HBV DNA and HBeAg followed by the appearance of anti-HBe[3]. This seroconversion from HBeAg to anti-HBe is usually followed by a fall of serum aminotransferases into the normal range, and gradual resolution of hepatic inflammation and necrosis. Often the seroconversion is preceded by a transient flare in the hepatitis, suggesting that a heightened immunological response to hepatitis antigens is causing the clearance of active viral replication[4]. Studies on liver tissue reveal that the seroconversion from HBeAg to anti-HBe is accompanied by a marked decrease in the levels of HBV DNA in liver and disappearance of the replicative forms of the virus[5]. Persistence of small amounts of integrated HBV DNA in liver probably accounts for the persistence of serum HBsAg.

Thus the transition from the replicative to the non-replicative phase of infection is a milestone in the natural history of chronic hepatitis B, in which the patient enters a remission and is left with HBsAg present in serum but with no serological evidence of viral replication (no HBV DNA in serum or replicative intermediates in liver) and no biochemical or histological evidence of liver injury; a condition referred to as the 'healthy' carrier state[6]. Seroconversion from HBeAg to anti-HBe is also the goal of most antiviral therapy in chronic hepatitis B. The majority of patients who clear HBeAg from serum with antiviral treatment will enter a long-term remission in disease. Indeed, follow-up of patients who become HBeAg negative as a result of antiviral therapy reveals that a high percentage eventually also become HBsAg negative and develop anti-HBs, suggesting a complete resolution and cure of the chronic infection.

THERAPY OF CHRONIC HEPATITIS B

A list of the agents that have been used to treat from hepatitis B is given in Table 1. Some of these agents have been shown to be ineffective; others are promising or have yet to be fully evaluated. The only agent on the list that has been repeatedly shown to be effective in inducing long-term remissions in chronic hepatitis B has been interferon-α.

The interferons are a group of host proteins that have antiviral effects on cells. They are usually separated into three forms: alpha, beta and gamma, based upon cell of origin and antigenicity. Interferon-α has been the most extensively studied form of interferon, and has shown the greatest promise as an antiviral agent. Although there are at least 24 forms of interferon-α, they all share extensive homology and are all interactive with the same surface cell receptor. For these reasons the different forms of interferon-α are thought to be similar in activity and toxicities. Several forms of interferon-α have been used in clinical trials, including human leucocyte-derived interferon[7,8], lymphoblastoid interferon (alfa-nl: 'Wellferon': Burroughs Well-

Table 1 Agents of potential usefulness as therapy of chronic hepatitis B

Interferon-α
Interferon-β
Interferon-γ
Interleukin 2
Granulocyte-macrophage colony-stimulating factor
Thymosin
Corticosteroids
Phyllanthus amarus
Levamisole
Adenine arabinoside (monophosphate)
Acyclovir (deoxyacyclovir)
Foscarnet
Suramin
Ribavirin
Azidothymidine
2′,3′-Dideoxynucleosides

come, UK), and two forms of recombinant human interferon-α (alfa-2a: 'Roferon-A': Hoffmann La Roche, Nutley, NJ and alfa-2b: 'Intron-A': Schering Corp., Kenilworth, NJ).

The initial studies of interferon therapy in chronic hepatitis B were carried out by Merigan and co-workers from Stanford University[7,8]. They demonstrated that buffy coat-delivered leucocyte interferon lowered serum levels of HBV transiently, and that prolonged therapy was sometimes followed with clearance of viral markers and subsequent remission in disease activity. Because of the difficulty in preparing adequate amounts of purified interferon at the time, few patients were treated and results of these early trials were promising but inconclusive.

When modern interferon-α became commercially available, several small pilot studies from the United States, Europe, Africa and Asia suggested that 3–6 month courses of interferon-α in doses of 3–18 million units (MU) given daily, every other day or three times weekly would induce remissions in disease in 25–50% of patients, and that a proportion of responders not only lost HBeAg, but also lost HBsAg and developed anti-HBs[9–11].

The promising pilot studies on interferon-α provided the groundwork for a large number of randomized, controlled trials which have been conducted on six continents and have involved hundreds of patients. To date only a few of these randomized, prospective controlled trials have been published in complete form[12–17]. Several other trials have been reported in abstracts and at scientific meetings[18]. However, the results of the trials have been remarkably consistent: between 25% and 50% of interferon-α-treated patients have responded to therapy with loss of HBV DNA and HBeAg from serum, and subsequent clinical and serum biochemical remission. In contrast, only 0–15% of untreated controls had a spontaneous remission in disease during a comparable follow-up period (Table 2). In these studies the optimal dose of interferon appeared to be 5–10 MU, given three times weekly by the subcutaneous route.

An example of a beneficial response to interferon-α therapy is shown in Figure 2. The patient shown was a middle-aged man with hepatitis B for 3 years, whose liver biopsy showed chronic active hepatitis and early (incomplete) cirrhosis. He received a 4-month course of recombinant human

Table2 Controlled trials of interferon-α therapy of chronic hepatitis B

		*Percentage responding**	
First author (ref.)	*Number of patients*	*Interferon*	*Controls*
Alexander[12]	46	26 (14)	0 (0)
McDonald[13]	37†	43 (18)	0 (0)
Hoofnagle[14]	45	32 (7)	7 (0)
Lok[15]‡	72	17 (0)	0 (0)
Lai[16]‡	24	0 (0)	0 (0)
Saracco[17]	64	70 (24)	39 (3)
Realdi[18]	80	31	17

* Response = rate of loss of HBeAg (in parentheses is rate of loss of HBsAg) from serum 8–12 months after therapy
† Anti-HIV negative patients only
‡ Controlled trials from Asia

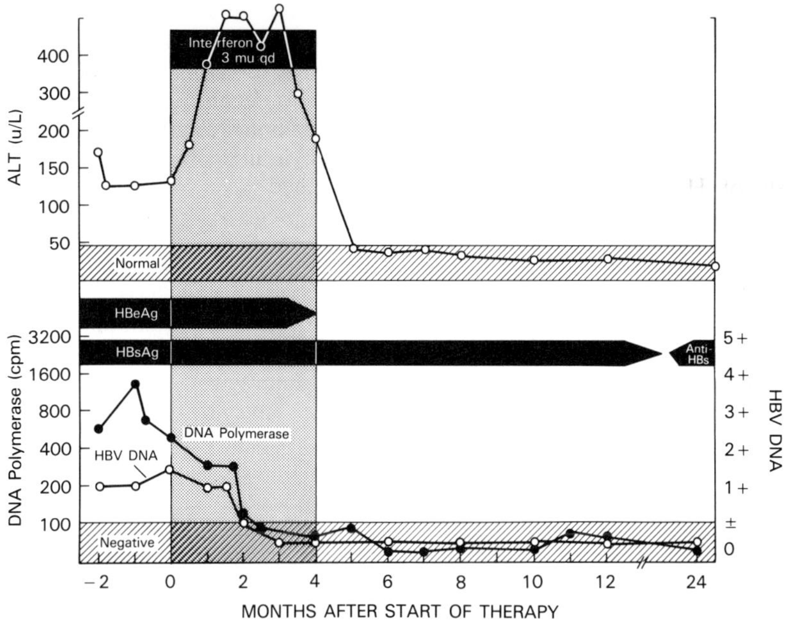

Figure 2 The clinical, serum biochemical and serological course of a patient with chronic hepatitis B who had a beneficial long-term response to treatment with recombinant human interferon-α. During therapy serum HBV DNA and DNA polymerase activity fell to undetectable levels. HBeAg became negative by the end of treatment and serum aminotransferase levels fell into the normal range. The patient lost all symptoms of hepatitis. Two years later, on routine follow-up, the patient was found to be HBsAg negative and anti-HBs positive

interferon-α given in a dose of 3 MU daily. Six weeks after starting interferon therapy he had a flare of hepatitis with serum aminotransferases increasing five-fold above the baseline pretreatment values. Simultaneously serum levels of HBeAg, HBV DNA and DNA polymerase fell and became negative. The patient had a long-term remission in disease, although he remained HBsAg positive. However, on routine follow-up 2 years after treatment he was found to be HBsAg negative and anti-HBs positive.

What was most typical of the patient shown in Figure 2 is the flare of hepatitis that occurs simultaneously with the clearance of HBV markers. A worsening of serum aminotransferases during interferon treatment is typical of a beneficial long-term response. Indeed, patients who have only partial inhibition of HBV levels usually have a slight improvement in serum aminotransferase levels with interferon therapy and relapse promptly when treatment is stopped. This flare of the underlying hepatitis that occurs with treatment suggests that interferon-α acts not only as an antiviral but also as an immunomodulatory agent in ameliorating the course of this disease.

Alpha-interferon therapy: unresolved issues

The early results of interferon-α therapy in chronic hepatitis B were promising and important. However, several problems with this therapy still exist.

Interferon is difficult to administer in the doses needed to treat chronic hepatitis B and has to be given for a prolonged period to obtain a sustained response. The response rate to interferon therapy alone has been somewhat disappointing. Furthermore, the side-effects of interferon can be problematic. How can one identify patients who are most likely to respond to treatment? How can the response rate be improved? How can side-effects be minimized?

Predictive determinants of response to interferon-α

Most large studies on therapy of chronic hepatitis B have attempted to analyse what features correlate with a successful outcome of treatment[11–14,19,20] (Table 3). The two major features that have been found to predict a response to interferon-α therapy in almost every study have been (1) high initial levels of serum aminotransferases and (2) low initial levels of HBV DNA. Thus, the patient with active disease and low levels of virus is most likely to respond to interferon-α therapy. Indeed, these two features of chronic hepatitis B – disease activity and level of viral replication – also constitute the major determinants in the natural history of this illness.

Other features that have been found to correlate with a beneficial response to interferon-α include the patient's age, sex, ethnic background, duration of disease and absence of complicating illnesses[20]. The age of patients may be important in that most studies conducted in children have yielded low response rates to interferon-α[16]. The children in these studies, however, were Asians who often had normal serum aminotransferase levels and high levels of HBV in serum. Thus the features of the disease, rather than the children's age, may have accounted for the poor response rate.

Chronic hepatitis B is less common in women than men and, as might be expected, women are more likely to have a beneficial response to interferon-α treatment. Ethnic background of patients may also determine the differences in response rates among different studies. Most studies conducted among Asian patients have yielded low rates of response, despite use of similar preparations and doses of interferon-α[15,16]. On the other hand, most Asian patients have had hepatitis B since childhood, and the duration of the HBV infection rather than ethnic background may account for the poor response rates.

Of major importance in determining the response of patients with chronic hepatitis B to interferon-α therapy is the effect of a complicating illness. Hepatitis B patients with other diseases such as renal insufficiency, diabetes mellitus, malignancies, immunosuppression, and particularly HIV infection

Table 3 Features that predict a response to interferon-α therapy of chronic hepatitis B

Disease activity (high serum aminotransferases)
Level of HBV (low levels of HBV DNA in serum)
Age (adults)
Sex (female)
Ethnic background (non-oriental patients)
Absence of other diseases (HIV positivity, renal disease, diabetes, immunosuppression)

From references 9–19

are unlikely to have a beneficial effect from interferon. These features are important as hepatitis B often complicates other illnesses such as acquired immunodeficiency syndrome, renal failure and organ transplantation. In these situations, interferon-α is unlikely to be of benefit.

Increasing the response rate to interferon-α

Several approaches have been taken to increase the response rate to interferon-α in chronic hepatitis B. Major efforts are being made in developing new antiviral agents that could be used alone or in combination with interferon-α.

Combinations of interferon-α with other antiviral agents such as adenine arabinoside, adenine arabinoside monophosphate, acyclovir, and interferon-γ have not met with much success[21–24]. Indeed, combination of agents often leads to a potentiation of side-effects rather than potentiation of antiviral effects[21].

Examples of new agents that hold some promise as therapeutic agents for hepatitis B include the plant extract *Phyllanthus amarus*[25]; immunomodulatory drugs such as levamisole[26], thymosin[27], granulocyte-macrophage colony stimulating factor (GM-CSF), and IL-2[28]; and antiviral compounds such as foscarnet[29] and the nucleoside analogues[30,31] (Table 1). Especially helpful in development of antiviral therapies have been recent identification of animal models of hepatitis B, such as the woodchuck hepatitis virus[30] and the duck hepatitis B virus[29,31–33] that can be used to screen antiviral compounds for activity against hepatitis B-like viruses. The further development of continuous cell lines that are transfected with HBV DNA[32], as well as techniques for primary hepatocyte cultures[33], will make screening of antiviral compounds even easier. A safe and easily administered antiviral agent for chronic hepatitis B is sorely needed, either as a single agent or as an agent to be used in combination with interferon-α.

Perhaps the most practical approach to increasing the response rate to interferon-α has been the use of a short course (pulse) of corticosteroids before starting interferon. The rationale for this approach arose out of the original observations by the Stanford investigators that concurrent corticosteroid therapy blocked the effects of interferon, but that withdrawal of corticosteroids immediately before starting interferon was associated with a high rate of response[7]. Retrospective and prospective studies showed that abrupt withdrawal of corticosteroid therapy in chronic hepatitis B led to a transient exacerbation of disease and accompanying decrease in serum HBV DNA and HBeAg levels that occurred 4–8 weeks afterwards[34–38].

Several small clinical trials were conducted evaluating a short course of prednisone by itself as treatment of chronic hepatitis B[34–37]. In some studies the pulse of prednisone was found to be harmful, being followed by a severe and, at times, prolonged exacerbation of disease without clearance of HBV DNA, HBeAg or HBsAg from serum[35]. This flare of hepatitis can be particularly severe in a patient with pre-existing cirrhosis, in whom variceal haemorrhage, hepatic encephalopathy or marked ascites can develop during the exacerbation[37].

Recent studies have evaluated the effects of a short course of prednisone immediately before starting interferon-α treatment of chronic hepatitis B[38]. By correct timing of treatment one could take advantage of the increase in serum aminotransferase activities and decrease in HBV levels that occurs after abrupt withdrawal of corticosteroids. The high aminotransferases and low HBV levels might predispose to a beneficial effect of interferon-α. In an uncontrolled study this approach to treatment yielded a high rate of response.

To evaluate fully the role of corticosteroid pretreatment and interferon-α, investigators from 12 US centres recently designed and carried out a large prospective, randomized controlled trial of interferon-α with and without a preceding course of prednisone[19]. Patients were randomized to receive either: (1) recombinant human interferon-α (alfa-2b) in a dose of 5 MU daily for 4 months; (2) interferon in a dose of 1 MU daily for 4 months; (3) prednisone in decreasing doses for 6 weeks followed 2 weeks later by interferon in a dose of 5 MU daily for 4 months; or (4) no therapy (Table 4). The results, that have been published in abstract form only[19], demonstrated that the short pulse of corticosteroids did not significantly increase the rate of response to interferon-α. However, 5 MU daily was superior to 1 MU daily. Furthermore, in the subset of patients with mild hepatitis there was a trend for a higher response rate in the group given the short course of prednisone. The results of this trial will be extremely important in elucidating the optimal dose of interferon-α therapy, and in clarifying the role of prednisone pretreatment in chronic hepatitis B.

Table 4 Results of a multicenter US trial of interferon-α therapy of chronic hepatitis B

		Percentage with loss of	
Group	No.	HBeAg	HBsAg
Interferon (1 MU)	39	17	2
Interferon (5 MU)	41	33	10
Pred/Interferon (5 MU)	42	38	12
No therapy	41	5	0

Abbreviations: HBsAg, hepatitis B surface antigen; HBeAg, hepatitis B e antigen; Pred, prednisone; MU, million units. From reference 19

THERAPY OF ATYPICAL CHRONIC HEPATITIS B

Most prospective trials of therapy in chronic hepatitis B have studied patients with compensated liver disease, no complicating illnesses, and the typical serological pattern of having HBV DNA and HBeAg in serum. Extrapolating results in this homogeneous group of patients to those with unusual features is not always possible. Three groups of patients deserve comment: those with extrahepatic manifestations, those with hepatic decompensation and those with atypical patterns of serological tests.

Extrahepatic manifestations of chronic hepatitis B include arthritis, mucocutaneous vasculitis, Raynaud's phenomenon, glomerulonephritis and polyarteritis nodosa. There have now been three studies of patients with HBV-related glomerulonephritis that have demonstrated that a high percentage of patients with this complication of HBV infection respond to interferon-α therapy with a loss of HBV markers as well as with improvement in the renal disease[39–41]. The temporal correlation between the amelioration of the glomerulonephritis and the loss of HBeAg supports the hypothesis that immune complexes of HBeAg and immunoglobulin account for the renal lesion. There have been no reported cases of polyarteritis nodosa due to HBV infection that have been treated with interferon. However, the poor prognosis of this condition when it is untreated compared to its good prognosis with prednisone indicates that antiviral therapy should be withheld until immunosuppressive treatment has been evaluated[42].

Patients with *decompensated chronic hepatitis B* represent a difficult group to evaluate in experimental trials of antiviral agents. The extremely poor prognosis of advanced cirrhosis due to chronic hepatitis B makes this group of patients prime candidates for some form of therapy short of liver transplantation[43]. Small numbers of patients with advanced chronic hepatitis B have been studied in uncontrolled trials of interferon-α[44]. In several cases therapy appeared to be dramatically beneficial. However, interferon therapy was almost always complicated by severe side-effects. Most patients experienced an immediate and clinically apparent exacerbation of the underlying chronic hepatitis B with start of therapy. The exacerbation, however, was accompanied by a decrease in serum levels of HBV DNA, and was sometimes followed by a long-lasting remission in disease activity and gradual improvement in the clinical and serum biochemical features of disease. Patients with clinically apparent cirrhosis usually tolerated interferon poorly, and the dose had to be decreased to one-half to one-tenth of the starting dose.

A final group of atypical patients with chronic hepatitis B that deserve comment are those who have active liver disease apparently due to HBV but who are *HBeAg negative*. The serological pattern of HBV DNA without HBeAg in serum is uncommon in the USA and UK, but is frequent in other areas of the world, especially in Mediterranean countries. Patients with antibody to HBeAg (anti-HBe) and chronic hepatitis B may have severe liver disease and warrant some form of intervention[45]. Results of antiviral therapy in a few patients in this category have yielded promising results; indeed the response rate among anti-HBe positive patients may be higher than among HBeAg positive patients. An important factor, however, has been a high rate of relapse or reactivation among such patients. Studies from Italy suggest that these patients benefit from therapy but may require multiple courses[44,45].

SIDE-EFFECTS OF INTERFERON

Side-effects of interferon-α are usually separated into two patterns: the early side-effects that occur during the first days of therapy, and the late side-effects that appear thereafter (Table 5).

Table 5 Side effects of interferon-α

Fatigue	Increased need for sleep
Fever and chills	Headaches
Muscle aches and pains	Nausea and vomiting
Anorexia	Weight loss
Abdominal pains and cramps	Diarrhoea
Hair loss	Sleep disturbance
Dizziness, vertigo	Anxiety
Difficulty concentrating	Irritability and depression
Emotional lability	Psychosis
Bone marrow suppression	Bacterial infections
Autoantibodies	Autoimmune conditions

At doses of interferon-α of 1 MU or greater, the first day of therapy is marked by the sudden onset of fever, chills, fatigue, muscle aches, headaches and nausea 4–8 h after the first injection[11–13]. The peak of fever may be 39 °C and accompanied by shaking chills. Some patients report abdominal cramps and diarrhoea. Because of these symptoms, patients should be kept in the hospital or at home for the first few days of therapy. This influenza-like syndrome usually lasts 4–12 h, and its severity is clearly dose-related. High doses of interferon (20 MU or greater) can be associated with severe fatigue as well as confusion, delirium, seizures, hypotension and cyanosis[11].

The early side-effects of interferon usually decrease after a few injections, but some symptoms may last and become chronic. The most troublesome chronic side-effects of interferon-α therapy are fatigue and muscle aches, which can be dose-limiting. Many patients also report a difficulty in concentrating, psychological effects, and poor sleep habits. In 5–10% of patients psychological side-effects such as irritability, depression and emotional lability are severe enough that therapy must be altered or discontinued[46,47]. All of these symptoms resolve within 3–5 days of discontinuation of treatment.

Severe side-effects from interferon-α are rare. The interferons are myelosuppressive, and bone marrow suppression can be a severe problem in patients with pre-existing abnormalities as often occurs in patients with cirrhosis and hypersplenism. Perhaps as a result of the leucopenia induced by interferon-α, patients receiving interferon-α have an increased frequency of bacterial infections, such as urinary tract infections, sinusitis, bronchitis and even pneumonia, septicaemia, abscesses, and bacterial peritonitis[10,14,46]. Infections are particularly common in patients with pre-existing cirrhosis. Any fever that appears after the first week of therapy should be quickly and carefully evaluated.

A further side-effect of interferon-α therapy has been the development of autoantibodies with or without autoimmune disease[48,49]. Autoantibodies develop frequently in patients treated with interferon-α and these are sometimes accompanied by the appearance of autoimmune conditions, the most common being autoimmune thyroid disease either hypo- or hyperthyroidism.

SUMMARY

Antiviral therapy for chronic hepatitis B is still experimental. Recent studies suggest that a 3–6-month course of interferon-α in doses of 5–10 MU three times weekly will result in a clinical, biochemical and serological remission in 25–50% of patients with well-compensated liver disease and HBV DNA and HBeAg in serum. Features that predict a beneficial response to treatment include high initial serum aminotransferase activities and low levels of circulating HBV DNA. Asian patients and children may be less likely to respond to treatment than Caucasian adults. Pretreatment of patients with a 4–6-week course of high doses of prednisone may help to increase the response rate to interferon-α alone, but this approach should be limited to patients with mild disease, and perhaps to patients who have previously failed to respond to interferon-α alone. The best approach to treatment of patients with complications of chronic hepatitis B and atypical serological patterns is still uncertain. The limited efficacy and the side-effects of interferon-α therapy should be carefully weighed in the decision to treat patients with chronic hepatitis B. Future studies should focus upon the use of newer antiviral agents alone or in combination with interferon-α.

References

1. Hoofnagle, J. H. and Alter, H. J. (1984). Chronic viral hepatitis. In Vyas, G. N., Dienstag, J. L. and Hoofnagle, J. H. (eds), *Viral Hepatitis and Liver Disease*, pp. 97–113. (New York: Grune & Stratton)
2. McQuillan, G. M., Townsend, T. R., Fields, H. A., Carroll, M., Leahy, M. and Polk, B. F. (1989). Seroepidemiology of hepatitis B virus infection in the United States, 1976 to 1980. *Am. J. Med.*, **87** (Suppl. 3A), 5S-10S
3. Hoofnagle, J. H., Dusheiko, G. M., Seeff, L. B., Jones, E. A., Waggoner, J. G. and Bales, Z. B. (1981). Seroconversion from hepatitis B e antigen to antibody in chronic type B hepatitis. *Ann. Intern. Med.*, **94**, 744–8
4. Liaw, Y. F., Chu, C. M., Su, I. J., *et al.* (1983). Clinical and histological events preceding hepatitis B e antigen seroconversion in chronic type B hepatitis. *Gastroenterology*, **84**, 216–19
5. Di Bisceglie, A. M., Waggoner, J. G. and Hoofnagle, J. H. (1987). Hepatitis B virus deoxyribonucleic acid in liver of chronic carriers. *Gastroenterology*, **93**, 1236–41
6. Hoofnagle, J. H., Shafritz, D. A. and Popper, H. (1987). Chronic type B hepatitis and the "healthy" HBsAg carrier state. *Hepatology*, **7**, 758–63
7. Greenberg, H. B., Pollard, R. B., Lutwick, L. I. *et al.* (1976). Effect of human leukocyte interferon on hepatitis B virus infection in patients with chronic active hepatitis. *N. Engl. J. Med.*, **295**, 517–22
8. Scullard, G. H., Pollard, R. B., Smith, J. L., Sacks, S. L., Gregory, P. B., Robinson, W. S. and Merigan, T. C. (1981). Antiviral treatment of chronic hepatitis B virus infection. I. Changes in viral markers with interferon combined with adenine arabinoside. *J. Infect. Dis.*, **143**, 772–83
9. Thomas, H. C. (1988). Treatment of hepatitis B viral infection. In Zuckerman, A. J. (ed.), *Viral Hepatitis and Liver Disease*, pp. 817–22. (New York: Alan R. Liss)
10. Dusheiko, G., Di Bisceglie, A., Boyer, A. *et al.* (1985). Recombinant leukocyte interferon treatment of chronic hepatitis B. *Hepatology*, **5**, 556–60
11. Dooley, J. S., Davis, G. L., Peters, M., Waggoner, J. G., Goodman, Z. and Hoofnagle, J. H. (1986). Pilot study of recombinant human alpha-interferon for chronic type B hepatitis. *Gastroenterology*, **90**, 150–7

12. Alexander, G. J. M., Brahm, J., Fagan, E. A. *et al.* (1987). Loss of HBsAg with interferon therapy in chronic hepatitis B virus infection. *Lancet*, **1**, 66–8
13. Brook, M. G., McDonald, J. A., Karayiannis, P., Caruso, L., Forster, G., Harris, J. R. W. and Thomas, H. C. (1989). Randomised controlled trial of interferon alfa 2A (rbe) (Roferon-A) for the treatment of chronic hepatitis B virus (HBV) infection: factors that influence response. *Gut*, **30**, 1116–22
14. Hoofnagle, J. H., Peters, M. G., Mullen, K. D. *et al.* (1988). Randomized controlled trial of a four-month course of recombinant human alpha interferon in chronic type B hepatitis. *Gastroenterology*, **95**, 1318–25
15. Lok, A. S. F., Lai, C. L., Wu, P. C. and Leung, E. K. Y. (1988). Long-term follow-up in a randomised controlled trial of recombinant alpha-2 interferon in Chinese patients with chronic hepatitis B infection. *Lancet*, **2**, 298–302
16. Lai, C. L., Lok, A. S. F., Lin, H. J. *et al.* (1987). Placebo-controlled trial of recombinant alpha2 interferon in Chinese HBsAg-carrier children. *Lancet*, **2**, 877–80
17. Saracco, G., Mazzella, G., Rosina, F. *et al.* (1989). A controlled trial of human lymphoblastoid interferon in chronic hepatitis B in Italy. *Hepatology*, **10**, 336–41
18. Realdi, G., Fattovich, G., Noventa, F. *et al.* (1989). Multicentric randomized controlled study of alfa-2a interferon (IFN) in chronic hepatitis type B. *J. Hepatol.*, **9** (Suppl. 1), S76
19. Perrillo, R., Schiff, E., Davis, G. L. *et al.* (1989). Multicenter randomized, controlled trial of recombinant alpha interferon (rIFNa 2-b), alone and following prednisone withdrawal, in chronic hepatitis B. *Hepatology*, **10**, 579
20. Brook, M. G., Karayiannis, P. and Thomas, H. C. (1989). Which patients with chronic hepatitis B virus infection will respond to alpha interferon therapy? A statistical analysis of predictive factors. *Hepatology*, **10**, 761–3
21. Garcia, G., Smith, C. I., Weissberg, J. I. *et al.* (1987). Adenine arabinoside monophosphate in combination with human leukocyte interferon in the treatment of chronic hepatitis B. A randomized, double-blind, placebo-controlled trial. *Ann. Intern. Med.*, **107**, 278–85
22. Bissett, J., Eisenberg, M., Gregory, P. *et al.* (1988). Recombinant fibroblast interferon and immune interferon for treating chronic hepatitis B virus infection. Patient's tolerance and the effect on viral markers. *J. Infect. Dis.*, **157**, 1076–80
23. Di Bisceglie, A. M., Kassianides, C., Lisker-Melman, M. *et al.* (1987). Treatment of chronic type B hepatitis with recombinant human alpha and gamma interferon in combination. A dose-finding study. *Hepatology*, **7**, 1116
24. Schalm, S. W., Heijtink, R. A., Van Buren, H. R. and de Man, H. (1985). Acyclovir enhances the antiviral effect of interferon in chronic hepatitis B. *Lancet*, **2**, 358–60
25. Thyagarajan, S. P., Subramantian, S., Thirunalasundari, T., Venkateswaran, P. S. and Blumberg, B. S. (1988). Effect of *Phyllanthus amarus* on chronic carriers of hepatitis B virus. *Lancet*, **2**, 764–6
26. Fattovich, G., Brollo, L., Pontisso, P. *et al.*, (1986). Levamisole therapy in chronic type B hepatitis: results of a double-blind randomized trial. *Gastroenterology*, **91**, 692–6
27. Mutchnick, M. G., Lee, H. H., Haynes, G. D., Hoofnagle, J. H. and Appelman, H. O. Thymosin treatment of chronic active hepatitis B. A preliminary report on a controlled, double-blind study. *Hepatology*, **8**, 1270
28. Nishioka, M., Kagawa, H., Shirai, M., Terada, S. and Watanabe, S. (1987). Effects of human recombinant interleukin 2 in patients with chronic hepatitis B. A preliminary report. *Am. J. Gastroenterol.*, **82**, 438–42
29. Hantz, O., Allaudeen, H. S., Ooka, T. and De Clerq, T. C. (1984). Inhibition of human and woodchuck hepatitis virus DNA polymerase by the triphosphates of acyclovir, 1-(2′deoxy-2′-fluoro-B-D-arabinofuranosyl)-5-iodocytosine and E-5-(2-bromovinyl)-2′-deoxyuridine. *Antiviral Res.*, **4**, 187–99
30. Sherker, A. H., Hirota, K., Omata, M. and Okuda, K. (1986). Foscarnet decreases serum and liver duck hepatitis B virus DNA in chronically infected ducks. *Gastroenterology*, **91**, 818–24
31. Kassianides, C., Hoofnagle, J. H., Miller, R. H., Doo, E., Ford, H., Broder, S. and Mitsuya, H. (1988). Effects of 2′,3′-dideoxycytidine on duck hepatitis B virus. *Gastroenterology*, **94**, A552
32. Sells, M. A., Chen, M.-L. and Acs, G. (1987). Production of hepatitis B virus in Hep G2 cells transfected with cloned hepatitis B virus DNA. *Proc. Natl. Acad. Sci., USA*, **84**, 1005–9

33. Tuttleman, J. S., Pugh, J. C. and Summers, J. W. (1986). In vitro experimental infection of primary duck hepatocyte cultures with duck hepatitis B virus. *J. Virol.*, **58**, 17–25
34. Scullard, G. H., Gregory, P. B., Robinson, W. S. and Merigan, T. C. (1981). The effect of immunosuppressive therapy on hepatitis B viral infection in patients with chronic hepatitis B. *Gastroenterology*, **81**, 987–91
35. Hoofnagle, J. H., Davis, G. L., Pappas, S. C. *et al.* (1986). A short course of prednisolone in chronic type B hepatitis. Report of a randomized double-blind, placebo controlled trial. *Ann. Intern. Med.*, **104**, 12–17
36. Rakela, J., Redeker, A. G. and Weliky, B. (1983). Effect of short-term prednisone therapy on aminotransferase levels and hepatitis B virus markers in chronic type B hepatitis. *Gastroenterology*, **84**, 956–60
37. Nair, P. V., Tong, M. J., Stevenson, D. *et al.* (1985). Effects of short-term, high-dose prednisone treatment of patients with HBsAg-positive chronic active hepatitis. *Liver*, **5**, 8–12
38. Perrillo, R., Regenstein, F., Peters, M. *et al.* (1988). Prednisone withdrawal followed by recombinant alpha interferon in the treatment of chronic type B hepatitis. A randomized controlled trial. *Ann. Intern. Med.*, **109**, 95–100
39. Garcia, G., Scullard, G., Smith, C. *et al.* (1985). Preliminary observations of hepatitis B-associated membranous glomerulonephritis after treatment with interferon. *Hepatology*, **5**, 317–20
40. Lisker-Melman, M., Webb, D., Di Bisceglie, A. M. *et al.* (1989). Glomerulonephritis caused by chronic hepatitis B virus infection: treatment with recombinant human alpha interferon. *Ann. Intern. Med.* **111**, 479–83
41. de Man, R. A., Schalm, S. W., van der Heijden, A. J., ten Kate, F. W., Wolff, E. D. and Heijtink, R. A. (1989). Improvement of hepatitis B associated glomerulonephritis after antiviral combination therapy. *J. Hepatol.*, **8**, 367–72
42. McMahon, B. J., Heyward, W. L., Templin, D. W., Clement, D. and Lanier, A. P. (1989). Hepatitis B-associated polyarteritis nodosa in Alaskan Eskimos: clinical and epidemiologic features and long-term follow-up. *Hepatology*, **9**, 97–101
43. Weissberg, J., Andres, L. L., Smith, C. I. *et al.* (1984). Survival in chronic hepatitis B. An analysis of 379 patients. *Ann. Intern. Med.*, **101**, 613–16
44. Kassianides, C., Di Bisceglie, A. M., Hoofnagle, J. H. *et al.* (1988). Alpha interferon therapy in patients with decompensated chronic type B hepatitis. In Zuckerman, A. J. (ed.), *Viral Hepatitis and Liver Disease*, pp. 840–3. (New York: Alan R. Liss)
45. Brunetto, M. R., Oliveri, F., Bonino, F. *et al.* (1989). Natural course and response to interferon of chronic hepatitis B accompanied by antibody to hepatitis B e antigen. *Hepatology*, **10**, 198–202
46. Renault, P. F., Hoofnagle, J. H., Park, Y. *et al.* (1987). Psychiatric complications of long-term interferon alfa therapy. *Arch. Intern. Med.*, **147**, 1577–80
47. McDonald, E. M., Mann, A. H. and Thomas, H. C. (1987). Interferons as mediators of psychiatric morbidity. An investigation in a trial of recombinant alpha-interferon in hepatitis B carriers. *Lancet*, **2**, 1175–7
48. Mayet, W.-J., Hess, G., Gerken, G., Rossol, S., Voth, R., Manns, M. and Meyer zum Buschenfelde, K.-H. (1989). Treatment of chronic type B hepatitis with recombinant alpha-interferon induces autoantibodies not specific for autoimmune chronic hepatitis. *Hepatology*, **10**, 24–8
49. Lisker-Melman, M., Di Bisceglie, A. M., Usala, S. J., Weintraub, B., Murray, L. M. and Hoofnagle, J. H. (1989). Autoimmune thyroid disease associated with recombinant human alpha interferon therapy in patients with chronic hepatitis B. *J. Am. Med. Assoc.* (In press)

21
Treatment of chronic hepatitis B with interferon-α-2b

R. MÜLLER, R. BAUMGARTEN, R. MARKUS, M. SCHULZ, H. WITTENBERG, B. HINTSCHE-KILGER, J.-D. FENGLER, P. v. WUSSOW, H. MEISEL, H. KLEIN, K. MALMUS and F. W. SCHMIDT

Abbreviations

HBV, hepatitis B virus; HBsAg, hepatitis B surface antigen; anti-HBs, antibodies to hepatitis B surface antigen; HBeAg, hepatitis Be antigen; anti-HBe, antibodies to hepatitis Be antigen; HBV DNA, hepatitis B virus-deoxyribonucleic acid; rIFN α-2b, recombinant interferon α-2b; ALP, alkaline phosphatase; ALT, alanine aminotransferase; AST, aspartate aminotransferase; CHE, cholinesterase; GLDH, glutamate dehydrogenase; GGT, gamma-glutamyltransferase.

INTRODUCTION

Interferons are endogenous glycoproteins which exhibit antiviral, immunomodulatory and antiproliferative properties. Since they can be produced by biotechnological methods they have been used in numerous clinical trials for the treatment of chronic viral hepatitis in different, mostly small numbers of patients who were reported to have response rates of 0 to 46%[1-5]. A randomized, controlled clinical trial in a Caucasian patient population was to evaluate the effect of well-tolerable low dose rIFN α-2b on inhibition of HBV replication and on transferring hepatitis into an inactive state.

PATIENTS

Between 1987 and 1989 a total of 58 patients (46 male and 12 female) aged 18–65 years were randomized to receive either rIFN α-2b ($n = 30$) or no treatment ($n = 28$). Those eligible were patients with histological confirmation of chronic hepatitis and seropositive findings of HBsAg and HBV DNA over more than 6 months. Patients with HDV and HIV infections, decompensated hepatocirrhosis, chronic renal insufficiency, or those requiring haemodialysis or immunosuppressive therapy, as well as patients with previous organ transplantations or in bad general condition, were excluded. Written informed consent was obtained from all patients. The presence of anti-HBe in the serum was not considered an exclusion criterion. Histological examination revealed a chronic persistent hepatitis in 27 patients, a chronic active hepatitis in 28 and the early onset of hepatocirrhosis in three. There were no group differences in respect to sex and age of the patients, duration of disease, activity of the aminotransferases, serum concentration of HBV DNA and histological findings. Twenty-eight patients treated (presence of HBeAg in 27) and 27 controls (presence of HBeAg in 26) completed the protocol. One patient of the treatment group and one patient of the control group dropped out due to lack of compliance. One female patient developed a psychosis while being treated with rIFN α-2b, which necessitated discontinuation of treatment.

METHODS

Blood samples were taken 3 months prior to initiation of therapy, during treatment and 6 months after completion of treatment in monthly intervals. Serum analysis included blood count, bilirubin, activities of ALT, AST, GGT, GLDH, CHE, ALP, electrophoresis, prothrombin time, HBsAg/anti-HBs, HBeAg/anti-HBe, HBV DNA and antibodies against IFN. The measurements were performed according to standardized methods. The HBV markers HBsAg/anti-HBs and HBeAg/anti-HBe were determined by radio-immunoassays (Ausria II^{R}, Ausab^{R}, Abbott-HBe^{R}, Abbott Laboratories, Chicago, Ill., USA), HBV DNA by HepProbe^{TM} (GIBCO/BRL, Life Technologies, Eggenstein-Leopoldshafen, FRG). In order to detect IFN antibodies an IFN binding test (ELISA), as well as the IFN neutralization test (bioassay), were used[6].

Treatment consisted of 3 megaunits of recombinant interferon-α-2b (Intron A^{R}, Essex Pharma GmbH, Munich, FRG) administered subcutaneously thrice a week over a period of 4 months. After initial hospitalization and observation the treatment was continued by the outpatient department.

The therapeutic response was assessed according to the following criteria:

Complete response: elimination of HBsAg, HBeAg and HBV DNA from the serum and normalization of ALT activity until completion of the follow-up period.

Partial response: elimination of HBeAg and HBV DNA, while HBsAg persisted, and normalization of ALT activity until completion of the follow-up period.

No response: no change or transient loss of HBV DNA and decrease in HBeAg titre.

STATISTICS

Evaluation of the therapeutic response was performed by using the chi-square test ($p < 0.05$). Biochemical and virological results were analysed by Wilcoxon's rank sum test.

RESULTS

Of 28 patients treated, one showed complete response, and another eight partial response. Within the same follow-up period three patients of the control group spontaneously lost their HBeAg and HBV DNA with seroconversion to anti-HBe. In contrast to the patients of the treatment group the decrease in HBV DNA activity below detection limits did not correlate with normalization of ALT serum activity. According to the definitions of complete and partial response the results differ significantly ($p < 0.05$); they are illustrated in Figure 1.

While only five of 23 male patients eliminated the HBeAg, four of five female patients treated responded to treatment. The only case of complete seroconversion from HBsAg to anti-HBs was observed in a 54-year-old female with chronic hepatitis, which persisted for over 2 years prior to initiation of therapy.

The baseline HBV DNA serum levels in the group of patients who successfully responded to treatment ($n = 9$) differed significantly (Table 1). There was no correlation between the therapeutic response and the following parameters: age; enzyme activities of AST, ALT, GGT, ALP, GLDH, CHE; concentrations of bilirubin and immunoglobulins; electrophoresis; duration of disease and anamnestic details of acute viral hepatitis.

The elimination of HBV markers in responders with HBeAg positive findings always occurred in a similar way. In general the decrease in HBV DNA below detection limits occurred rapidly and within the first 4 weeks after initiation of treatment. HBeAg was eliminated later after a mean interval of 5.9 ± 0.84 months, seroconversion to anti-HBe was observed at a mean of 6.6 ± 0.81 months after initiation of therapy. At 21 days after the onset of treatment HBV DNA was no longer detectable in the patient who initially showed the presence of anti-HBe. The elimination of HBeAg was followed by normalization of ALT activity, which was preceded by a transient increase in ALT activity by 2 to 3 times the baseline values in seven of nine responders.

At the time of documentation all patients had been followed up for 6 to

Table 1 Comparison of HBV DNA serum concentrations (*mean values of the past 3 months prior to initiation of therapy) in responders and non-responders to treatment with rIFN α-2b

	Number of patients	*HBV DNA* (*genomes/ml* × 10^8) ($x \pm$ SEM)
Complete and partial response	9	1.17* ± 0.19
No response	19	1.91* ± 0.22

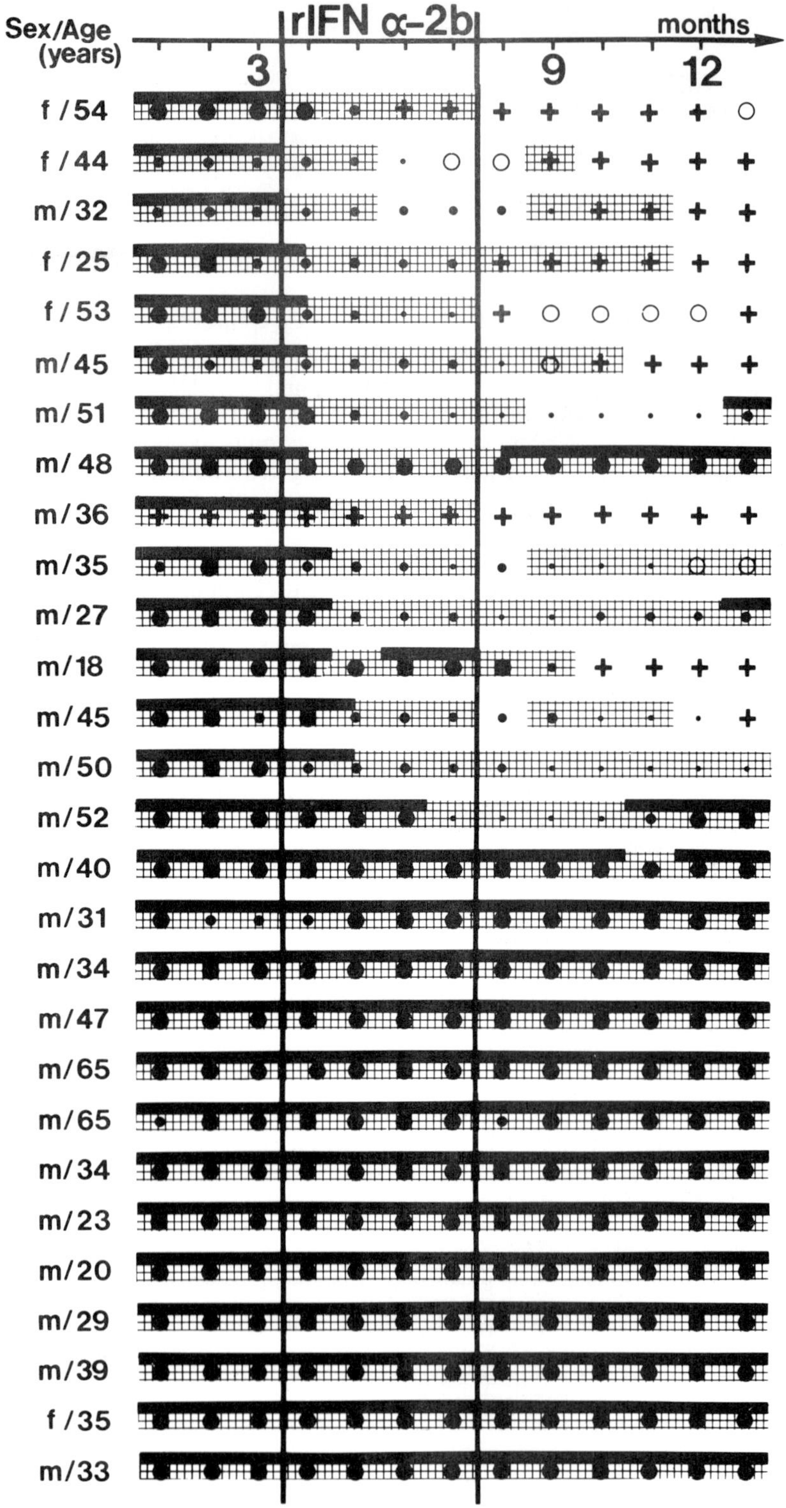

Sex/Age
(years)
rIFN α-2b
months
3
9
12
f / 54
f / 44
m/32
f / 25
f / 53
m/45
m/51
m/48
m/36
m/35
m/27
m/18
m/45
m/50
m/52
m/40
m/31
m/34
m/47
m/65
m/65
m/34
m/23
m/20
m/29
m/39
f / 35
m/33

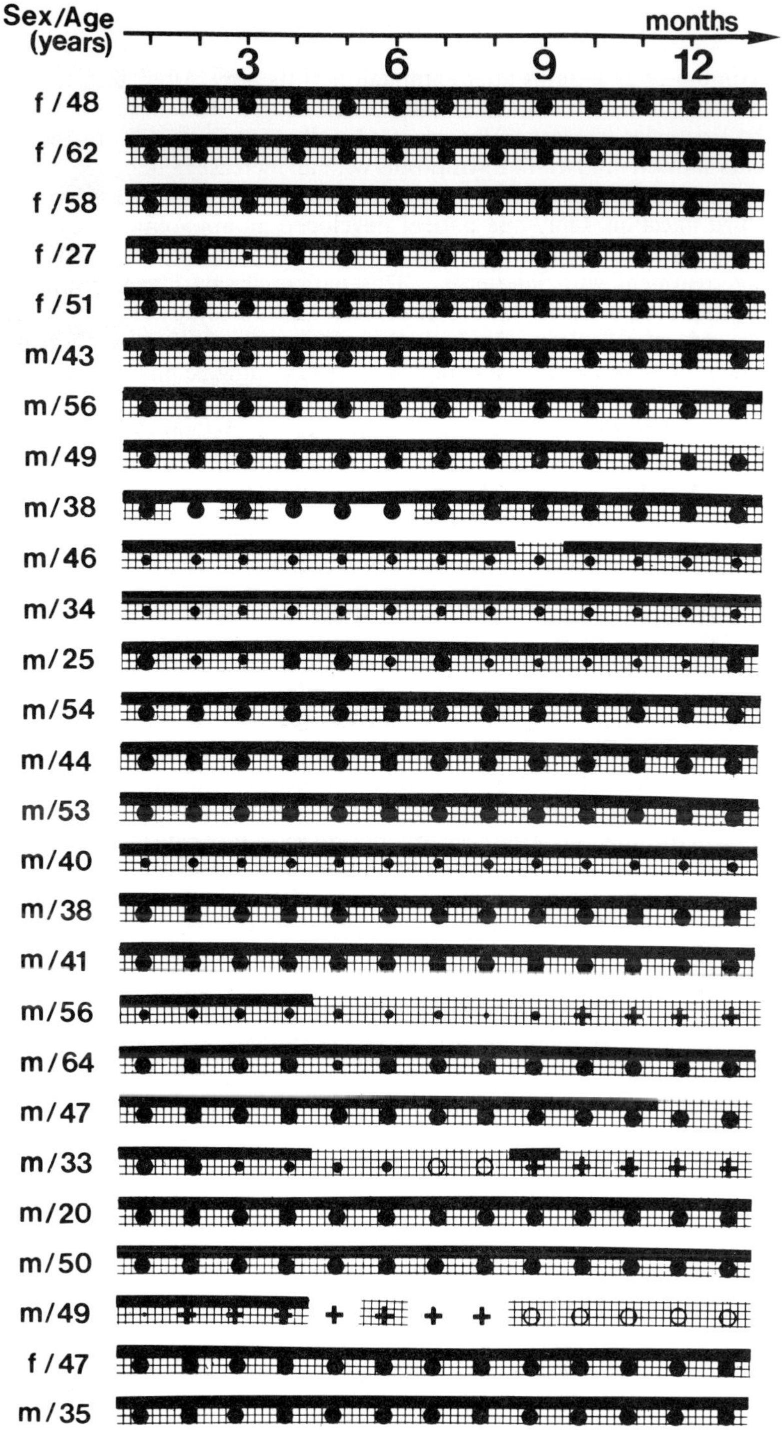

Figure 1 Recombinant interferon-α-2b for treatment of chronic hepatitis B: on the left: patients treated; on the right: control patients with no treatment. *Legend to symbols*: HBV-DNA positive, ▬; HBeAg titre: 1:10 000, ●; 1:100, ●; 1:10 ●; 1:1 •; HbeAg negative, ○; anti-HBe positive, +; increased ALT activity, ⊞

a maximum of 24 months after completion of therapy. After seroconversion to anti-HBe no reactivation has been observed.

The treatment was generally tolerated well. At the onset of treatment all patients showed mild flu-like symptoms with an increase in body temperature to a maximum of 38.5 °C, which in the majority of patients disappeared after the third injection. Only one patient developed an apparently latently pre-existing climacteric depressive psychosis which may manifest more frequently during treatment with interferon[7]. This patient discontinued treatment in the sixth week; 6 weeks later HBV DNA was no longer detectable, at a further 3.5 months later she had also eliminated the HBeAg. Since the treatment cycle had not been completed, these data were not included in the final analysis. Two patients developed neutralizing antibodies to interferon after 2 and 4 months of treatment. At least in one patient the formation of antibodies did not affect the therapeutic results. This patient eliminated HBeAg 4 months after the occurrence of antibodies to interferon which had been persisting for over 5 months.

DISCUSSION

The results show that with 3 megaunits rIFN α-2b administered three times weekly over a period of 4 months a positive response can be achieved in 32% of Caucasian patients with chronic hepatitis B without immunosuppression. The response rate is comparable with the results of other studies, which have been performed with various interferons in different dose regimens and with different treatment durations[1–3,4,8–16].

None of the previously used treatment protocols succeeded in considerably increasing the effectiveness even by numerous modifications and combinations with other antiviral agents[17–21]. In the majority of patients HBV replication cannot be permanently influenced by treatment with interferon. Our results, as well as those of other authors, indicate that patients with low HBV DNA serum concentrations – as in four of five female patients treated in our study – benefit most from treatment with interferon[2]; the reasons are not yet fully understood. In general the HBV DNA concentration can be affected by host- or pathogen-specific factors. Against the influence of virulence factors is the fact that in our patient population the HBV DNA concentration was lower in women than in men. The latter seems to depend largely on the immunoreactivity of the host.

It is known, for example, that markers for viral replication, namely serum levels of HBV DNAp and HBV DNA, are in concordance with drug-induced immunosuppression, and that immunocompromised patients are characterized by specifically high HBV DNA levels[22–26].

These observations suggest that the levels of HBV DNA serum concentration are substantially influenced by the responses of the immune system. The antiviral and immunomodulatory properties of IFN will only exert a clinically beneficial effect in patients with a previously stimulated immune system, which has already caused an inhibition of the viral replication to a certain degree. If HBV DNA baseline values are high, and therefore the reactivity of the immunological defence mechanisms can be assumed to be low, an elimination of the virus by IFN alone can hardly be expected. A potential increase in the response rate may be achieved by additional immunomodulation.

SUMMARY

A total of 58 patients with histologically confirmed chronic viral hepatitis B and presence of HBsAg and HBV DNA in the serum were randomized in a prospectively controlled trial. Thirty patients were treated with 3 megaunits of rIFN α-2b s.c. thrice weekly for 4 months; 28 controls received no treatment. The post-treatment follow-up period consisted of 6 months. Twenty-eight patients treated and 27 controls completed the protocol. One female patient of the treatment group showed a complete response (loss of HBsAg, HBeAg and HBV DNA), eight other patients (32%) revealed a partial response to therapy (loss of HBeAg and HBV DNA). Three patients of the control group (11%) lost HBeAg and HBV DNA spontaneously. This finding is statistically significant ($p < 0.05$). The elimination of HBV markers from the serum was associated with a normalization of aminotransferase activities in the serum. A reactivation of hepatitis was not observed after seroconversion.

References

1. Carreno, V., Porres, J. C., Mora, I., Bartolome, J., Bas, C., Gutiez, J., Cortes, J. and Hernandez Guso, C. (1987). Prolonged (6 months) treatment of chronic hepatitis B virus infection with recombinant leukocyte A interferon. *Liver*, **7**, 325–32
2. Hess, G., Weber, C., Rossol, S., Voth, R., Drees, N. and Meyer zum Büschenfelde, K. H. (1988). Behandlung der Hepatitis-B-surface-antigen (HBsAg)-positiven chronischen Hepatitis mit rekombinantem alpha-A-Interferon. Ergebnisse einer Phase-II-Studie. *Z. Gastroenterol.*, **26**, 380–7
3. Hoofnagle, J. H., Peters, M., Mullen, K. D., Jones, D. B., Rustgi, V., diBisceglie, A. M., Hallahan, C., Park, Y., Meschievitz, C. and Jones, E. A. (1988). Randomized, controlled trial of recombinant human alpha-interferon in patients with chronic hepatitis B. *Gastroenterology*, **95**, 1318–25
4. Mazella, G., Villanova, N., Abdu-Ahmed, M., Barbara, L., Saracco, G., Rizzetto, M., Cancellieri, C. and Roda, E. (1988). Treatment of chronic hepatitis B with human lymphoblastoid interferon: results of a controlled trial. *Chemioterapia*, **7**, 12–14
5. Müller, R., Klein, H. and Niehoff, G. (1988). Virostatische Therapie der chronischen Hepatitis. *Z. Gesamte Inn. Med.*, **43**, 705–10
6. von Wussow, P., Freund, M., Hartmann, F., Diedrich, H., Poliwoda, H. and Deicher, H. (1988). Clinical significance of neutralizing antibodies in patients with chronic myelogenic leukemia. In Huhn, D., Hellriegel, K. P. and Niederle, N. (eds), *Chronic Myelocytic Leukemia and Interferon*, pp. 91–101. (Berlin: Springer Verlag)
7. McDonald, E. M., Mann, A. H. and Thomas, H. C. (1987). Interferons as mediators of psychiatric morbidity. *Lancet*, **2**, 1175–7
8. Carreno, V., Porres, J. C., Mora, I., Gutiez, J., Ouiroga, J. A., Ramon y Cajal, S., Oliva, H., Compernolle, C. and Bartolome, J. (1987). A controlled study of treatment with recombinant interferon alpha in chronic hepatitis B virus infection: induction and maintenance schedules. *Antiviral Res.*, **8**, 125–37
9. Dusheiko, G. M., Paterson, A. C., Pitcher, L., Kassianides, C., DiBisceglie, A. M., Song, E.

and Kew, M. C. (1986). Recombinant leukocyte interferon treatment of chronic hepatitis B. An analysis of two therapeutic trials. *J. Hepatol.*, **3** (Suppl. 2), S199–S207
10. Dusheiko, G. M., DiBisceglie, A. M., Bowyer, S., Sacks, E., Ritchie, M., Schoub, B. and Kew, M. C. (1985). Recombinant leukocyte interferon treatment of chronic hepatitis B. *Hepatology*, **5**, 556–60
11. Franco, A., Barnaba, V., Levrero, M., Ruberti, G., van Dyke, A., Bonavita, M. S. and Balsano, F. (1986). Effect of 28 consecutive days lymphoblastoid interferon alpha (alpha-IFN) administration on hepatitis B virus related chronic liver disease. *J. Hepatol.*, **3** (Suppl. 2), S239–S243
12. Lai, C. L., Lok, A. S., Lin, H. J., Wu, P. C., Yeoh, E. K. and Yeung, C. Y. (1987). Placebo-controlled trial of recombinant alpha 2-interferon in Chinese HBsAg-carrier children. *Lancet*, **2**, 877–80
13. Lok, A. S., Lai, C. L. and Wu, P. C. (1986). Interferon therapy of chronic hepatitis B virus infection in Chinese. *J. Hepatol.*, **3** (Suppl. 2), S209–S215
14. Müller, R., Klein, H., Vido, I., Niehoff, G., Lautz, H. U., Gebel, M. and Schmidt, F. W. (1986). Antiviral treatment in chronic hepatitis B. Data of 5 prospectively controlled randomized trials. *J. Hepatol.*, **3** (Suppl. 2), S217–S223
15. Müller, R. (1987). Antivirale Therapie bei chronischer Hepatitis B. *Med. Klin.*, **82**, 414–19
16. Thomas, H. C., Scully, L. J. and McDonald, J. A. (1986). Lymphoblastoid and recombinant alpha interferon therapy of chronic hepatitis B virus infection. The Royal Free Hospital experience. *J. Hepatol.*, **3** (Suppl. 2), S193–S197
17. Carreno, V. and Mora, I. (1987). Combination of recombinant interferons alpha and gamma in treatment of chronic hepatitis B. *Lancet*, **2**, 1086
18. Garcia, G., Smith, C. I., Weissberg, J. I., Eisenberg, M., Bissett, J., Nair, P. V., Mastre, B., Rosno, S., Roskamp, D., Waterman, K., Pollard, R. B., Tong, M. J., Brown, B. W., Robinson, W. S., Gregory, P. B. and Merigan, T. C. (1987). Adenine arabinoside monophosphate (vidarabine phosphate) in combination with human leukocyte interferon in the treatment of chronic hepatitis B. A randomized, double-blind, placebo-controlled trial. *Ann. Intern. Med.*, **107**, 278–85
19. deMan, R. A., Schalm, S. W., Heijtink, R. A., Beik, L., den Ouden, J., ten Kate, F. J., Chamuleau, R. A. and Reesink, H. W. (1988). Long term follow-up of an antiviral combination therapy in chronic hepatitis B. *Am. J. Med.*, **85**, 150–4
20. Scullard, G. H., Pollard, R. B., Smith, J. L., Gregory, P. B., Robinson, W. S. and Merigan, T. C. (1981). Antiviral treatment of chronic hepatitis B virus infection. 1. Changes in viral markers with interferon combined with adenine arabinoside. *J. Infect. Dis.*, **143**, 772–83
21. Smith, C. J., Kitchen, L. W., Scullard, G. H., Robinson, W. S., Gregory, P. B. and Merigan, T. C. (1982). Vidarabine monophosphate and human leukocyte interferon in chronic hepatitis B infection. *J. Am. Med. Assoc.*, **247**, 2261–5
22. Fagan, E. A., Guarner, P., Perera, S. D., Trowbridge, R., Rolando, N., Davison, F. and Williams, R. (1985). Quantitation of hepatitis B virus DNA (HBV-DNA) in serum using the spot hybridization technique and scintillation counting. *J. Virol. Methods*, **12**, 251–62
23. Hoofnagle, J. H. (1982). Chronic hepatitis: the role of corticosteroids. In Szmuness, W., Alter, H. J. and Maynard, J. E. (eds), *Viral Hepatitis*, p. 573. (Philadelphia: Franklin Institute Press)
24. Müller, R., Vido, I. and Schmidt, F. W. (1981). Rapid withdrawal of immunosuppressive therapy in chronic active hepatitis B infection. *Lancet*, **1**, 1323
25. Nair, P. V., Tong, M. J., Stevenson, D., Roskamp, D. and Boone, C. (1986). A pilot study on the effects of prednisone withdrawal on serum hepatitis B virus DNA and HBeAg in chronic active hepatitis B. *Hepatology*, **6**, 1319–24
26. Scullard, G. H., Smith, C. I., Merigan, T. C., Robinson, W. S. and Gregory, P. B. (1981). Effects of immunosuppressive therapy on viral markers in chronic active hepatitis B. *Gastroenterology*, **81**, 987–91

22
Prospects in immune prophylaxis of hepatitis B

W. H. GERLICH, R. DEEPEN, K.-H. HEERMANN, B. KRONE, R. THOMSSEN and A. UY

Immune prophylaxis against hepatitis B includes passive administration of hepatitis B immune globulin (HBIG) or active immunization using hepatitis B surface antigen.

Passive immunization is still important for persons who are not able to develop an active immune response against HBsAg or if acute exposure occurs in a non-immune person. A problem of passive immunization is that it requires repeatedly high doses of HBIG and is consequently very expensive. Moreover, protection is still far from being complete. Usually, HBIG does not prevent HBV infection but attenuates it[1]. Thus, it leads to a passive–active immunization. At first glance this may seem to be a perfect mode to acquire immunity, but it is too unreliable and cannot work in immunodeficient persons.

For continuous treatment of immunodeficient persons an antibody preparation more effective against HBV than the current HBIG would be required. The titre of total anti-HBs is very high in HBIG (>200 units/ml), if one considers that 1 unit is theoretically able to bind 10^{11} HBsAg particles or 10^{10} HBV particles[2]. Unfortunately, it appears that conventional anti-HBs titre does not really reflect high protective potency. Feasible *in vitro* neutralization assays are urgently needed to define protective titres against HBV, but such assays are not available for human HBV.

Neutralization assays have been performed with some selected antibody preparations and natural HBV of known titre, using suspectible chimpanzees as indicators of HBV replication. By this approach a monoclonal antibody, RF1, against an epitope of dimer small HBs protein[3] and antisera against preS2(1–29) and preS1 peptide(12–48) have been found to neutralize[4]. RF1 cross-reactive antibodies are found in recipients of a recombinant hepatitis B vaccine[5], but it is not known if significant titres of such an antibody specificity occur in HBIG.

Our own unpublished data (R. Deepen) suggest that several commercially available HBIG preparations contain only traces of anti-preS1 and anti-preS2. Since the neutralization assays mentioned above, and theoretical considerations (see below), suggest that antibodies against selected preS epitopes would be more useful than the majority of S epitopes, it appears desirable to prepare future HBIG preparations from good responders to preS containing vaccines. Even more promising could be the production of human monoclonal antibodies against preS attachment sites of HBV. Such antibodies would be the therapy of choice to prevent reinfection in HBV carriers who required liver transplantation. Currently, only those HBV positive recipients of livers can be protected against reinfection who did not have high HBV titres before transplantation, and even then the passive anti-HBs titre has to be maintained higher than 100 mU/ml (R. Müller, personal communication). The costs for this immune prophylaxis exceed all other costs for liver transplantation.

Recently it has been observed that HBIG given after intravenous inoculation of HBV cannot prevent experimental infection in chimpanzees[6], whereas active immunization in a similar setting was highly protective[7]. These findings are not in accordance with studies in newborns from HBV carrier mothers[8]. Even there active immunization was superior to passive immunization, and the best results were found if active and passive immunization were combined[9]. In cases of post-exposure prophylaxis a combination of one dose HBIG and a full active immunization cycle should be started, since the passive immunization does not disturb active anti-HBs production[10]. A rapid course of active immunization with doses at 0, 2 and 6 weeks seems to be preferable for this purpose[11].

Current hepatitis B vaccines have been shown to be protective in many experimental and epidemiological settings. The development of efficient recombinant HB vaccines from transfected yeast is one of the major contributions of modern gene technology to human medicine. The large amount of HB vaccine now available will make it possible to control HBV infection on a worldwide level, provided such a vaccination campaign is properly funded and organized[12]. Currently the HB vaccine is offered only to high-risk groups and to newborns in regions of high endemicity. It is doubtful if limitation to these groups will allow for long-term eradication of HBV. Vaccination of the whole population would be the final goal of a multi-stage vaccination campaign against HBV. A short-term goal is to increase the acceptance and compliance for HB vaccines in medical staff and other high-risk groups, and to make the vaccine available to all children in highly endemic regions. While vaccination campaigns should be immediately enhanced on a worldwide scale, laboratory research should go on to create even more efficient and more protective HB vaccines.

A drawback of the current HB vaccines is the mode of immunization. As a non-replicating antigen it has to be injected several times, together with adjuvants. Three injections are required to protect more than 90% of the healthy population and an optimal antibody response requires intervals of several weeks between first and second injections, and several months up to 1 year between second and third injection[13] (also unpublished observations). The last injection is very often missed by vaccinees! In many regions of high endemicity people have a nomadic lifestyle, which makes it additionally difficult to reach the vaccine recipients.

Injections themselves can be a problem in underdeveloped countries. Reuse of injection needles and syringes without proper disinfection is still widely practised. A HB vaccination campaign which does not reliably prevent such malpractice would possibly do more harm than good by spreading hepatitis C, D, HIV and other blood-borne diseases. For this reason HB vaccines should always be supplied in non-reusable single-dose injection devices, together with containers for safe disposal of the used devices.

Currently, *costs of HB vaccines* are still too high for large-scale vaccination programmes in poor countries. Production costs of recombinant HB vaccines would, however, allow much lower prices provided a very large number of doses could be sold. The costs of injection per dose, in contrast, cannot be reduced much. Thus, a mode of vaccination would be desirable which could reduce the number of injections from three to two or one, or make injection unnecessary at all by using the oral route. Possibly this goal can be reached by developing more immunogenic HB vaccines and/or by using better adjuvants or vectors.

The second reason why *more efficient HB vaccines* should be developed is the considerable number of non- or low-responders. Patients with reduced immune reactivity are often at high risk of HBV infection but approximately one-half or more of them cannot be protected by HB vaccines. The detectable but weak response in the remaining patients suggests that vaccination against HBV is not hopeless in these high-risk groups.

A certain proportion of healthy persons is also unable to develop anti-HBs after vaccination. Although this group constitutes only a small percentage, this insecurity requires serological control of anti-HBs production in vaccinees. A reduction of the non-responders to less than 1% among healthy subjects would make this control unnecessary.

Possibilities to improve the immune response are manifold. While the standard dosage of three times 5–20 μg HBsAg is good for the majority of vaccinees, an increased amount of HBs antigen may be helpful for weak or non-responders. Provided the purity of the vaccines is good enough one might consider doses of 100 or 200 μg HBsAg[14].

Repeated injections are certainly a way to improve the seroconversion in chronic dialysis patients (Trepo, personal communication), but they are too costly and uncomfortable for persons who are not under constant medical supervision. Change of immunization intervals or injection sites is not helpful. Use of adjuvants other than aluminium hydroxide or phosphate is problematic. However, the immune response may be non-specifically increased by injecting interleukin 2 together with the vaccine[15]. This type of modern adjuvant is helpful in those who suffer from a functional monocyte or T-helper cell defect. None of these approaches are suitable for the general population.

The *mode of protection* induced by current vaccines is not well understood. The general assumption is that HBsAg induces anti-HBs, and that this prevents an invading HBV from replication. As pointed out above, this concept has no solid theoretical basis. The anti-HBs response may be only a secondary marker for the establishment of T-cell-dependent immunity.

Neutralizing antibodies usually prevent a virus from attachment to its target cell. No attachment site has been clearly defined in the small HBs protein. Thus, the mode of neutralization by conventional anti-HBs is unclear, if it occurs at all.

It has been known for several years that the *envelope of HBV* is formed by three related proteins, called large (L), middle (M) and small (S) HBs protein. LHBs protein contains three domains: preS1, preS2 and S. MHBs lacks preS1, while SHBs consists of only the S domain[16]. The old plasma-derived HB vaccines (in particular that from Pasteur Vaccines) contained traces of LHBs and MHBs, but SHBs was clearly the predominant component. The preS1 and preS2 domains of these vaccines induced weak but detectable antibody responses[17]. Given the fact that major epitopes of preS1 and preS2 are neutralization-specifying, these weak responses are not negligible. Even more important may be the observation that most HBs-specific T-helper cell clones from good responders to a plasma-derived vaccine were directed against the preS1 domain[18].

The most widely used recombinant vaccines contain only SHBs which has been produced in yeast. The protective effect of these materials has been shown in chimpanzees[5] and in newborns of HBV carrier mothers[19]. Adding further B and T cell epitopes of the viral surface to HBs particles would be an essential improvement. This can be done in various ways. The most obvious way would be to copy the natural biosynthesis of HBs filaments. The protein composition of these HBs filaments is very similar to that of the HBV envelope. In contrast to the HBs spheres, they contain much more LHBs and consequently preS1[16]. There are two obstacles against using LHBs alone, for vaccination. One is that pure LHBs does not expose the known B-cell epitopes of HBs spheres, which are considered (whether justified or not) to be essential components[20]. The other obstacle is that pure LHBs is not secreted by the cells[21]. With yeast as host organism this is not considered a problem, because yeast does not secrete HBs spheres either[22]. In animal cells coexpression of LHBs with SHBs is required to obtain secreted HBs filaments[23]. Most non-hepatic cells do not start transcription from the natural promoter (SPI) of LHBs, but the promoter SPII for MHBs and SHBs works in all cell types[24]. This is probably the reason why permanent mouse L cells or Chinese hamster ovary (CHO) cells do not produce LHBs. The CHO vaccine from Pasteur Vaccines consists in fact only of MHBs and SHBs, although the preS1 was also brought into the transfected CHO cells[25]. Positioning of a heterologous strong promoter upstream of LHBs may lead to the above-mentioned problems. A problem arising in yeast is the aberrant glycosylation[26]. The S domain is not glycosylated at all, but the preS2 domain is overglycosylated. While the first lack is apparently irrelevant the second phenomenon is probably important, because identified neutralizing regions become covered by glycoside. This problem can be circumvented by mutating the glycosylation signals away, or by using a hypoglycosylating yeast strain[27].

An alternative approach is to place short DNA segments which code for neutralizing preS1 and preS2 sequences into genes of carrier particles. SHBs particles themselves have been used as a carrier because they already carry protective epitopes[28,29]. Another possibility is to attach a protective preS1 peptide to HBs particles by hydrophobic interaction[30]. Chemically synthesized peptides are useful to identify neutralizing B cell or T-helper cell epitopes, but they work only in combination with carrier particles and/or strong adjuvants. Suitable particles are antigens which have been licensed as vaccines, HBs spheres being the natural choice[29].

SHBs particles are not, however, very immunogenic carriers. Compared to isometric particles such as hepatitis A virus[31] 10–50 times more HBs is necessary to reach a detectable anti-HBs titre. HBV core particles are also highly immunogenic, and have been successfully used as carriers for B cell epitopes including preS1 and preS2 epitopes[32]. Moreover, HBcAg is able to confer partial protection[33,34]. Since anti-HBc is probably non-protective the protection must rely on cellular immunity. Anti-HBc may even be deleterous[35]. Using truncated HBc protein one can generate particulate HBe in *E. coli*[36], which still has high immunity and can carry foreign epitopes even better. Such a truncated HBc particle does not package RNA (M. Melegari, unpublished observations). Besides being an excellent B cell immunogen, HBc protein has also strong T cell epitopes which help to enhance the B cell response[37].

Using non-replicating immunogenic carrier particles would still require injections. A more far-reacting goal is the development of a life vaccine against HBV. Vaccinia vectors are very useful for research purposes but probably not for practical application[38]. A promising possibility is the use of recombinant adenovirus vaccine strains which carry the gene for SHBs[39]. A disadvantage of living virus vectors is that their replication cannot be controlled in an immunodeficient host. A living bacterial vector could be used in a less attenuated state because intervention by antibiotic therapy would be possible. Strains of oral typhoid vaccine have been suggested. For bacterial vector only sequential epitopes of HBV seem to be suitable. PreS2 sequences have been inserted into the hypervariable region of flagellin[40] or into heat-labile enterotoxin[41].

In *summary*, many approaches are investigated to create more practical and more efficient hepatitis B vaccines. In the future HBs particles carrying preS1 and preS2 epitopes will be introduced. Even more pressing, however, is the need to bring down the price of HB vaccination to a level which allows large-scale vaccination in hyperendemic regions.

References

1. Dienstag, J. L. (1989). Passive–active immunoprophylaxis after percutaneous exposure to hepatitis B virus. *Hepatology*, **10**, 385–7
2. Stamm, B., Gerlich, W. H. and Thomssen, R. (1980). Quantitative determination of antibody against hepatitis B surface antigen: measurement of its binding capacity. *J. Biol. Stand*, **8**, 59–68
3. Iwarson, S., Tabor, E., Thomas, H. E., Goodall, A., Waters, J., Snoy, P., Shih, J. W.-K. and Gerety, R. J. (1985). Neutralization of hepatitis B virus infectivity by a murine monoclonal antibody: an experimental study in chimpanzee. *J. Med. Virol.*, **16**, 89–96
4. Neurath, A. R., Strick, N., Kent, S. B. H., Parker, K., Seto, B. and Girard, M. (1988). Design of synthetic peptides mimicking the immunologic and biologic functions of the pre-S1

sequence of the hepatitis-B virus envelope protein. In Ginsberg, H., Brown, F., Lerner, R. A. and Chanock, R. M. (eds), *Vaccines*, **88**, pp. 229–234. (Cold Spring Harbor Laboratory)
5. Hauser, P., Thomas, H. C., Waters, J., Simoen, P., Voet, P., De Wilde, M., Stephenne, J. and Petre, J. (1988). Induction of neutralising antibodies in chimpanzees and in humans by a recombinant yeast-derived hepatitis B surface antigen particle. In Zuckerman, A. J. (ed), *Viral Hepatitis and Liver Disease*, pp. 1031–7. (New York: Alan R. Liss)
6. Wahl, M., Iwarson, S., Snoy, P. and Gerety, R. J. (1989). Failure of hepatitis B immune globulin to protect against exp infection in chimpanzees. *J. Hepatol.*, **9**, 198–203
7. Iwarson, S., Wahl, M., Ruttiman, E., Snoy, P., Seto, B. and Gerety, R. J. (1988). Successful post-exposure vaccination against hepatitis B in chimpanzees. *J. Med. Virol.*, **25**, 433–9
8. Beasley, R. P., Hwang, L. Y., Stevens, C. E., Lin, C. C., Hsieh, F., Wang, J., Sun, K. Y. and Szmuness, W. (1983). Efficacy of hepatitis B immune globulin for prevention of perinatal transmission of the hepatitis B virus carrier state. Final report of a randomized double-blind, placebo-controlled trial. *Hepatology*, **3**, 135–41
9. Beasley, R. P., Hwang, L. Y., Lee, G. C. Y., Lan, C. C., Roan, C. H.,Huang, F. Y. and Chen, C. L. (1983). Prevention of perinatally transmitted hepatitis B virus infections with hepatitis B immune globulin and hepatitis B vaccine. *Lancet*, **2**, 1099–1102
10. Stamm, B., Gerlich, W. and Thomssen, R. (1979). Modellversuche zur Entwicklung einer Hepatitis B Vaccine: Immunogenität von HBsAg im Meerschweinchen. *Med. Microbiol. Immunol.*, **167**, 83–97
11. Iwarson, S. (1989). Post-exposure prophylaxis for hepatitis B: active or passive? *Lancet*, **1**, 146–7
12. WHO (1988). Progress in the control of viral hepatitis. Memorandum from a WHO meeting. *Bull. WHO*, **66**, 433–55
13. Papaevangelou, G. and Hennessen, W. (eds) *Viral Hepatitis: Standardization in immunoprophylaxis of infections by hepatitis viruses.* Developments in Biological Standardization, Vol. 54. (Basel: Karger)
14. Desmyter, J. and Leuwen, B. (1988). Recombinant vaccines. Symposium on Current Trends in Chronically-evolving Viral Hepatitis, Fiuggi, Italy
15. Meuer, S. C., Dumann, H., Meyer zum Büschenfelde, K.-H. and Köhler, H. (1989). Low-dose interleukin-2 induces systemic immune responses against HBsAg in immunodeficient non-responders to hepatitis B vaccination. *Lancet*, **1**, 15–17
16. Heerman, K.-H., Goldmann, U., Schwartz, W., Seyffarth, T., Baumgarten, H. and Gerlich, W. H. (1984). Large surface proteins of hepatitis B virus containing the pre-S sequence. *J. Virol.* **52**, 396–402
17. Tron, F., Degos, F., Brechot, C., Courouce, A.-M., Goudeau, A., Marie, F.-N., Adamowicz, P., Saliou, P., Laplanche, A., Benhamou, J.-P. and Girard, M. (1989). Randomized dose range study of a recombinant hepatitis B vaccine produced in mammalian cells and containing the S and preS2 sequences. *J. Infect. Dis.*, **160**, 199–204
18. Ferrari, C., Penna, A., Bertoletti, A., Cavalli, A., Valli, A., Schianchi, C. and Fiaccadori, F. (1989). The preS1 antigen of hepatitis B virus is highly immunogenic at the T cell level in man. *J. Clin. Invest.*, **84**, 1314–19
19. Poovorawan, Y., Sanpavat, S., Pongpunlert, W., Chumdermpadetsuk, S., Sentrakul, P. and Safary, A. (1989). Protective efficacy of a recombinant DNA hepatitis B vaccine in neonates of HBeAg-positive mothers. *J. Am. Med. Assoc.*, **261**, 3278–81
20. Heermann, K.-H., Kruse, F., Seifer, M. and Gerlich, W. H. (1987). Immunogenicity of the gene S and pre-S domains in hepatitis B virons and HBsAg filaments. *Intervirology*, **28**, 14–25
21. Marquardt, O., Heermann, K.-H., Seifer, M. and Gerlich, W. H. (1987). Cell-type dependent expression and secretion of hepatitis B virus pre-S1 surface antigen. *Postgrad. Med. J.*, **63**, 41–50
22. Kniskern, P. J., Hagopian, A., Burke, P., Dunn, N. R., Yamazaki, S., Emmi, E. A., Miller, W. J. and Ellis, R. W. (1988). A candidate vaccine for hepatitis B containing the complete viral surface protein. *Hepatology*, **8**, 82–7
23. Standring, D. N., Ou, J.-H. and Rutter, W. J. (1986). Assembly of viral particles in Xenopus oocytes: Pre-surface-antigens regulate secretion of the hepatitis B viral surface envelope particle. *Proc. Natl. Acad. Sci., USA*, **83**, 9338–42
24. Chang, H.-K., Wang, B.-Y., Yuh, C.-H., Wei, C.-L. and Ting, L.-P. (1989). A liver specific

nuclear factor interacts with the promoter region of the large surface protein gene of human hepatitis B virus. *Molec. Cell. Biol.*, **9**, 5189–97
25. Michel, M.-L., Pontisso, P., Sobczak, E., Malpiece, Y., Streeck, R. E. and Tiollais, P. (1984). Synthesis in animal cells of hepatitis B surface antigen particles carrying a receptor for polymerized human serum albumin. *Proc. Natl. Acad. Sci., USA*, **81**, 7708–12
26. Rutgers, T., Cabezon, T., Harford, N., Vanderbrugge, D., Descurieux, M., Van Opstal, O., Van Wijnendaele, F., Hauser, P., Voet, P. and De Wilde, M. (1988). Expression of different forms of hepatitis B virus envelope proteins in yeast. In Zuckerman, A. J. (ed.), *Viral Hepatitis and Liver Disease*, pp. 304–8. (New York: Alan R. Liss)
27. Gerety, R. J. (1988). Recombinant hepatitis B vaccines. In Zuckerman, A. J. (ed.), *Viral Hepatitis and Liver Disease*, pp. 1017–24. (New York: Alan R. Liss)
28. Thoma, H. A. and Hemmerling, A. E. (1988). Recombinant pre-S1 and pre-S2 containing hepatitis B particles as third generation hepatitis B vaccines. Current Trends in Chronically-Evolving Viral Hepatitis, Fiuggi, Italy
29. Delpeyroux, F., Chenciner, N., Lim, A., Malpiece, Y., Blondel, B., Crainic, R., Van der Werf, S. and Streeck, R. E. (1986). A poliovirus neutralization epitope expressed on hybrid hepatitis B surface antigen particles. *Science*, **233**, 472–5
30. Neurath, A. R., Strick, N. and Girard, M. (1989). Hepatitis B virus surface antigen (HBsAg) as carrier for synthetic peptides having an attached hydrophobic tail. *Molec. Immunol.*, **26**, 53–62
31. Flehming, B., Heinricy, U. and Pfisterer, M. (1989). Immunogenicity of a killed hepatitis A vaccine in seronegative volunteers. *Lancet*, **1**, 1039–41
32. Stahl, S. J., Murray, K. (1989). Immunogenicity of peptide fusions to hepatitis B virus core antigen. *Proc. Natl. Acad. Sci. USA*, **86**, 6283–7
33. Murray, K., Bruce, S. A., Hinnen, A., Wingfield, P., van Erd, P. M. C. A., de Reus, A. and Schellekens, H. (1984). Hepatitis B virus antigens made in microbial cells immunise against viral infection. *EMBO J.*, **3**, 645
34. Iwarson, S., Tabor, E., Thomas, H. C., Snoy, P. and Gerety, R. J. (1985). Protection against hepatitis B virus infection by immunization with hepatitis B core antigen. *Gastroenterology*, **88**, 763
35. Pignatelli, M., Waters, J., Lever, A. M. L., Iwarson, S., Gerety, R. and Thomas, H. C. (1987). Cytotoxic T-cell responses to the nucleocapsid proteins of HBV in chronic hepatitis. *J. Hepatol.*, **4**, 15–21
36. Gallina, A., Bonelli, F., Zentilin, L., Rindi, G., Muttini, M. and Milanesi, G. (1989). A recombinant hepatitis B core antigen polypeptide with the protamine-like domain deleted self-assembles into capsid particles but fails to bind nucleic acids. *J. Virol.*, **63**, 4645–52
37. Milich, D. R., McLachlan, A., Thornton, G. B. and Hughes, J. L. (1987). Antibody production to the nucleocapsid and envelope of the hepatitis B virus primed by a single T-cell site. *Nature*, **239**, 547–9
38. Purcell, R. H. and Gerin, J. L. (1987). Hepatitis B vaccines, past, present and future: Lessons for AIDS vaccine development. In Robinson, W., Koike, K. and Will, H. (eds), *Hepadna Viruses*, pp. 465–79. (New York, Alan R. Liss)
39. Lubeck, M. D., Davis, A. R., Chengalvalva, M., Natuk, R. J., Morin, J. E., Molnar-Kimber, K., Mason, B. B., Bhat, B. M., Mizutani, S., Hung, P. P. and Purcell, R. H. (1989). Immunogenicity and efficacy testing in chimpanzees of an oral hepatitis B vaccine based on live recombinant adenovirus. *Proc. Natl. Acad. Sci. USA*, **86**, 6763–7
40. Wu, J. Y., Newton, S., Stocker, B. and Robinson, W. S. (1988). Presentation of HBV epitopes in *Salmonella* flagellin. Meeting on Molecular Biology of Hepatitis B Viruses, San Diego, USA
41. Schödel, F. and Will, H. (1989). Construction of a plasmid for expression of foreign epitopes as fusion proteins with subunit B of *Escherichia coli* heat-labile enterotoxin. *Infect. Immun.*, **57**, 1347–50

23
Hepatitis delta infection

M. RIZZETTO and A. SMEDILE

INTRODUCTION

The particular nature of the delta antigen was first reported in 1979 at the Falk Symposium 28 on Virus and the Liver[1]. Experimental studies in chimpanzees, carried out at the National Institute of Health in 1978 and 1979[2] had shown that the delta antigen, originally described as an immunofluorescence reactivity associated with the hepatitis B virus (HBV), was expression of a transmissible agent that might be either a modified form of HBV or a non-A-non-B agent requiring replication of HBV for its own replication. The subsequent discovery, in the autumn of 1979, that the hepatitis delta virus (HDV) possessed a very minute RNA genome different from the DNA genome of the HBV[3] led to the hypothesis that the new virus might be a defective agent resembling the satellite RNAs of higher plants[4]. These are incomplete RNA pseudoviruses belonging to the family of the viroids. They become infectious in the presence of a mature vegetable virus and are capable of altering the expression of symptoms caused by infection with the competent helper[5]; as the satellite RNAs derive their capsid from the helper virus coinfecting the plant, HDV obtains from HBV the capsid of HBsAg by which it becomes transmissible through the vectors and modes of transmission of the ubiquitous helper.

MOLECULAR BIOLOGY

The analogy between HDV and the viroids has been confirmed by the cloning and mapping of its RNA genome; the data indicate that the conformational characteristics of the human pseudovirus are more similar to the plant viroids than to conventional RNA viruses of animals.

In 1986 Kos *et al.* in Holland[6] and Wang *et al.* in the USA[7] showed that HDV adapted in animals has a genome of about 1700 nucleotides, conformed as a circular single-stranded RNA molecule within which are extensive areas of base-pair complementarity that fold the native molecule into a pseudolinear structure.

Human derived HDV RNA has been sequenced by Makino *et al.* in the USA[8] and by Saldahna *et al.* in the UK[9]. Both in the human- and animal-adapted genome there are at least five open reading frames that could potentially encode for protein; to date only a reading frame in the antigenomic strand has been shown to code for a polypeptide immunologically reactive as the HD-antigen[10], indicating that HDV is a RNA virus of negative polarity.

The structure of HDV revealed by molecular studies is different from the structure of conventional RNA viruses of animals. It is smaller than the smallest of the picornaviruses and its circular conformation differs from the linear structure typical of animal RNA viruses. These features are instead similar to the conformational properties of the satellite RNAs and the satellite viruses of plants[5]; like HDV, viroids and related satellites have very inconspicuous genomic sizes and are in general conformed as circular single-stranded RNAs folded together, due to extensive base pairing. *In situ* hybridization studies have shown that HDV RNA is located predominantly in the liver cell nuclei[11], a feature again reminescent of the nuclear localization of the viroids. Most important both in the animal-adapted and human-derived genomes, two small domains have been identified which are analogous to two oligonucleotide sequences maintained in the viroids throughout evolution[7,8].

INFECTION AND REPLICATION STRATEGIES

Two unanswered questions concern the nature of the helper function provided by the HBV and how the HDV replicates in the infected host. Although successful natural infection with HDV requires the presence of infection with a hepadnavirus, transfection experiments[12] and studies in primary cultures of hepatocytes of woodchucks[13] have shown that the intracellular replication cycle of HDV can occur in the absence of hepadnavirus sequences; thus the hepadnavirus may be needed only to initiate infection and to assemble (and export?) the virion.

Studies of the intracellular replication of HDV RNA have shown that this is not accomplished via reverse transcription but through the copying of the RNA genome into complementary (antigenomic) RNA which provides the template to synthesis of new genomic RNA[14]. In infected cells genomic RNA is found in excess of antigenomic RNA with as many as 300 000 copies detectable in single liver cells[14]. Possibly HDV replicates by the rolling circle mechanism proposed for the viroids[15], involving the cleavage of linear, multimeric RNA strands to form monomeric-size RNA that is circularized into the genomic form; circular forms of genomic and antigenomic RNA were found in livers of HDV-infected chimpanzees, some of which are twice the length of virion RNA or in form of double-stranded RNA[14] and *in vitro* experiments have shown that a subgenomic segment of HDV can undergo self-cleavage and self-ligation[16]. However, the enzymatic process duplicating the RNA molecule is not understood. As no polymerase gene or RNA-dependent RNA polymerase was found in the HD virion, and this function is not a property of the helper virus or of the infected host, HDV might subvert to its own advantage the normal replicative machinery of the hepatocyte in a manner similar to that postulated for the viroids.

DISEASE

The current interpretation of the pathobiology of hepatitis D rests on two postulates extrapolated from infectivity studies in chimpanzees: (1) that infection with HDV requires the presence of overt infection with HBV and (2) that expression of HDV is associated with liver damage. Accordingly, HDV infection is thought to occur only in two circumstances: when the defective virus coinfects normal persons together with HBV (coinfection) or when it superinfects chronic carriers of the HBV (superinfection)[17].

Though the concepts of coinfection and superinfection have provided diagnostic frames to interpret the clinical course of hepatitis D, the natural history of HDV infection may be more complex and involve a previously unrecognized transmission pattern. Low-grade replication of HDV has continued without liver damage in half of the HBsAg carrier chimpanzees superinfected at the National Institute of Health[18] and an atypical mode of reinfection was observed in patients transplanted for terminal HDV cirrhosis[19,20]. Among patients transplanted in Belgium and Italy[19], five (three of them under cover with anti-HBs immune globulins) became reinfected with HDV but did not experience hepatitis D.

In these patients serum or liver tests for HDV were positive in the absence of markers of HBV reinfection; they have been followed up for 11–38 months without evidence of recurrence of HBV or of hepatitis, and in all of them the IgM antibody to HDV has declined rapidly following transplantation.

In many of the reinfected patients who also experienced recrudescence of liver disease, the HDV has recurred very early without simultaneous recurrence of HBV. Disease has returned only if and when HBV has also returned to the graft. Coincident with the return of HBV and of hepatitis, HDV has spread within the liver and IgM anti-HD has increased in titre.

The data in the model of liver transplantation would indicate that HDV is capable of establishing infection independently from the HBV and separate from disease expression, and that it is not in itself pathogenic, but activation to disease expression requires interactions with HBV.

Thus hepatitis D might result not only from coinfection with HBV or superinfection of HBV carriers, but also from activation of a latent HDV infection by HBV superinfection.

References

1. Purcell, R. H. (1980). Round table discussion non A, non B hepatitis. In Bianchi, L., Gerok, W., Sicklinger, K. and Stalder, G. A. (eds), Virus and the liver, *Falk Symposium no. 28*, p. 125. (Lancaster: MTP Press)
2. Rizzetto, M., Canese, M. G., Gerin, J. L. *et al.* (1980). Transmission of hepatitis B virus associated delta antigen to chimpanzees. *J. Infect. Dis.*, **121**, 590–602

3. Rizzetto, M., Hoyer, B., Canese, M. G. *et al.* (1980). Delta antigen: the association of delta antigen with hepatitis B surface antigen and ribonucleic acid in the serum of delta infected chimpanzees. *Proc. Natl. Acad. Sci., USA*, **77**, 6124–28
4. Rizzetto, M., Gerin, J. L. and Purcell, R. H. (1981). Delta antigen: evidence for a variant of hepatitis B virus or a defective non A, non B agent. In Pollard, M. (ed.), *Perspective in Virology*, XI, pp. 195–217. (New York: Alan R. Liss)
5. Diener, T. O. (1987). Autonomous and helper-dependent small pathogenic RNAs of plants: viroids and satellites. In Rizzetto, M., Gerin, J. L. and Purcell, R. H. (eds.), *The Hepatitis Delta Virus and its Infection*, Prog. Clin. Biol. Res., vol. 234, pp. 3–18. (New York: Alan R. Liss)
6. Kos, A., Dijkema, R., Arnberg, A. C., van der Meide, P. H. and Schellekens, H. (1986). The hepatitis delta (δ) virus possesses a circular RNA. *Nature*, **323**, 558–60
7. Wang, K. S., Choo, Q. L., Weiner, A. J. *et al.* (1986). Structure, sequence and expression of the hepatitis delta (δ) viral genome. *Nature*, **323**, 508–13
8. Makino, S., Chang, M. F., Shieh, C. K. *et al.* (1987). Molecular cloning and sequencing of a human hepatitis delta virus RNA. *Nature*, **329**, 343–6
9. Saldanha, J. A., Thomas, H. C. and Monjardino, J. P. (1987). Cloning and characterization of delta virus cDNA sequence derived from a human source. *J. Med. Virol.*, **22**, 323–31
10. Weiner, A. J., Loo, Q. L., Wang, K. S. *et al.* (1987). A single antigenomic open reading frame of the hepatitis delta virus encodes the epitope(s) of both hepatitis delta antigen polypeptides p.24 and p.27. *J. Virol.*, **62**, 622–9
11. Gowans, E. J., Baroudy, B. M., Negro, F. *et al.* (1988). Evidence for replication of hepatitis delta virus RNA in hepatocyte nuclei after in vivo infection. *Virology*, **167**, 274–8
12. Mason, W. S. and Taylor, J. M. (1989). Experimental system for the study of hepadnaviruses and hepatitis delta virus infections. *Hepatology*, **9**, 635–45
13. Taylor, J., Mason, W., Summers, J. *et al.* (1987). Replication of human hepatitis delta virus in primary cultures of woodchuck hepatocytes. *J. Virol.*, **61**, 2891–5
14. Chen, P. J., Kalpana, G., Goldberg, J. *et al.* (1986). The structure and replication of hepatitis delta virus genome. *Proc. Natl. Acad. Sci., USA*, **83**, 8774–8
15. Wu, H. N. and Lai, M. M. C. (1989). Reversible cleavage and ligation of hepatitis delta virus RNA. *Science*, **243**, 652–4
16. Branch, A. D. and Robertson, H. D. (1984). A replication cycle for viroids and other small infectious RNAs. *Science*, **223**, 450–5
17. Rizzetto, M., Verme, G., Gerin, J. L. and Purcell, R. H. (1986). Hepatitis delta virus disease. In Popper, H. and Schaffner, E. (eds), *Progress in Liver Disease*, Vol. VIII, pp. 417–31. (New York: Grune & Stratton)
18. Negro, F., Bergman, K. F., Baroudy, B. M. *et al.* (1988). Chronic hepatitis delta virus (HDV) infection in hepatitis B virus carrier chimpanzees experimentally superinfected with HDV. *J. Infect. Dis.*, **158**, 151–9
19. Ottobrelli, A., Salizzoni, M., Cornù, C. *et al.* (1989). Patterns of HDV reinfection in liver transplantation. *J. Hepatol.*, **9** (Suppl. 1), S68
20. Zignego, A. L., Samuel, D., Gentilini, P. *et al.* (1989). Hepatitis D virus (HDV) RNA in patients with acute delta hepatitis and in liver graft recipients. *J. Hepatol.*, **9** (Suppl. 1), S98

24
Non-A, non-B hepatitis: Infections by the enteral and parenteral route

K.-P. MAIER

INTRODUCTION

Epidemiological and clinical studies have led to the conclusion that there are at least two types of hepatitis non-A, non-B (HNANB): one type is associated with the tranfusion of blood and blood products. The virus of this parenterally transmitted HNANB(p) has been termed hepatitis-C virus (HCV)[1].

The term 'enterically transmitted' HNANB(e) derives from the presumed enteric route of infection in humans. New findings strongly suggest that a single-stranded, 8.5 kb RNA virus, tentatively called hepatitis-E virus (HEV) is responsible for epidemic outbreaks of acute hepatitis in various parts of the world (India, Burma, Mexico and the Soviet Union)[2–5].

This article reviews some aspects of the epidemiology and natural course of both diseases, as well as new data on the approach to treatment.

HNANB(e)

HNANB(e) has been shown to occur epidemically or endemically in India, Nepal, Burma, Africa and the Soviet Union, mostly due to faecal contamination of drinking water[4,5]. So far the disease is rarely found in the western hemisphere. Most of the cases in the US and in Europe are spread by travellers infected in endemic areas[6].

Analysis of the clinical features of this disease disclosed an average incubation period of 35–40 days and a low case-fatality rate, except among pregnant women[7,8]. Tables 1 and 2 list some of the epidemiological features of acute HNANB(e) which usually does not become chronic[9]. Clinically, acute HNANB (e) largely resembles hepatitis A.

Symptoms of the disease include nausea (84%), dark urine (92%), fever (54%), abdominal pain (75%) and itching (55%). During the last epidemic

Table 1 NHANB(e)–epidemiology (I)

'HAV-like' epidemological features:
Causative agent: HEV (32–34 nm RNA virus)
Epidemic and endemic (Asia, Africa)
In populations immune to HAV
Spread by the fecal–oral route ('waterborne')

Table 2 HNANB(e)–epidemiology (II)

Rarity of secondary cases
Mostly affecting young adults (20–40 years)
High case fatality rate in pregnant women (10–20%)
No progression to chronic liver disease

in Nepal in summer of 1987, 87% had a moderate elevation of GPT and mild icteric illness.

As in the case of hepatitis A, there is no effective treatment in patients with acute waterborne HNANB(e). In the absence of effective therapy the need for prevention assumes even greater importance. This is especially true in the case of pregnant women, who are confronted with the problem of severe acute illness or even death due to liver failure. Unfortunately, however, the effectiveness of immunoprophylaxis in reducing the severity of HNANB(e) has not been convincingly demonstrated.

HNANB(p)

By contrast, HNANB(p) is a world-wide problem, affecting 3–10% of transfused patients. Obviously, HCV accounts for most cases of post-transfusion hepatitis, as recently demonstrated in patients undergoing open-heart surgery[10].

Anti-HCV could be detected in 85% of prospectively followed patients with non-A, non-B post-transfusion hepatitis, as well as in a substantial number of haemophiliacs and i.v. drug users, whereas among healthy subjects without such risk factors the overall prevalence of anti-HCV was very low[11]. Interesting and still unexplained is the finding that nearly half of the patients whose liver disease is currently attributed to non-viral causes, are positive for anti-HCV (Table 3). However, HCV is a major cause of hepatitis not only in haemophiliacs and drug addicts but also in haemodialysis patients[12]. Some cases also seem to be transmitted perinatally[13,14]. Remarkably, only a few homosexual men (91% positive for anti-HIV) were positive for anti-HCV[11].

Table 3 Hepatitis C virus antibodies in liver disease

	No. of sera tested	*Anti-HCV positive (%)*
HNANB(p)	54	85
Haemophiliacs	97	64
Intravenous drug abusers	83	70
Autoimmune CAH; PBC	34	44
Cirrhosis (cryptogenic and alcoholic)	26	38
Healthy pregnant women	241	1.2

Their NANBH(p) annual attack rate ranges between 3 and 4%, which is below the incidence of HAV (5%) and HBV (18%) in this group[15].

The clinical features of acute HNANB(p), which occurs after a mean incubation period of 50–60 days, tend to be less severe than hepatitis A or hepatitis B. The rate of icteric cases is much lower than in post-transfusion hepatitis B (25% vs. 60%) and the peak serum aminotransferase activities are lower[13]. Further, the frequency of asymptomatic cases is high in HNANB(p). In the latest study comprising 53 patients with acute HNANB(p) 45% were asymptomatic, 55% were symptomatic and serum bilirubin was elevated in only 9%[16]. Therefore the disease often remains undetected unless liver tests are monitored in regular intervals.

Patients with acute HNANB(p) face three major problems:

1. fulminant liver failure;
2. chronicity and progression to liver cirrhosis;
3. development of liver carcinoma.

Fulminant hepatic failure may occur as a result of HNANB(p) infection. However, the rate of this fatal complication seems to be rare in the post-transfusion setting: no case of fulminant hepatitis was observed in 515 patients with acute post-transfusion hepatitis[13]. Fatalities have been reported in instances of sporadic hepatitis NANB, accounting for 27–44% of cases in England and the US, respectively[13]. These data, however, represent the maximal proportion of cases attributable to HCV. The exact number of HCV infections in the case of fulminant viral liver disease still awaits clarification.

The rate of progression seems to be different in different parts of the world, with the lowest in Canada (36%) and the highest in Spain (67%)[16,17]. To date, the factors determining the rate of chronicity (?viral, ?host), are unknown.

Clinically patients are often asymptomatic. Fatigue is the predominant complaint. Transaminases tend to fluctuate, bilirubin values rarely exceed 3 mg/dl and are normal in nearly half of the patients (see Table 4). Thus by the time the patient experiences symptoms he or she may already have

Table 4 Long-term follow-up of chronic HNANB(p) (clinical data)[18]

Asymptomatic 13/77 patients (35%)
Fluctuating transaminases 22/37 patients (59%)
Normal bilirubin values 21/37 patients (57%)

histologically advanced chronic liver disease or even cirrhosis. Therefore, information on both, liver histology and follow-up time is mandatory.

In the case of blood-transfusion acquired hepatitis NANB, the follow-up period can be calculated with certainty. Tables 5 and 6 summarize the histological outcome in 37 patients with HNANB(p) 15 and 30 months, respectively, from acute onset[18]. It is evident from these data that an increasing duration of follow-up is associated with an increasing number of patients who develop liver cirrhosis as a consequence of post-transfusion hepatitis. Additionally, long-term follow-up (average nearly 5 years) disclosed liver cirrhosis in 46% in the post-transfusion group as compared to 23% in a group of patients with sporadic NANB hepatitis[19].

What is the risk of developing hepatocellular carcinoma (HCC) in association with long-standing liver cirrhosis due to HCV infection? Again, the exact answer is not yet known; however, indirect evidence for an association between HNANB and HCC is beginning to accumulate. Single cases of HCC following non-A, non-B post-transfusion hepatitis are described[20].

In Japan, 40% of 108 cases of HCC had a history of blood transfusion about 20 years before the diagnosis of liver cancer was established[21]. In the Far East, hepatitis B-unrelated cases of HCC are increasingly observed[22]. In Italy, more than half of the patients with HCC are infected with HCV, as are many patients with chronic HNANB(p) (see Table 7)[23,24]. Anti-HCV positivity seems not to be related to the presence or absence of HBsAg. These data, and the well-known aetiological link between hepatitis B virus (HBV) and HCC suggest that both viruses, HBV and HCV, may be implicated in the development of HCC.

Table 5 Histological findings in chronic HNANB (first biopsy*)[18]

Acute hepatitis	*CPH*	*CAH*	*CAH/Ci*
1	14	10	12
2%	38%	27%	33%
		60% (CAH + CAH/Ci)	

* 15 (4–54) months from acute onset (n = 37 patients)

Table 6 Histological findings in chronic HNANB (second biopsy*)[18]

Progression	8/16 (50%)
Improvement	1/16 (12.5%)
Unchanged	6/16 (37.5%)

* 30 (11–97) months from acute onset (n = 16)

Table 7 Anti-HCV in patients with HCC[24]

n	*Anti-HCV positive* (%)	*Anti-HBc positive* (%)
HCC 132	65	70
HNANB(p) 19	84	—

In patients with established chronic HNANB(p) many therapeutic modalities have been used including corticosteroids, interferons and acyclovir. Steroids are known to be highly effective in autoimmune hepatitis. A beneficial effect of corticosteroids in cases of chronic HNANB[25] was observed in one study in Italy. By contrast, our group failed to confirm these data in a small series of patients who were followed histologically[26]. It cannot be excluded that some cases of HNANB are mis-diagnosed as autoimmune chronic hepatitis and treated appropriately. However, since steroids have been shown to be ineffective or even harmful in chronic hepatitis B[27] it would be prudent to withhold this form of therapy in the case of proven chronic HCV infection.

Acyclovir has been tested in a pilot study in a few patients in a dosage of 5 mg/kg every 8 h for 10 days[28]. During treatment, serum enzyme activities decreased (two patients), remained unchanged (two patients) or rose (1 patient). None of the five patients showed clinical or biochemical improvement during the follow-up period of 1 year. Following the initial report of a favourable response of recombinant interferon-α in 10 patients with symptomatic chronic HNANB[29], many studies have been conducted. However, most of them are very heterogeneous with respect to treatment schedule, duration of therapy (4, 6, 9, 12, 18 months), daily application of IFN or administration every other day, fixed dosage or adaptation of the IFN dosage to serum enzymes. Despite these discrepancies some common findings have emerged.

Confirming earlier uncontrolled studies, the first controlled trial[30] disclosed that in most patients serum enzymes fall rapidly to normal, usually within 4–8 weeks after starting IFN treatment. Treatment with interferon-α (IFN-α) in patients with chronic HNANB induces a biochemical remission in 36–80% in current, mostly uncontrolled, studies. However, after termination of treatment, relapse rates are high. Sustained response can be achieved in 13–60% of successfully treated patients. This may be due to the fact that many important issues regarding IFN therapy of chronic HNANB are still unresolved. These include:

(a) The problem of correctly diagnosing HNANB, which up till now is a diagnosis of exclusion in most institutions. Interestingly, however, this information seems not to discriminate between responders and non-responders to IFN therapy, at least in patients with post-transfusion hepatitis[31].
(b) The optimal dose of IFN-α is not yet known. The majority of patients seem to respond to a dosage of 1–3 million units three times weekly. Higher doses increase the frequency of side-effects without additional beneficial effect upon the induction of a biochemical remission.
(c) The optimal duration of IFN therapy remains an open question. Most results, although widely uncontrolled, seem to indicate that prolonged therapy (9–12 months) is necessary in most patients to suppress disease activity.
(d) The problem of the patients relapsing after successful therapy is still unresolved. Should long-term, low-dose IFN be administered in this

special group of patients?

(e) Since many patients with acute HNANB develop chronic hepatitis, should IFN therapy be evaluated in acute HNANB, as has been stressed by some authors?[32]

SUMMARY

Enterically transmitted non-A, non-B hepatitis ('hepatitis E') occurs in either endemic or epidemic form in various parts of the world as a disease, which is clinically indistinguishable from acute hepatitis A. The infection runs a benign course in most patients; fulminant hepatic failure, however, remains a remarkable threat to pregnant women in the third trimester. It has been discussed that combined infection with HEV and HBV may be responsible for the high case fatality rate (up to 22%) in this situation – not surprisingly in countries where B-carrier rates amount to 10% and more. So far, however, the pathogenetic background of fulminant hepatitis in acute HEV infection in pregnancy is not known. Specific control measures in the form of immunoprophylaxis will have to await the exact characterization of the causative virus, especially its genomic structure.

Parenterally transmitted non-A, non-B hepatitis ('hepatitis C') is still the most common complication of blood transfusion, clinically characterized by a lack of symptoms in the acute as well as in the chronic stage of the disease.

Most acute infections run a subclinical course; therefore, clinical diagnosis is difficult, if not impossible. Not only acute hepatitis non-A, non-B, but also the chronic form, is an insidious, progressive disease. The high rate of chronicity, the progression to cirrhosis in about one-fifth of the patients with chronic liver disease and an assumed association with HCC represent some of the complications encountered by patients in the post-transfusion situation.

The recently developed assay for circulating antibodies to hepatitis C virus (anti-HCV) clearly demonstrated a causative relationship between parenteral exposure and acute and chronic hepatitis. This breakthrough will open the way for screening of blood and blood products, as well as for the development of specific immunoprophylaxis. At present, however, there are no means to prevent or treat the acute infection or to prevent chronicity. It is not at present known which patients with acute hepatitis non-A, non-B are prone to develop chronic liver disease. Fortunately, however, IFN-α shows great promise as a beneficial therapeutic agent in patients with chronic non-A, non-B hepatitis, inducing a biochemical remission in up to 80% of cases during therapy. We urge inclusion of all these patients into controlled, prospective studies in order to gain insight into the many problems still associated with this therapeutic strategy.

References

1. Choo, Q. L., Kuo, G., Weiner, A. J., Overby, L. R., Bradley, D. W. and Houghton, M. (1989). Isolation of a cDNA clone derived from a blood-borne non-A, non-B hepatitis genome. *Science*, **244**, 359–62
2. Bradley, D. W., Krawczynsi, K., Cook, E. H., McCaustland, K. A., Humphrey, C. D.,

Spielbring, J. E., Myint, H. and Maynard, J. E. (1987). Enterically transmitted non-A, non-B hepatitis: Serial passage of disease in cynomolgus macaques and tamarins and recovery of disease-associated 27- to 34 nm viruslike particles. *Proc. Natl. Acad. Sci.*, **84**, 6277–81

3. Bradley, D. W. (1989). The viruses of non-A, non-B hepatitis, enterically and parenterally transmitted. *J. Hepatol.* (Suppl 1), 16
4. Arankalle, V. A., Sreenivasan, M. A., Popper, H., Ticehurst, J., Kapikian, A. Z., Pavri, K. M. and Purcell, R. H. (1988). Aetiological association of a viruslike with enterically transmitted non-A, non-B hepatitis. *Lancet*, **1**, 550–3
5. Balayan, M. S., Andjaparidze, A. G., Savinskaya, S. S., Ketiladze, E. S., Braginsky, D. M., Savinov, A. P. and Poleschuk, V. F. (1983). Evidence for a virus in non-A, non-B hepatitis transmitted via the fecal oral route. *Intervirology*, **20**, 23–31
6. Cock, K. M., Bradley, D. W., Sandford, N. L., Govindarajan, S., Maynard, J. E. and Redeker, A. G. (1987). Epidemic non-A, non-B hepatitis in patients from Pakistan. *Ann. Intern. Med.*, **106**, 227–30
7. Ramalingaswami, V. and Purcell, R. H. (1988). Waterborne non-A, non-B hepatitis. *Lancet*, **1**, 571–3
8. Wong, D. C., Purcell, R. H., Sreenivasan, M. A., Prasad, S. R. and Pavri, K. M. (1980). Epidemic and endemic hepatitis in India: Evidence for a non-A, non-B hepatitis virus aetiology. *Lancet*, **2**, 876–8
9. Khuroo, M. S., Saleem, M., Teli, M. R. and Sofi, M. A. (1980). Failure to detect chronic liver disease after epidemic non-A, non-B hepatitis. *Lancet*, **1**, 97–8
10. Poel, van der C. L., Reesink, H. W., Lelie, P. N., Leentvaar-Kuypers, A., Choo, Q.-L. and Kuo, G. (1989). Anti-hepatitis C antibodies and non-A, non-B post-transfusion hepatitis in the Netherlands. *Lancet*, **2**, 297–9
11. Esteban, J. I., Viladoumio, L., Roget, M., Genesca, J., Esteban, R., Lopez-Talavera, J. C., Hernandez, J. M., Vargas, V., Buti, M. and Guardia, J. (1989). Hepatitis C virus antibodies among risk groups in Spain. *Lancet*, **2**, 294–7
12. Roggendorf, M., Deinhardt, F., Rasshofer, R., Eberle, J., Hopf, U., Möller, B., Zachoval, R., Pape, G., Schramm, W. and Rommel, F. (1989). Antibodies to hepatitis C virus. *Lancet*, **2**, 324–5
13. Dienstag, J. L. (1983). Non-A, non-B hepatitis. I. Recognition, epidemiology and clinical features. *Gastroenterology*, **85**, 439–62
14. Tong, M. J., Thrusby, M., Rakela, J., McPaek, C., Edwards, V. M. and Mosley, J. W. (1981). Studies on maternal–infant transmission of the viruses which cause acute hepatitis. *Gastroenterology*, **80**, 999–1004
15. Szmuness, W., Stevens, C. E. and Harley, E. J. (1980). Hepatitis B vaccine: demonstration of efficacy in a controlled clinical trial in a high-risk population in the United States. *N. Engl. J. Med.*, **303**, 833–41
16. Feinman, S. V., Berris, B. and Bojarski, S. (1988). Posttransfusions Hepatitis in Toronto Canada. *Gastroenterology*, **95**, 464–9
17. Barcena, R., Suarez-Garcia, E. and Gill, L. Post transfusion non A, non B hepatitis. A prospective study. *Liver*, **5**, 71–6
18. Mattsson, L., Weiland, O. and Glaumann, H. (1988). Long-term follow-up of chronic post-transfusion non-A, non-B hepatitis: clinical and histological outcome. *Liver*, **8**, 184–8
19. Mattsson, L., Weiland, O. and Glaumann, H. (1989). Chronic non-A, non-B hepatitis developed after transfusions, illicit self-injections or sporadically. Outcome during long-term follow-up – a comparison. *Liver*, **9**, 120–7
20. Kiyosawa, K., Akahane, Y., Nagata, A. and Furuta, S. (1984). Hepatocellular carcinoma after non-A, non-B posttransfusion hepatitis. *Am. J. Gastroenterol.*, **79**, 777–81
21. Ohbayashi, A., Tanaka, S., Ohthke, H., Harada, H., Komachiya, K., Kodama, T., Okada, Y., Takahashi, K. and Tanaka, N. (1983). Clinico-pathological observations on relationship of blood transfusion to liver cirrhosis and hepatocellular carcinoma. *Acta Hepatol. Jpn.*, **24**, 521–5
22. Okuda, K., Fujimoto, I., Hanai, A. and Urano, Y. (1987). Changing incidence of hepatocellular carcinoma in Japan. *Cancer Res.*, **47**, 4967–72
23. Colombo, M., Kuo, G., Choo, L., Houghton, M., Tommasini, M. A., Rumi, M. G., Dioguardi, M. L., Donato, M. F. and Ninno, Del E. (1989). High prevalence of antibody to hepatitis C virus in patients with hepatocellular carcinoma (HCC). *J. Hepatol.* (Suppl. 1), 20

24. Donato, M. F., Kuo, G., Choo, L., Houghton, M., Tommasini, M. A., Bargiggia, S., Piva, A., Oldani, S., Dioguardi, M. L., Del-Ninno, E. and Colombo, M. (1989). High prevalence of antibody to hepatitis (virus in patients with hepatocellular carcinoma (HCC). VIII International Congress of Liver Diseases, Basel, Switzerland, 12–14 October (abstract)
25. Realdi, G., Alberti, A. and Rugge, M. (1982). Long-term follow-up of acute and chronic non-A, non-B post-transfusion hepatitis-evidence of progression to liver cirrhosis. *Gut*, **23**, 270–5
26. Maier, K. P., Blum, H., Gerok, W., Herz, R. and Berthold, H. (1981). Liver histology in patients with and without immunosuppressive therapy due to non-A, non-B chronic active hepatitis. *Hepatology*, **1**, 529 (abstract)
27. EASL trial-group (1986). Steroids in chronic B-hepatitis, a randomized, double blind trial on the effect of low-dose, long-term treatment on survival. *Liver*, **6**, 227–31
28. Pappas, S. C., Hoofnagle, J. H., Young, N., Straus, S. E. and Jones, E. A. (1985). Treatment of chronic non-A, non-B hepatitis with acyclovir: pilot study. *J. Med. Virol.*, **15**, 1–9
29. Hoofnagle, J. H., Mullen, K. D. and Jones, D. B. (1986). Treatment of chronic non-A, non-B hepatitis with recombinant human alpha interferon. A preliminary report. *N. Engl. J. Med.*, **315**, 1575–8
30. Jacyna, R. M., Brooks, M. G., Loke, R. H. T., Main, J., Murray-Lyon, I. M. and Thomas, H. C. (1989). Randomized controlled trial of interferon alpha (lymphoblastoid interferon) in chronic non-A, non-B hepatitis. *Br. Med. J.*, **298**, 80–2
31. Saccaro, G., Houghton, M., Kuo, G., Choo, Q. L., Rossina, F., Lattore, V., Torrani, M. R., Chiandussi, L., Bonino, F. and Rizzetto, M. (1989). Anti-hepatitis C virus in non-A, non-B hepatitis responding and non-responding to alpha-ZA interferon. *J. Hepatol* (Suppl 1), 219
32. Viladomju, L., Esteban, J. I., Gonzalez, A., Lopez-Talavera, J. C., Sanchez, C., Quer, J., Caragol, I., Hernandez, J. M., Esteban, R., Guardia, J., Kuo, G. and Houghton, M. (1989). Efficacy of alfa-interferon to prevent chronicity in patients with acute post-transfusion non-A, non-B hepatitis: a randomized, controlled trial. *J. Hepatol.* (Suppl. 1), 241

25
Isolation and characterization of hepatitis E virus (HEV)

D. W. BRADLEY

INTRODUCTION

The enterically and parenterally transmitted forms of non-A, non-B hepatitis (ET-NANBH and PT-NANBH, respectively) have long been recognized as important causes of morbidity and mortality in man. Until recently, however, little was known about the aetiology of either ET-NANBH or PT-NANBH except that viral agents were strongly suspected on the basis of the epidemiological, clinical, and histological features of each disease. The development of sensitive and specific serological assays for markers of acute infection by hepatitis A virus (HAV)[1,2] and hepatitis B virus (HBV)[3,4] led to the realization that many epidemics of hepatitis associated with faecally contaminated water were not caused by HAV[5] and that the majority of post-transfusion hepatitis was due to infection with an agent other than HBV[6]. Laboratory studies of both ET-NANBH and PT-NANBH were largely unsuccessful until suitable primate models of human disease were identified and developed in the late 1970s and early-to-mid 1980s. The following discussion chronicles research conducted at the US Centers for Disease Control that led to the discovery of the virus responsible for the majority of ET-NANBH worldwide. More extensive general reviews of ET-NANBH can be found elsewhere[7–13].

ENTERICALLY TRANSMITTED NON-A, NON-B HEPATITIS

Natural history; geographical distribution; clinical features

A significant proportion of acute viral hepatitis occurring in young to middle-age adults in Asia and the Indian subcontinent appears to be caused by an agent that is serologically unrelated to either HAV or HBV[5]. Disease has been shown to occur in both epidemic and sporadic–endemic forms and is primarily associated with the ingestion of faecally contaminated drinking water. The term enterically transmitted NANBH (ET-NANBH) has evolved from the waterborne mode of virus transmission and presumed route of natural infection in humans[14]. ET-NANBH was first documented in New Delhi, India, in 1955, when 29 000 cases of icteric hepatisis were identified following widespread faecal contamination of the city's drinking water[15]. A similar epidemic of viral hepatitis occurred between December 1975 and January 1976 in Ahmedabad City, India, again due to contaminated water supplies[16]. Both outbreaks were originally thought to be caused by HAV; however, retrospective serological analysis of paired serum specimens from documented cases revealed that neither HAV nor HBV could be implicated as the causative agent[5]. Large epidemics of enterically transmitted viral hepatitis have also been observed in the Kirgiz Republic, USSR[17]. Between 1955 and 1956 more than 10 800 cases of acute viral hepatitis were documented in young to middle-aged (15–40-year-old) adults; approximately 18% of infected pregnant women died as a result of acute disease. The clinical and epidemiological features of these outbreaks are remarkably similar to those associated with the 1955–56 New Delhi outbreak. Subsequent outbreaks of epidemic and acute, sporadic NANBH were documented in North India[18], and in Kashmir, India[19]. Outbreaks of epidemiologically similar NANBH have also been reported in Southeast Asia, including Burma[20] and Nepal[21], and were associated with an unusually high mortality rate in infected pregnant women. Between June 1976 and August 1977 more than 20 000 icteric cases occurred in Mandalay, Burma, with a case fatality ratio of 18% in pregnant women (Schreeder, unpublished data). An epidemic of viral hepatitis involving 10 000 cases in the Kathmandu Valley, Nepal, in 1973 was also reported to be associated with a high mortality rate in infected pregnant women[22]. The occurrence of ET-NANBH in Pakistan has also been inferred from the observation of multiple cases (Pakistani nationals) imported into the United States[23].

Outbreaks of ET-NANBH have also been reported in Africa, including Algeria[24], Ivory Coast[25], Eastern Sudan[26], and Somalia[26]. Between October 1980 and January 1981 more than 780 cases of NANBH were documented in Algeria and linked to the use of faecally contaminated drinking water. Mostly young adults were affected, and all nine infected pregnant women died as a direct result of NANBH. A similar number of NANBH cases (623) in Tortiya, Ivory Coast, was observed between 1983 and 1984[25]. Although no precise figure was given, a high mortality rate among infected pregnant women was noted. More recently, large outbreaks of ET-NANBH have been documented in Eritrean and Tigrean (Ethiopian) refugees encamped in Eastern Sudan[26]. More than 2000 cases occurred in these refugees between August and September 1985, again due to the use of faecally contaminated drinking water. Several thousand cases of ET-NANBH were also noted in Ethiopian refugees residing in Tug Wajale and other refugee camps in northwest Somalia[26]; these cases accounted for the majority of acute viral hepatitis observed between 1985 and 1986. The mortality rate among ET-NANBH infected pregnant women was greater than 17% and a faecally contaminated environment was again implicated as the vehicle for virus transmission.

ET-NANBH does not appear to be confined to Asia, the Soviet Union, and North Africa, however. In fact, outbreaks of ET-NANBH associated with faecally contaminated drinking water have recently been documented in Borneo (Lubis and Wuryadi, personal communication), and in two rural villages located south of Mexico City, Mexico[27].

More than 90 cases of presumed ET-NANBH were recorded in Huitzililla, Mexico, between June and October of 1986. Additional cases of NANBH were seen in Telixtac, Mexico, shortly thereafter. There was no evidence that the disease was either imported or resulted from inter-village traffic. Virological and serological studies of case stool and serum specimens, respectively, suggested that the aetiological agent responsible for disease in North America might be very similar or identical to that associated with ET-NANBH in other regions of the world. Tables 1 and 2 summarize the major epidemiological and clinical features of ET-NANBH.

Development of primate models

Transmission of ET-NANBH to non-human primates was first reported by Balayan and co-workers in 1983[28]. Two cynomolgus macaques ('cynos') were intravenously inoculated with a 10% w/v suspension of a human volunteer stool that was positive by IEM for 27–30 nm diameter VLPs. These animals developed elevations in ALT activity between 24 and 36 days after inoculation, excreted 27–30 nm VLPs in their pre-acute phase stools, and seroconverted to morphologically similar VLPs in the inoculum. Andjaparidze and co-workers later reported the successful transmission of ET-NANBH to African green monkeys, as well as cynos using ET-NANBH case stool specimens positive by IEM for 27–30 nm VLPs[29]. Although ET-NANBH was serially passaged in the latter animals, a decreased efficiency of transmission was observed during each successive passage. Intravenous inoculation of four

Table 1 Epidemiological features of ET-NANBH

1.	Outbreaks may involve tens of thousands of cases in developing countries of world, particularly in India and Indian subcontinent
2.	Sporadic cases and smaller outbreaks involving hundreds of cases occur in endemic areas
3.	To date, cases in Western countries related to travel to endemic areas
4.	Disease transmitted by faecally contaminated drinking water or contact with faecally contaminated environment
5.	Peaks of epidemics occur approximately 6 weeks after primary exposure
6.	Low secondary attack rate among exposed household members
7.	High case fatality ratio in infected pregnant women (average: 20%)

Table 2 Clinical features of ET-NANBH

1.	Incubation period ranges between 2 and 9 weeks (average 6 weeks)
2.	Self-limiting disease resembling hepatitis A; chronic liver disease or persistent viraemia has not been observed
3.	Extremely high mortality rate in infected pregnant women
4.	Highest attack rate observed in young to middle-aged (15–40-year-old) adults
5.	Subclinical cases in younger individuals suspected but not documented

Saguinus mystax (tamarins) with another acute-phase stool suspension obtained from a case of ET-NANBH in Nepal resulted in biochemical evidence of liver dysfunction in three; 27–30 nm VLPs were observed in several early acute-illness phase stool specimens of one animal studied in detail[21]. The latter animal also seroconverted to 27–30 nm VLPs contained in the original stool inoculum.

More recently, animal transmission studies have been conducted in cynos, tamarins, chimpanzees, and rhesus monkeys using highly characterized inocula[30–32]. Our studies at the CDC have specifically employed the use of tamarins, cynos, and colony-born chimpanzees for the purpose of developing a reliable source of infected stools and liver tissue. These same studies have provided preinoculation, acute-phase, and convalescent sera for use in coded serum panels, immunofluorescent antibody assays (see below), and in immunoscreening studies of lambda gt11 cDNA libraries. Intravenous inoculation of four tamarins with a 1982–83 Burma outbreak stool pool (positive by IEM for 32–34 nm VLPs) caused elevated serum isocitrate dehydrogenase (SICD) activity in three animals with peak values occurring between 70 and 80 days after inoculation[32]. Three of four cynos inoculated i.v. with the same material developed elevated ALT activity after an average incubation period of 38 days[32]. ET-NANBH was passaged in cynos using pre-acute-phase stool suspensions from animals exhibiting elevations of ALT activity. The incubation period at each passage level appeared to be shorter, and all animals became infected. Third passage of ET-NANBH in five cynos, for example, resulted in elevated ALT activity in all animals, with an average incubation period of 20 days (Figure 1). Additional passage of disease in cynos using either liver or stool resulted in incubation periods as short as 5 days (D. Bradley, unpublished data). Intravenous inoculation of four cynos with a partially purified virus preparation (Mexico case stool; see below for details) containing a relatively large number of 32–34 nm VLPs resulted in elevated ALT activity after incubation periods of 5, 5, 8, and 12 days, respectively (Figure 2) (D. Bradley, unpublished data). Intravenous inoculation of colony-born chimpanzees with this same inoculum resulted in relatively severe disease and liver histopathology consistent with a diagnosis of viral hepatitis (K. Krawczynski and D. Bradley, unpublished data). It is interesting to note that inoculation of other chimpanzees with ET-NANBH case stools obtained from outbreaks in geographical areas other than Mexico, or containing either fewer numbers of 32–34 nm VLPs (or smaller VPLs) demonstrated less severe disease or no disease at all. The stools used in these studies were derived from cases of ET-NANBH occurring in India[31], the USSR (A. Andjaparidze and D. Bradley, unpublished data), and Burma (D. Bradley, unpublished data).

Although we were able to demonstrate reliable and efficient transmission of ET-NANBH to cynos, tamarins, and chimpanzees using inocula containing 32–34 nm VLPs, we were unable to consistently recover VLPs with a similar or identical morphology from proven-infectious stool pools. These findings indicated that either the virus of ET-NANBH was normally present in small numbers in infected stools, or that it was so labile that passage through the gut resulted in significant particle degradation. The latter presumption was

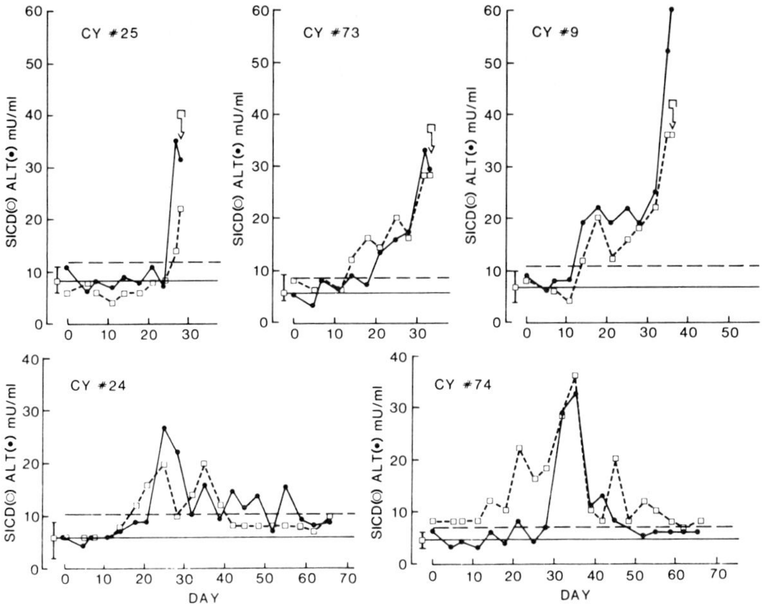

Figure 1 Third passage of ET-NANBH virus (HEV) in cynomolgus macaques (cynos) after i.v. inoculation of a second-passage animal pre-acute-phase stool pool. The solid horizontal lines represent the mean value of ALT activity in at least 12 preinoculation sera; the vertical bars indicate the range of preinoculation ALT values; the dashed horizontal lines represent the 95% confidence limit for the upper level of normal ALT activity. Arrows indicate day of necropsy

favoured in view of the observed instability of virus in stored stool suspensions and the lack of virus particles in a high percentage of well-documented cases of severe disease. As a result, in order to demonstrate a serological relationship between ET-NANBH in experimentally infected primates and virus particles associated with human disease, we had to screen more than 2000 case stools in order to find several that contained sufficient numbers of virus particles to facilitate meaningful IEM studies (M. Balayan, A. Anjaparidze and D. Bradley, unpublished findings of early collaborative studies). Table 3 summarizes the results of one study showing a consistent and specific relationship between ET-NANBH in primates (and humans) and 32–34 nm VLPs recovered from case stools in Mexico and the Soviet Union[33]. Earlier IEM studies in our laboratory relied on the use of pairs of pre-inoculation and *convalescent* sera from experimentally infected primates in order to show a serological relationship between disease and the putative viral agent of ET-NANBH. However, many of our results were inconsistent or unconvincing, since some of the convalescent sera failed to react with reagent virus particles. Further studies using stools containing large numbers of 32–34 nm VLPs revealed that acute-phase sera from both human cases and experimentally infected primates were much more likely to aggregate virus

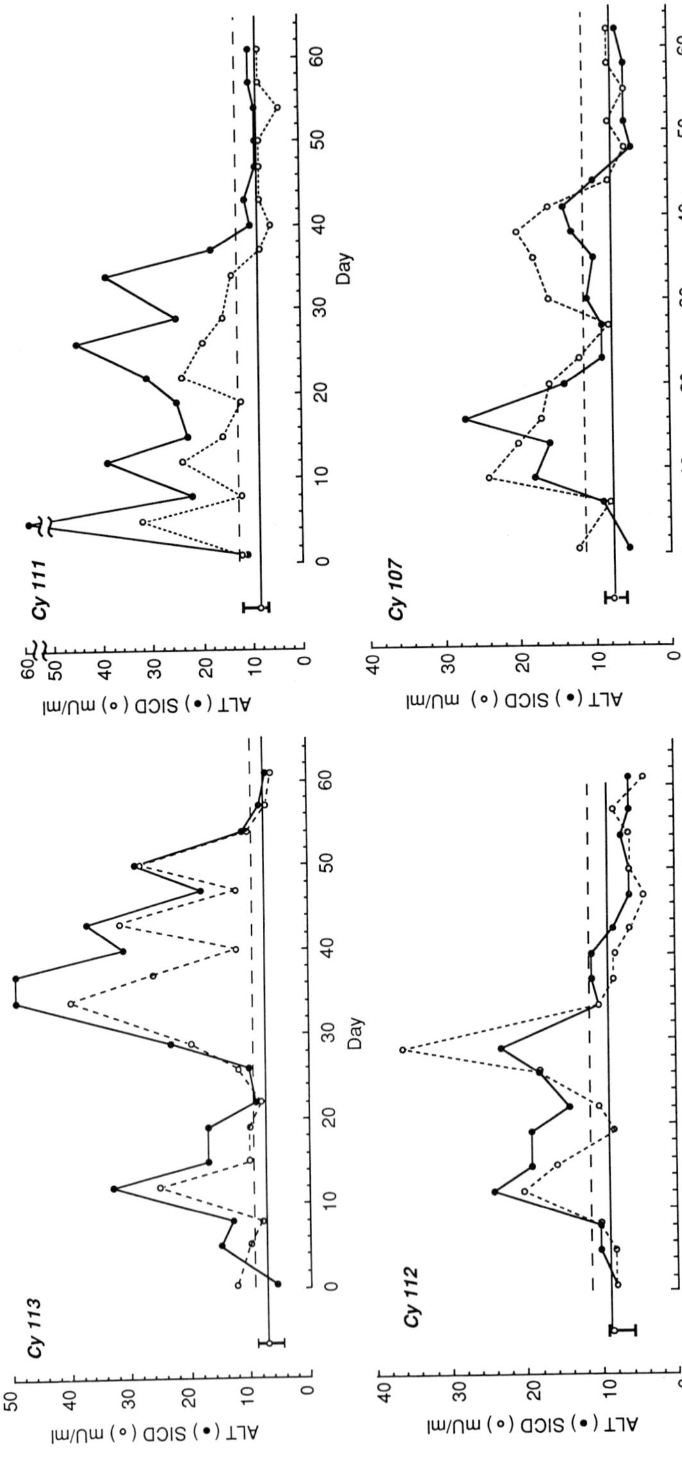

Figure 2 First passage of ET-NANBH virus (HEV) in cynos after i.v. inoculation of partially purified virus from a Mexican case stool specimen (see text for details). Very short incubation period disease was observed and biphasic pattern of ALT was seen during course of disease

Table 3 Immunoreactivity of 32 nm VLPs in case stools from Soviet Asia and North America

Antiserum (1:60 final dilution)	*Tashkent no. 1435 (USSR)* Crude, 10% w/v suspension VLPs/3sq.	Aby	*Tashkent no. 1435 (USSR)* Partially purified VLPs/3sq.	Aby	*Telixtac no. 14 (Mexico)* Partially purified VLPs/3sq.	Aby
PBS, pH 7.6	0	0	0	0	0	0
NHS no. 1 (USA)	0	0	0	0	0	0
NHS no. 2 (USA)	0	0	NT		NT	
Anti-HAV (USA)	0	0	0	0	0	0
HV (USSR) pre-inoculation	0	0	NT		NT	
HV (USSR) acute	176	4+	58		387	4+
Pak no. 1 acute	236	4+	42		96	4+
Nepal acute pool no. 1	38 (1:5)	3–4+	NT	3+	39	4+
Burma acute pool no. 1	35 (1:5)	2+	NT	2–3+	9	4+
Sudan acute pool no. 1	23 (1:5)		NT		NT	
Somalia acute pool no. 1	45 (1:5)	2+	NT		NT	
Mexico acute pool no. 2	96 (1:2)	2–3+	63		NT	
Mexico acute no. 4	NT	4+	NT	4+	168	4+
CY no. 191 (P1) pre-inoculation	0	0	NT		NT	
CY no. 191 (P1) acute	158	2–3+	NT		NT	
CY no. 17 (P1) pre-inoculation	0	0	NT		0	0
CY no. 17 (P1) boosted	163	2+	NT		24	4+
CY no. 29 (P2) pre-inoculation	NT		NT		0	0
CY no. 29 (P2) acute	NT		NT		51	4+
CY no. 74 (P3) pre-inoculation	NT		NT		0	0
CY no. 74 (P3) acute	NT		NT		15	4+
MY no. 43 (P1) pre-inoculation	0 (1:5)	0	0	0	0	0
MY no. 43 (P1) acute	49 (1:5)	3+	54	2+	168	4+

than convalescent sera from the same individuals. This finding was considered to be significant in that it allowed us to consistently demonstrate a clear serological relationship between 32–34 nm VLPs and experimentally induced disease in non-human primates (see below).

IEM for disease-associated virus particles

Although several reports of 27–30 nm VLPs associated with ET-NANBH have appeared in the literature, independent confirmation of the specificity of these candidate viruses for disease has been complicated by the limited availability of reagent stool and the relative instability of the virus. Our initial IEM studies of stool specimens for VLPs were initiated in 1982 when stools from cases of ET-NANBH occurring in Kathmandu Valley, Nepal were examined using convalescent serum as a source of antibody. One of nine stools was found to be positive for 27–32 nm VLPs; many particles appeared to have characteristic surface features, including indentations and projections. Convalescent (but not pre-inoculation) serum from a tamarin that had developed NANBH after inoculation of this stool specimen was shown to have antibody against these virus particles[21]. This finding suggested that the animal had specifically seroconverted to VLPs contained in the inoculum and further indicated that these particles (or a related particle) might be aetiologically related to disease. Subsequent serological studies with these virus particles were compromised by the diminished number of particles found in stored and freeze-thawed stool suspensions. Stools from another outbreak of ET-NANBH occurring in 1982–83 in Rangoon, Burma, were made available to the CDC through collaboration with the Ministry of Health (H. Myint)[20,32]. Four of 31 case stools were found to be positive by IEM for 27–30 and 32–34 nm VLPs. Both sets of particles appeared to possess surface features that were morphologically similar to those found on the Nepal case stool particles described above. One perplexing aspect of these studies was the notable discrepancy in the antibody coating of 27–30 and 32–34 nm VLPs; the smaller particles appeared to be minimally reactive with antibody contained in case sera, whereas the larger virus particles were found to be heavily coated. Unfortunately, the lack of 'pedigreed' serum panels containing pre-infection and pre-inoculation sera from human cases and experimentally infected primates precluded further serological analyses of the unexpectedly large virus particles found in these case stools. In addition, freeze-thawing and/or storage of these stools as 10% w/v suspensions was found to result in a complete loss of intact, 32–34 nm VLPs, although some 27–30 nm particles could still be visualized by IEM.

More extensive IEM studies have recently been performed using case stools obtained from outbreaks in the Soviet Union and Mexico. One stool recovered from a case of ET-NANBH occurring in Tashkent, USSR (1982–83 epidemic) was found to contain large numbers of 32–34 nm diameter virus particles. These particles specifically reacted with acute-phase and convalescent sera from well-documented cases occurring in other regions of the world, including Burma, Pakistan, Nepal, Somalia, Sudan, Borneo and Mexico[33]. More convincing evidence for the association between 32–34 nm VLPs and disease, however, derived from the demonstrated seroconversion of primates experimentally infected with ET-NANBH (see Table 3). Cynos infected with Soviet or Burma ET-NANBH case stools (positive for 32–34 nm VLPs) were shown to develop antibody to 32–34 nm VLPs in the Tashkent no. 1435 stool suspension (Table 3). One tamarin infected with the Burma isolate was also shown by IEM to have antibody against the larger, 32–34 nm VLPs. Partially purified 32–34 nm VLPs derived from the stool of a case of ET-NANBH occurring in Telixtac, Mexico, were also shown to react with acute-phase antibody in sera from humans and primates infected with NANBH[33]. Sera from cases in the Soviet Union, Pakistan, Nepal, Burma, Borneo, Somalia and Mexico were all capable of aggregating 32–34 nm VLPs in the Telixtac no. 14 stool; antibody coating on these particles was very heavy and was rated 4+ (scale: 0–4+). Seroconversion of experimentally infected primates was also clearly documented, since all animals tested developed acute-phase antibody to the above particles (all pre-inoculation sera were negative). It is equally important to note that selected cynos from the first, second and third passage of a Burma ET-NANBH isolate were shown to acquire virus-specific antibody, thus reinforcing the notion that human-origin ET-NANBH can be successfully passaged in this species of non-human primate and that animals infected with one isolate readily develop antibody against another geographically distinct isolate[33].

Although our studies show that the larger, 32–34 nm VLP is responsible for all or nearly all cases of ET-NANBH, an inconsistency in reported particle diameters is evident. The smaller, 27–30 nm VLP found associated with some cases of ET-NANBH may either be a degradation product of the larger 'parent' particle or a coinfecting or coexisting virus that is unrelated to the infectious agent. Proteolytic digestion or denaturation of the 32–34 nm virus during its passage through the gut may be responsible for some of the discrepancies in reported particle diameter. For example, a calicivirus that infects naval orangeworms has been shown to undergo a reduction in particle diameter from 35–38 nm to 27–30 nm after treatment with trypsin, a common enzyme found in the frass (excreta) of orangeworms and in the gut of man[34]. Proteolytic degradation of the virus responsible for ET-NANBH may also account for the unexpectedly low numbers of VLPs found in acute-phase case stools. Furthermore, these particles may be inherently unstable (labile) and may readily succumb to mild proteolysis or to some other denaturing process in the gut. In any case it is clear that one virus or class of serologically related viruses is responsible for disease worldwide, including Soviet Asia, Asia, Southeast Asia, North Africa, and North America. Limited cross-challenge studies conducted in cynos further suggest that animals convalescent from a bout of ET-NANBH induced by an Asian isolate are protected from reinfection by a second (North American) isolate (D. Bradley, unpublished data). The latter finding is in agreement with the serological (IEM) data showing that geographically distinct virus isolates react with antisera from a variety of ET-NANBH outbreaks. Figure 3 shows antibody-aggregated 32–34 nm VLPs typical of those found in stools of ET-NANBH cases in Borneo, Burma, Mexico, Pakistan, Somalia and the Soviet Union.

Physicochemical properties of ET-NANBH-associated 32–34 nm VLPs

Table 4 summarizes what is known to date about the major aetiological agent of ET-NANBH. The virus appears to be extremely labile and will not tolerate exposure to high concentrations of salt, including CsCl. Pelleting of the virus from stool suspensions or gradient fractions frequently results in loss of detectable virus. It is interesting to note that isopycnically banded Norwalk virus, a morphologically similar virus with calicivirus-like properties, can only be recovered from CsCl density gradient fractions if they are first dialyzed to remove salt (S. Monroe, personal communication). Rate-zonal banding of 32–34 nm VLPs in linear, preformed sucrose gradients was found to yield partially purified virus suitable for further IEM studies[33] (Figure 4). It is of interest to note that 32–34 nm VLPs contained in both the Tashkent no. 1435 and Telixtac (Mexico) no. 14 stool suspensions described above sedimented significantly faster in rate-zonal gradients than did HAV run in parallel gradients. The computed sedimentation coefficient

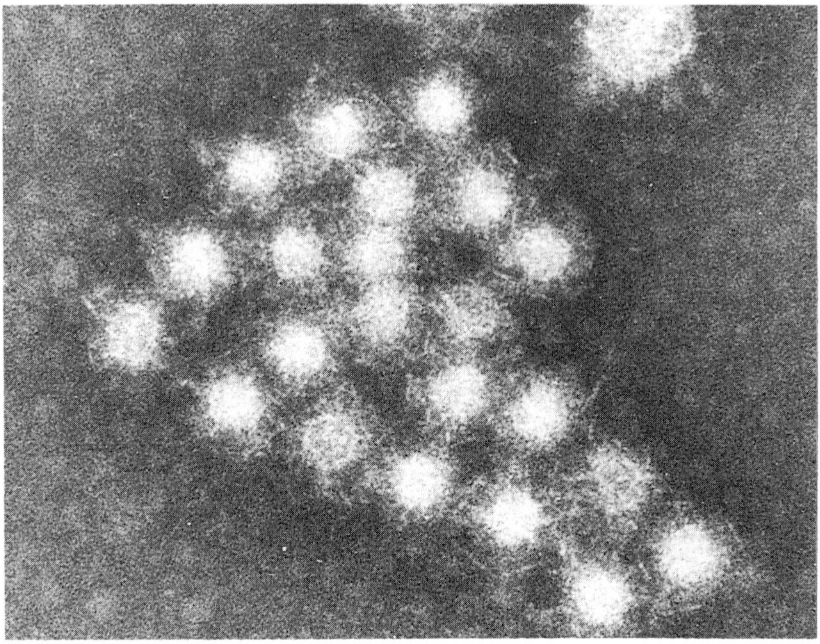

Figure 3 Electron micrograph of typical 32–34 nm virus particles recovered from stool of ET-NANBH case occurring in Telixtac, Mexico during 1986 outbreak of disease. Particles are morphologically indistinguishable from those recovered from cases in Borneo, Burma, India, Somalia and Tashkent

Table 4 Properties of hepatitis E virus (HEV)

1. *Size*: 32–34 nm in diameter (80% of virus particles visualized by IEM; 32.2 nm mean (x) diameter [range: 27–38 nm])
2. *Morphology*: spherical, non-enveloped particle; spikes and indentations visible on surface of virus; sensitive to CsCl, freeze–thawing, pelleting
3. *Biophysical properties*: Sedimentation coefficient = 183S (defectives, 165S). Buoyant density = 1.29 g/cm^3 in KTar/Gly.
4. *Genome*: single-stranded, polyadenylated RNA of approx. 8.0 kb
5. In vitro *propagation*: unsuccessful (FRhK-4, AGMK, HEK, BSC-1, etc.)
6. In vivo: no effect on suckling mice inoculated i.c. with numerous case stool suspensions (10% w/v)

for the ET-NANBH-associated virus was approximately 183S, in contrast to 157S for that of HAV, a member of the Picornaviridae. ET-NANBH-associated virus particles sedimenting at 165S were sometimes found; these particles are presumed to be defective and probably lack a complete viral genome. Isopycnic banding of an aliquot of the Telixtac no. 14 stool suspension in a potassium-tartrate/glycerol (KTar/Gly) gradient revealed 32–34 nm VLPs at a buoyant density of 1.29 g/cm^3. These biophysical properties are consistent with the notion that the major agent of ET-NANBH is calicivirus-like, since many caliciviruses sediment at approximately 183S and band at 1.29 g/cm^3 in KTar/Gly gradients. Like caliciviruses, the 32–

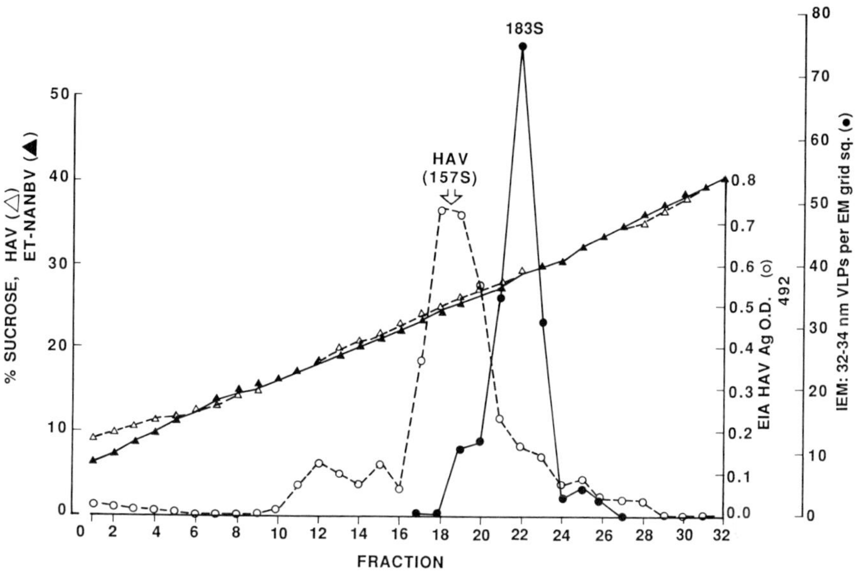

Figure 4 Sedimentation analysis of 32–34 nm virus particles (HEV) present in Mexican case stool suspension. HAV (strain HAS-15) was run in a parallel gradient. The total number of antibody-coated 32–34 nm virus particles seen in three EM grid squares of each gradient fraction were used to plot the sedimentation profile of the virus. More than 90% of the virus was found in aggregates containing five to 50 particles

34 nm VLPs described here are also sensitive to freeze-thawing, storage in liquid suspensions at temperatures between −70 °C and +8 °C, and pelleting from solutions of sucrose or buffer. Figure 5 is a histogram showing, in a comparative fashion, the range of HAV and ET-NANBH-associated virus particle diameters. HAS-15 HAV, partially purified from tissue culture lysates, and ET-NANBH-associated virus particles contained in case stools from Burma, Mexico, Somalia and the Soviet Union were independently measured by three individuals. HAV was found to have a mean diameter of 27.8 nm and the ET-NANBH-associated virus was found to have a mean diameter of 32.2 nm; the majority of the latter particles (78%) had diameters between 31 and 35 nm, and there were no statistically significant differences in mean (x) particle diameters of any of the four isolates.

Serological assays and immune response

Attempts to develop a conventional radioimmunoassay (RIA) or enzyme-linked immunoassay (EIA) for ET-NANBH-associated antigen using acute-phase or convalescent-phase IgM or IgG, respectively, have met with failure in our laboratory. Analysis of stools and sucrose gradient fractions rich in

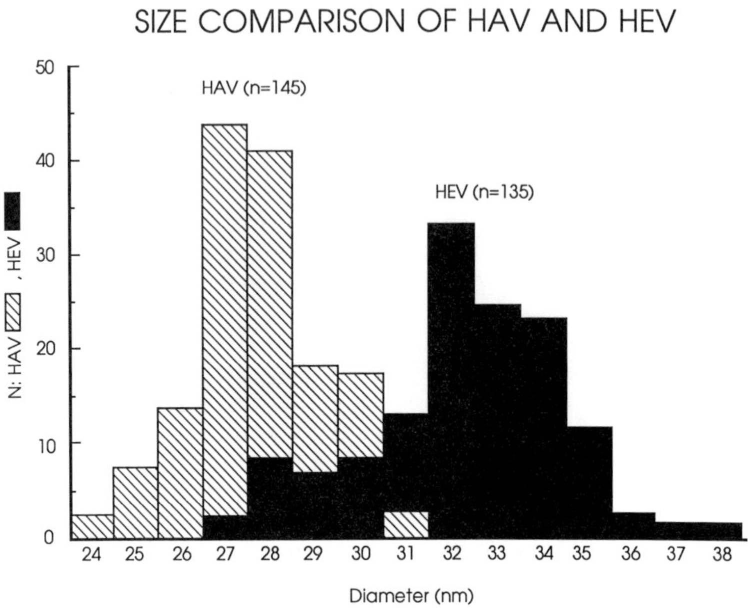

Figure 5 Histogram showing size distribution of HAV and HEV particles

virus particles has not revealed any specific, positive result to date. The reproducibility of our results may have been complicated by the lability of the virus, although even stools and sucrose gradient fractions rich in particles failed to give a positive signal in our tests. In fact, RIA analysis of separate gradient fractions containing equal numbers of HAV and ET-NANBH-associated virus particles (by IEM) showed that HAV could be easily detected using a conventional antibody 'sandwich' assay, while no ET-NANBH-associated antigen could be found by this method. These results indicated that while antibody in some sera may be adequate for IEM or immunofluorescent antibody (FA) analysis, these same antibodies lack the avidity to function in RIA or EIA assays. This presumption was further supported by the finding that an IgG fraction of a convalescent serum obtained from a case of ET-NANBH in Mexico could be labelled with FITC and used to detect ET-NANBH-associated antigen in liver tissue of infected cynos[35]. The latter assay was subsequently used to titre many acute-phase and convalescent human and primate sera in order to identify those with the highest reactivity and potential to function in prototype RIAs and EIAs. Unfortunately, none of these latter sera, when used in antibody sandwich or direct capture assay configurations, was able to consistently detect virus-specific antigen in known positive stool and liver preparations. Our combined findings suggest that individuals who are infected with the virus of ET-NANBH usually develop a vigorous acute-phase (IgM) antibody response but generally fail to develop high-titre, high-affinity convalescent antibody, in contrast to individuals who are infected with HAV.

Molecular cloning of the viral genome

Successful molecular cloning of the genome of the virus of ET-NANBH has been a major goal of our laboratory studies. Although we had previously tried to clone the genome from stool concentrates or sucrose gradient fractions rich in virus particles, none of our efforts resulted in a virus-specific clone. Clearly, a high-titred preparation of virus lacking the nucleic acid complexity of stool or liver was needed in order to achieve our goal. Since virus particles recovered from stool were also frequently found to be degraded or in the process of degradation, it was apparent that molecular cloning of the virus could not be achieved unless it could first be stabilized or another, more plentiful source of virus be identified. In consideration of the probable deleterious effects of proteases or inhospitable environment on the integrity of the virus during its transit through the small intestine, it seemed reasonable to assume that large amounts of virus could be present in gall bladder bile *prior* to its discharge into the duodenum. In fact, aspiration of bile from gallbladders of several ET-NANBH-infected cynos during the early acute phase of disease yielded one aspirate with a very high virus particle count (>1000 VLP per EM grid square). Virus particles contained in gallbladder bile were found to have a diameter of 32–34 nm and were morphologically indistinguishable from those recovered from stool (D. Bradley, manuscript in preparation).

Molecular cloning of the viral genome of the 32–34 nm VLPs described above was carried out in collaboration with Genelabs, Inc., Redwood City, California[36]. Briefly, cDNA libraries were made from RNA extracted from bile collected from cynos infected with a third-passage Burma ET-NANBH isolate. Libraries (in lambda gt10) were screened by differential hybridization with cDNA probes prepared from RNA extracted from uninfected and infected bile preparations. Several candidate clones were identified that hybridized only to the infected bile cDNA probe. One molecular clone, termed ET 1.1, was further characterized and shown to be approximately 1.3 kb in size. This clone did not hybridize to DNA extracted from normal stools or normal or infected cyno livers (or to normal human placental DNA), nor did it hybridize to RNA extracted from normal cyno liver tissue or three normal human stool suspensions. This clone, however, did hybridize to cDNA prepared from RNA extracted from ET-NANBH-infected case stools from Somalia, Borneo, Pakistan and the Soviet Union. Also, ET 1.1 hybridized to an approximately 8.0 Kb single-stranded, polyadenylated RNA species in infected cyno livers. The latter finding is in keeping with our presumption that the major agent of ET-NANBH is calicivirus-like, since caliciviruses possess an RNA genome with similar properties. In view of the combined data linking the above-described 32–34 nm VLPs to ET-NANBH, it is suggested that this agent now be called hepatitis E virus, or HEV.

References

1. Bradley, D. W., Maynard, J. E., Hindman, S. H. *et al.* (1977) Serodiagnosis of viral hepatitis A: Detection of acute phase IgM anti-HAV by radioimmunoassay. *J. Clin. Microbiol.*, **5**, 521–30
2. Bradley, D. W., Fields, H. A., McCaustland, K. A. *et al.* (1979). Serodiagnosis of viral hepatitis A by a modified competitive binding radioimmunoassay for immunoglobulin M anti-hepatitis A virus. *J. Clin. Microbiol.*, **9**, 120–7
3. Walsh, J. H., Yalow, R. and Beeson, S. A. (1970). Detection of Australia antigen and antibody by means of radioimmunoassay techniques. *J. Infect. Dis.*, **121**, 550–4
4. WHO Bulletin (1970). Viral hepatitis and tests for the Australia (hepatitis-associated) antigen and antibody. *Bull. WHO*, **42**, 957–62
5. Wong, D. C., Purcell, R. H., Sreenivasan, M. A. *et al.* (1980). Epidemic and endemic hepatitis in India: Evidence for non-A/non-B hepatitis virus etiology. *Lancet*, **2**, 876–8
6. Alter, H. J., Purcell, R. H., Holland, P. V. *et al.* (1975). Clinical and serological analysis of transfusion-associated hepatitis. *Lancet*, **2**, 838–41
7. Dienstag, J. L. (1983). Non-A, non-B hepatitis. II. Experimental transmission, putative virus agents and markers, and prevention. *Gastroenterology*, **85**, 743–68
8. Fagan, E. A. and Williams, R. (1984). Non-A, non-B hepatitis. *Sem. Liv. Dis.*, **4**, 314–35
9. Bradley, D. W. (1985). The agents of non-A, non-B viral hepatitis. *J. Virol. Methods*, **10**, 307–19
10. Bradley, D. W. and Maynard, J. E. (1986). Etiology and natural history of posttransfusion and enterically-transmitted non-A, non-B hepatitis. *Sem. Liv. Dis.*, **6**, 56–66
11. Bradley, D. W., Krawczynski, K. and Kane, M. A. (1988). Enterically-transmitted non-A, non-B hepatitis: biology and etiology of disease. In *Proceedings, First Asia-Pacific Congress of Medical Virology*, 6–11 Nov. Singapore (In press)
12. Bradley, D. W., Krawczynski, K. and Kane, M. A. (1989). Enterically-transmitted non-A, non-B hepatitis. In Belshe, R. B. (ed.), *Textbook of Human Virology*. (Littleton, MA: PSG Publishing, 2nd edn) (In press)
13. Feinstone, S. H. (1989) Parenterally transmitted non-A, non-B hepatitis. In Belshe, R. B. (ed.), *Textbook of Human Virology*. (Littleton, M. A.: PSG Publishing Co.), 2nd edn (In press)
14. Bradley, D. W., Krawczynski, K., Cook, E. H. *et al.* (1988). Enterically transmitted non-A, non-B hepatitis: Etiology of disease and laboratory studies in nonhuman primates. In Zuckerman, A. J. (ed.), *Viral Hepatitis and Liver Disease*, pp. 138–47. (New York: Alan R. Liss)
15. Viswanathan, R. (1957). Infectious hepatitis in Delhi (1955–56): a critical study: epidemiology. *Indian J. Med. Res.*, **45**, 1–30
16. Sreenivasan, M. A., Banerjee, K., Pandya, P. G. *et al.* (1978). Epidemiological investigations of an outbreak of infectious hepatitis in Ahmedabad city during 1975–76. *Indian J. Med. Res.*, **67**, 197–206
17. Sergeev, N. W., Paktoris, E. A., Ananev, W. A. *et al.* (1957). General characteristics of Botkin's disease occurring in Kirgiz Republic of USSR in 1955–1956. *Soviet Healthcare Kirgizii*, **5**, 16–23
18. Tandon, B. N., Joshi, Y. K., Jain, S. K. *et al.* (1982). An epidemic of non-A, non-B hepatitis in North India. *Indian J. Med. Res.*, **75**, 739–44
19. Khuroo, S. M., Duermeyer, W., Zargar, S. A. *et al.* (1983). Acute sporadic non-A/non-B hepatitis in India. *Am. J. Epidemiol.*, **118**, 360–4
20. Myint, H., Soe, M. M., Khin, T. *et al.* (1985). A clinical and epidemiological study of an epidemic of non-A, non-B hepatitis in Rangoon. *Am. J. Trop. Med. Hyg.*, **34**, 1183–9
21. Kane, M. A., Bradley, D. W., Shrestha, S. M. *et al.* (1984). Epidemic non-A, non-B hepatitis in Nepal: recovery of a possible etiologic agent and transmission studies in marmosets. *J. Am. Med. Assoc.*, **252**, 3140–5
22. Hillis, A., Shrestha, S. M. and Saha, N. K. (1973). An epidemic of infectious hepatitis in the Kathmandu Valley. *J. Nepal Med. Assoc.*, **11**, 145–51
23. De Cock, K. M., Bradley, D. W., Sandford, N. L. *et al.* (1987). Epidemic non-A, non-B hepatitis in patients from Pakistan. *Ann. Intern. Med.*, **106**, 227–30
24. Bellabes, H., Benatallah, A. and Bourguermouh, A. (1984). Non-A/non-B epidemic viral hepatitis in Algeria: Strong evidence for its water spread. In: Vyas, G. N., Dienstag, J. L.

and Hoofnagle, J. H. (eds), *Viral Hepatitis and Liver Disease*, p. 637. (New York: Grune & Stratton)

25. Sarthou, J. I., Budkowska, A., Sharma, M. D. *et al.* (1976). Characterization of an antigen-antibody system associated with epidemic non-A, non-B hepatitis in West Africa and experimental transmission of an infectious agent to primates. *Ann. Inst. Pasteur/Virol.*, **137E**, 225–232
26. Centers For Disease Control (1987). Enterically transmitted non-A, non-B hepatitis–East Africa. *Morbid. Mortal. Weekly Rep.*, **36**, 241–4
27. Centers For Disease Control (1987). Enterically transmitted non-A, non-B hepatitis-Mexico. *Morbid. Mortal. Weekly Rep.*, **36**, 597–602
28. Balayan, M. S., Andjaparidze, A. G., Savinskaya, S. S. *et al.* (1983). Evidence for a virus in non-A, non-B hepatitis transmitted via the fecal-oral route. *Intervirology*, **20**, 23–31
29. Andjaparidze, A. G., Balayan, M. S., Savinov, A. P. *et al.* (1986). Fecal–orally transmitted non-A, non-B hepatitis induced in monkeys. *Voprosy Virusol.*, **1**, 73–80
30. Datta, R., Panda, S. K., Tanden, B. N. *et al.* (1987). Acute sporadic non-A, non-B viral hepatitis of adults in India-Epidemiological and immunological studies. *J. Gastroenterol. Hepatol.*, **2**, 333–45
31. Arankalle, V. A., Ticehurst, J., Sreenivasan, M. A. *et al.* (1988). Etiological association of a virus-like particle with enterically-transmitted non-A, non-B hepatitis. *Lancet*, **2**, 550–4
32. Bradley, D. W., Krawczynski, K., Cook, E. H. *et al.* (1987). Enterically transmitted non-A, non-B hepatitis: Serial passage of disease in cynomolgus macaques and tamarins and recovery of disease-associated 27–34 nm viruslike particles. *Proc. Natl. Acad. Sci.*, **84**, 6277–81
33. Bradley, D. W., Andjaparidze, A., Cook, E. H. *et al.* (1988). Aetiological agent of enterically transmitted non-A, non-B hepatitis. *J. Gen. Virol.*, **69**, 731–8
34. Hillman, B., Morris, T. J., Kellen, W. R. *et al.* (1982). An invertebrate calici-like virus: Evidence for partial virion disintegration in host excreta. *J. Gen. Virol.*, **60**, 115–23
35. Krawczynski, K. and Bradley, D. W. (1989). Enterically transmitted non-A, non-B hepatitis: Identification of virus-associated antigen in experimentally infected cynomolgus macaques. *J. Infect. Dis.*, **159**, 1042–9
36. Reyes, G. R., Purdy, M. A., Luk, K.-C. *et al.* (1990) Molecular cloning of the enterically transmitted non-A, non-B hepatitis virus genome. *Science* (In press)

26
The liver in acquired immunodeficiency syndrome (AIDS)

N. BACH, S. N. THUNG and P. D. BERK

INTRODUCTION

With retrospective data dating back to early 1978, and the onset of an epidemic in 1981, acquired immunodeficiency syndrome (AIDS) has become a serious health crisis[1,2]. As of December 1988, in the United States alone, 80 538 cases of AIDS have been reported to the Centers for Disease Control; 45 164 have died[3]. Around the world, especially in Africa, North and South America and Western Europe, the impact of this epidemic is increasingly recognized, as the numbers of cases continue to multiply. This epidemic has affected almost all sub-specialities of medicine including hepatology. Since the explosion of AIDS cases, about 25% of the consultations done by the Division of Liver Diseases at the Mount Sinai Hospital, New York, have involved AIDS/AIDS-related complex (ARC) patients. Although frequent changes in diagnostic coding make precise figures difficult to obtain, we estimate that Mount Sinai has treated approximately 1500 inpatient cases of AIDS/ARC, with ~900 deaths, over the past decade. Interestingly, despite an increase in hospital admissions for AIDS patients, the percentage of liver biopsies performed on these patients at our institution has remained constant between 3% and 7%. However, recommendations regarding liver biopsy have varied throughout the years and are discussed below.

The liver is a common site of involvement for opportunistic infections and neoplasms in individuals with AIDS. Hepatomegaly, confirmed at autopsy, occurs in 62–91% of HIV-infected persons[4–10]. Abnormalities in biochemical hepatic tests have been reported in 67–93% of cases[7,8,10–12]. However, despite being a frequent site of involvement, the liver does not often alter morbidity and mortality in these patients[5,7,9,12,13].

VIRAL INFECTIONS

Suggestions that human immunodeficiency virus-I (HIV) itself can produce liver disease have not been substantiated. Examination of liver biopsies, including electron microscopic studies, have not yielded any pathognomonic or specific features attributable to HIV. Most studies have noted prominence of macrovesicular steatosis[6,9,13]. Pre-existing conditions including chronic debilitating illness, malnutrition, weight loss, disseminated infection, concomitant alcohol abuse or total parenteral nutrition may be contributory[6]. Other features frequently noted in individuals with AIDS include small, non-caseating granulomas (Figure 1), focal hepatic necrosis (Figure 2), sinusoidal cell hyperplasia and sinusoidal dilatation[6,7,9–11,14,15]. When chronic hepatitis is present the histological pattern of chronic active hepatitis is uncommon; a mild lymphocyte infiltrate in the portal tracts has been noted.

Peliosis hepatis has also been noted, although the exact pathogenesis remains an enigma[7,14,15]. Some have speculated that HIV infection may injure the endothelial cells directly or indirectly, thus leading to the development of these sinusoidal lesions[14]. The same pathogenesis may be responsible for the development of Kaposi's sarcoma[16].

Viral hepatitis

Epidemiological differences among subgroups of AIDS populations are responsible for the variations in diseases reported in these patients. However, those at greatest risk for the development of AIDS, namely intravenous drug abusers, male homosexuals, haemophiliacs and the spouses and children of these groups are all also at great risk for the development of viral hepatitis.

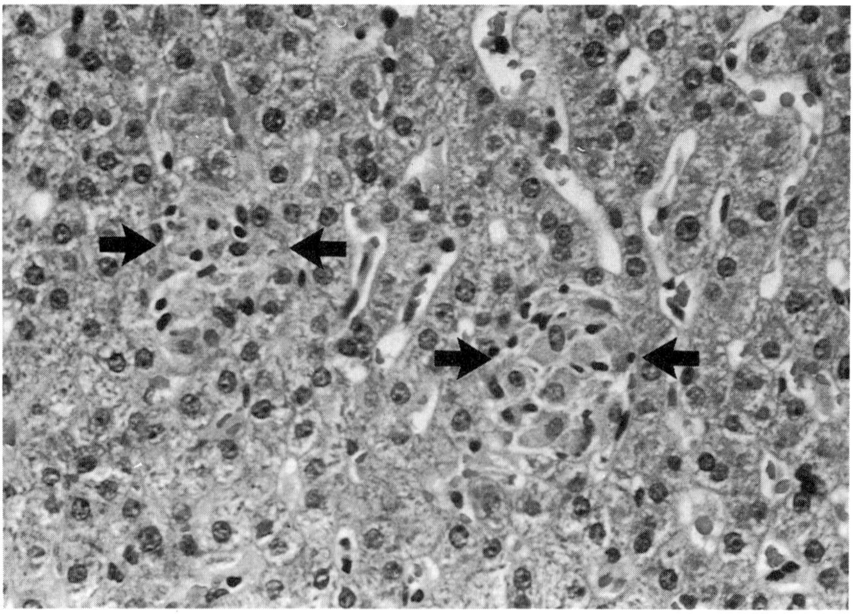

Figure 1 Two small poorly formed epithelioid granulomata (arrows) in liver biopsy of a patient with AIDS (H&E, ×250)

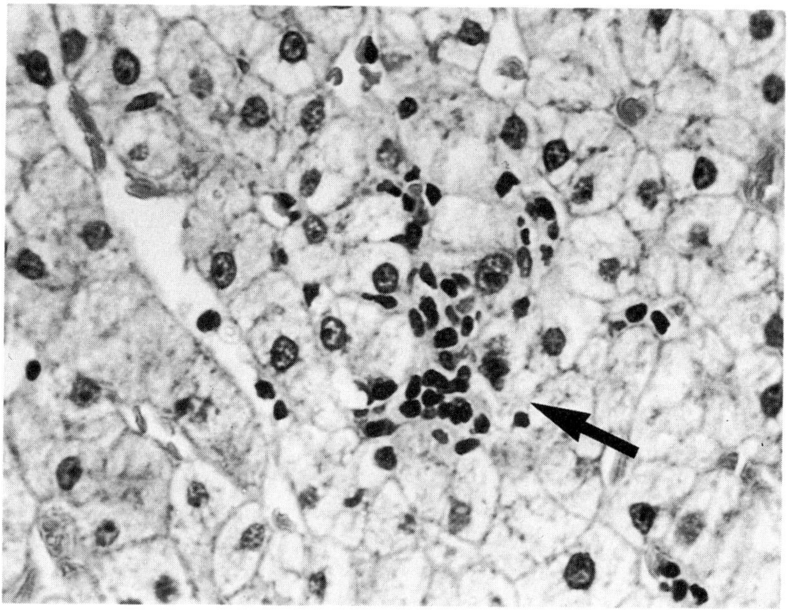

Figure 2 Liver biopsy specimen from a patient with AIDS showing focal parenchymal necrosis (H&E, ×400)

Not surprisingly, the incidence of concomitant hepatitis in individuals with AIDS is increased[12]. Thus, we begin our discussion with the impact of HIV infection on the various forms of viral hepatitis.

Hepatitis A (HAV)

A prior history of exposure to HAV or anti-HAV is common amongst HIV seropositive individuals[17]. The role of HIV in the natural history of HAV, however, has not been studied.

Hepatitis B (HBV)

Considerable attention has been paid to the association between HBV and HIV infection[18]. Transmission routes of HBV and HIV are similar, although HBV is at least ten times as infectious as HIV. This is illustrated by a case report of an accidental needlestick to a physician from an HBsAg and HIV positive patient. Acute HBV infection occurred without the development of anti-HIV or T4:T8 ratio inversion[19].

HBV markers are frequently identified in HIV-infected individuals. With the exception of one study, 76–96% of persons infected with AIDS display at least one serological marker of HBV[5,6,7,12,16,20]. In contrast to these numbers was a study in Mexico which found only 2 out of 77 HIV infected individuals with HBV markers[20].

A virus other than HIV has been suggested to be a co-factor in the pathogenesis of AIDS. This other virus may interact with or activate the host's immune system, and thus contribute to the development of clinically overt disease[21–24]. HBV may play such a role. HBV-specific DNA has been identified by dot blot hybridization in peripheral blood mononuclear cells of almost all patients with AIDS virus infection[22,24]. This finding has been noted even in the absence of HBV markers. Also, a 3.2 kb DNA has been identified in peripheral blood mononuclear cells of HIV-infected individuals. This extrachromosomal DNA may represent a natural recombinant between these two viruses[24].

HIV infection may also modify the natural course of liver disease in chronic carriers of HBV[7,12,25,26]. Clinical flare-ups are uncommon; however, viral replication, assessed by the activity of HBeAg, HBV DNA and HBV DNA polymerase, is increased or accentuated by HIV[25,27,28]. Immunofluorescent and immunoperoxidase staining show an increase in HBeAg and HBcAg in the nuclei of hepatocytes of HIV positive HBV carriers (Figure 3)[29]. This is further evidence of an increase in viral replication.

HBV hepatotoxicity is believed to be immune-mediated. It therefore follows that suppression of the immune system by HIV would decrease the necro-inflammatory process of HBV. Indeed, histologically less severe disease is seen[25–27]. Immunological deficiencies may also make HBsAg positive individuals less responsive to HBV antigens and therefore less likely to

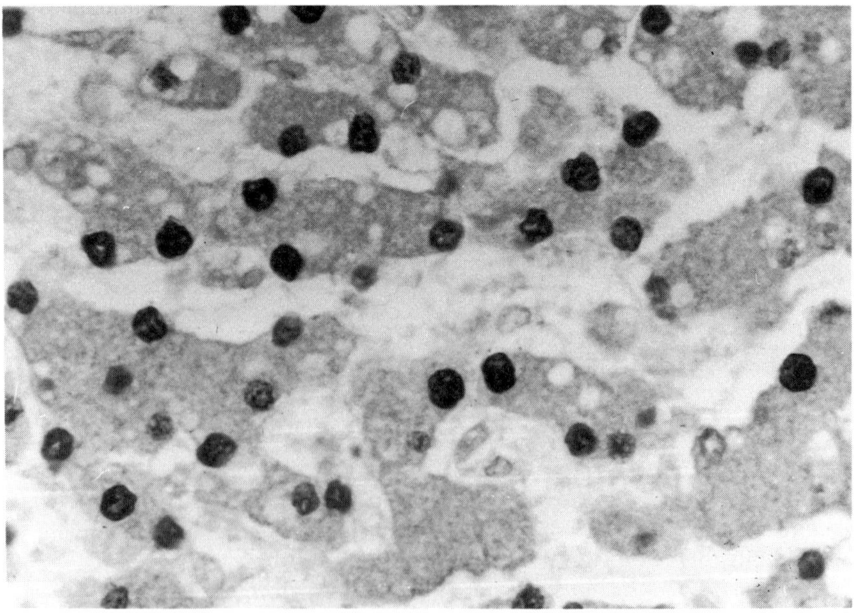

Figure 3 Hepatitis B core antigen in nuclei of almost all hepatocytes in a biopsy from a case of AIDS. Some of the hepatocytes contain microvesicular fat droplets (immunoperoxidase method using biotinylated anti-HBc, counterstained with methylene blue, ×400)

convert to anti-HBs and anti-HBe. Thus, an increased carrier rate for hepatitis B has been noted in individuals already infected with HIV[30].

An accelerated loss of anti-HBs has been observed in HIV seropositive individuals[31,32]. Reactivation to HBsAg was also reported in three individuals who were positive for anti-HBc and either anti-HBs or anti-pre S2 prior to infection with HIV[33]. We have also seen reversion from anti-HBe to HBeAg. Additionally, studies of vaccination with hepatitis B vaccine have correlated HIV positivity with a suboptimal response or inability to develop anti-HBs after vaccination[31,32,34].

Lastly, irrational fears and concerns that HIV may be transmitted with the plasma-derived hepatitis B vaccine have led some individuals not to be vaccinated[35,36]. When treated with formalin, using the same conditions as the manufacturer of the plasma-derived vaccine, HIV is denatured[37,38].

Hepatitis D (HDV)

Epidemiological studies have previously reported that HDV infection occurs in a significant percentage of HBsAg positive intravenous drug users[39–41]. HDV infection, however, is less common in homosexual men, the other large group affected by AIDS[42]. These differences in the incidence of HDV have also been reported in HIV-infected individuals[39,40]. In one study of HDV-infected intravenous drug users, indices of hepatic function were not significantly different in either the HIV seropositive or seronegative patients[40,41]. Further study of these two viruses is necessary in order to determine whether or not HIV affects the usual course of HDV infection.

HDV antigenaemia, which is usually transient, may be prolonged in HIV seropositive individuals. Persistence of HDV antigenaemia has been reported in HIV seropositive individuals[43]. As has been suggested for HBV, the underlying immunodeficiency state may sustain HDV replication, allowing increased pathogenicity of the virus[43]. Additionally, an intravenous drug user who had been a chronic carrier of HBV and HDV reactivated HDV following infection with HIV[44].

Hepatitis C (HCV)

Along with the other viral hepatitides, HCV affects the same epidemiological group as does HIV. As testing for HCV has recently become available, the exact role of HIV in HCV will be further elucidated. HCV, rapidly progressing to severe and symptomatic cirrhosis, has been observed in some HIV positive individuals. Based on this observation, one group has suggested that HIV permits increased viral replication of HCV, thus promoting increased liver, injury[45]. A case of fulminant hepatitis secondary to HCV was reported in an HIV seropositive male; the authors interpreted this finding as evidence of a direct cytopathic effect of HCV on the liver[46].

Other causes of viral hepatitis

Cytomegalovirus (CMV)

CMV is probably the most common organism found in individuals with AIDS at autopsy[47,48]. Most series report CMV as either the first or second most common infectious pathogen seen in the liver[5,9]. Identification of CMV in the liver, however, almost always reflects dissemination from other organs. Conversely, when extrahepatic CMV is identified, the liver is involved 5–44% of the time[5,7,49–51].

CMV has been implicated in causing at least two clinical entities within the hepatobiliary system. CMV hepatitis and more recently CMV-related biliary tract disease have been described. The latter entity is discussed under AIDS-related biliary disease.

Hepatic infection with CMV may present (1) asymptomatically, (2) as a mononucleosis-like syndrome or (3) as a life-threatening illness. CMV hepatitis may cause a slight elevation in aminotransferase activity[7]. As with HBV, the lack of an inflammatory response in individuals with HIV explains why only a slight elevation in serum aminotransferase activity is seen.

Diagnosis is made on liver biopsy with either identification of cytomegalic inclusion bodies, immunohistochemical staining, *in-situ* hybridization or viral culture. Histologically, CMV is characterized by large intranuclear and cytoplasmic inclusions found within bile duct epithelium, endothelial cells or hepatocytes (Figure 4)[16]. As CMV hepatitis alone is not considered to be associated with appreciable morbidity or mortality, treatment with ganciclovir (DHPG) is generally not indicated for CMV hepatitis alone[7,52].

Epstein–Barr virus (EBV)

EBV infection is not included as a diagnostic criterion for immunodeficiency in AIDS, nor has it been reported to be a major cause of disease in adults with AIDS[53]. The spectrum of disease in this population ranges from a self-limited mononucleosis to the development of EBV-related lymphomas (discussed later). Chronic active hepatitis has been described in pediatric populations with AIDS but not in adults[54–56]. EBV was suggested to be the cause of hepatic inflammation and chronic active hepatitis in four children with AIDS[54].

Herpes simplex virus (HSV)

Disseminated HSV may cause a fulminant hepatitis in immunosuppressed patients[57]. Fever, leucopenia, elevation of serum bilirubin and aminotransferase activity may be evident. Fulminant hepatitis with fatal acute liver failure has been reported in individuals with AIDS. Necrotic haemorrhagic foci have been seen in the liver, as well as in other organs[57]. Evidence that herpes simplex virus type I can reactivate transcription of latent HIV has added interest to the role of the herpes virus in the pathogenesis of symptomatic AIDS[58].

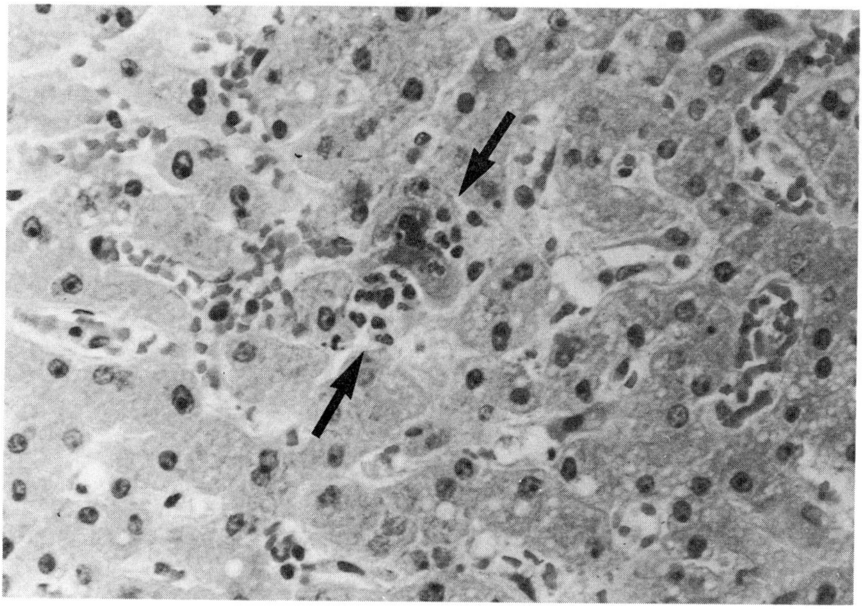

Figure 4 Cytomegalo (CMV) viral inclusions within the nucleus and cytoplasm of an infected cell, which is surrounded by polymorphonuclear cells (arrows). (H&E, ×250; biopsy from an AIDS patient)

Bacterial infections

Mycobacteria

The most common mycobacteria to affect HIV seropositive individuals are *M. tuberculosis* (MTB), *M. avium intracellulare* (MAI) and *M. kansasii*[17]. Of these, MAI is the most common and most frequent infectious organism diagnosed on liver biopsy[5,13,16,17,59,60]. Disseminated MAI, which occurs in 25–50% of individuals with AIDS, involves the liver in 10–57% of these cases[7,9,13]. Increasing rates of MTB have also been reported, affecting similar groups as those infected with AIDS[61]. A recent study of 520 intravenous drug users found similar prevalence and incidence rates in HIV seropositive and seronegative groups. However, the risk of active tuberculosis was increased only in the HIV-infected group[62].

Infection with any mycobacteria may produce a non-specific 'wasting syndrome' consisting of fever, malaise, anorexia, weight loss, weakness, night sweats and sometimes abdominal pain. Hepatomegaly has also been observed. However, MAI may be diagnosed even in the absence of any signs or symptoms of disease[6]. An atypical presentation of MTB, with extrapulmonary or disseminated disease, is now common in HIV-infected individuals. Rarely, MTB has led to tuberculous liver abscesses in HIV-seropositive individuals[63,64]. The most common laboratory finding is an elevation of serum alkaline phosphatase activity, often reflecting concomitant bone involvement. Elevated lactate dehydrogenase activity and/or mild increases of aminotransferase activity may be seen; jaundice is rare[7,16,59].

Diagnosis, made by liver biopsy, most commonly reveals poorly formed, non-caseating granulomas, large foamy macrophages and a paucity of lymphocytes[5,7,9,11,59]. A granulomatous response may not be elicited by the mycobacterium; therefore special stains, including the Ziehl–Nielsen stain, periodic acid Schiff reaction after diastase digestion (D-PAS) and culture should be performed on all specimens. Aside from culture, MAI may be differentiated from MTB by D-PAS positive staining; MAI is positive while MTB is not. Hundreds of acid-fast organisms in granulomas, sinusoidal lining cells, sinusoids and foamy cells are seen with MAI (Figure 5) while stains for MTB show only rare acid-fast bacilli.

No effective therapy for MAI is available. Although *in vitro* activity of rifabutin, clofazimine, ciprofloxacin, cycloserine and amikacin may be demonstrated, *in vivo* clinical benefits have not been reported to date. Recommended therapy for MTB is similar to that for non-HIV infected individuals: 9 months of therapy with isoniazid and rifampicin, often supplemented with pyrazinamide, streptomycin or both. Disseminated disease may be fatal.

Other bacterial infections

An increased frequency of bacterial infections has been noted in HIV-infected individuals but such infections of the liver are uncommon[61]. There have been scattered case reports suggesting unusual presentations of bacterial-related liver disease.

Pre-existing liver disease is thought to be a predisposing factor for infection with *Vibrio vulnificus*. In HIV-infected individuals with liver disease, an increased susceptibility to develop overwhelming sepsis from this invasive organism has been seen[65]. *Salmonella enteritidis* also led to bacterial peritonitis in one HIV-infected individual with cirrhosis[66].

FUNGAL INFECTIONS

Disseminated cryptococcus, histoplasmosis, candidiasis and coccidiomycosis have been reported to involve the liver in AIDS. Hepatic involvement for the most part is secondary to disseminated disease, although primary fungal involvement of the liver has been reported[7,59]. Disseminated histoplasmosis and coccidiomycosis involving the liver have been reported in individuals coming from areas in which these fungi are endemic[67–69]. Unlike patients receiving cancer chemotherapy, candida fungaemia has rarely been reported in patients with AIDS[61].

Fever, hepatomegaly and elevated serum alkaline phosphatase and gamma glutamyl transferase activities may be noted. When fungal abscesses are of sufficient size they can be detected on ultrasound or CT scan. Diagnosis is usually made by identification of the organism on liver biopsy or fine-needle aspiration.

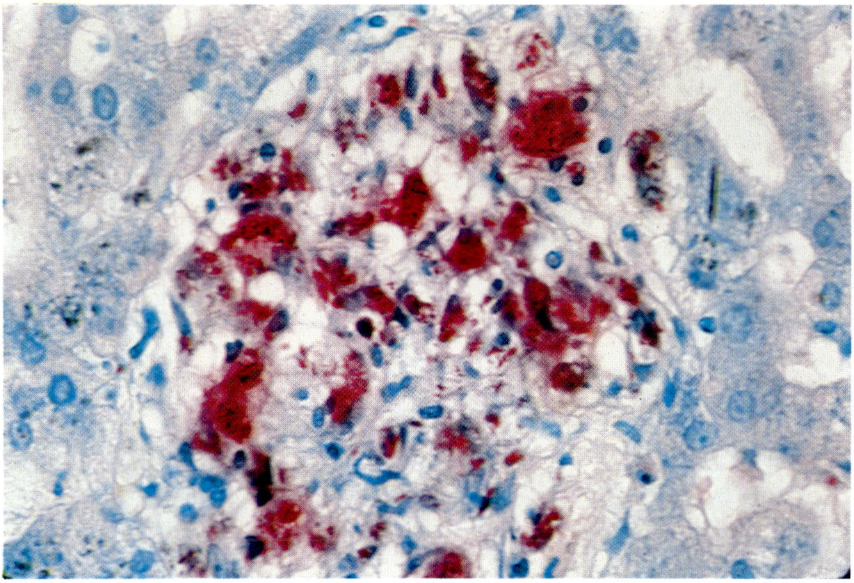

Figure 5 Abundant intracellular acid-fast bacilli within a granuloma in a case of AIDS. Culture of this specimen grew *Mycobacterium avium-intracellulare* (Ziehl-Nielsen stain, × 400)

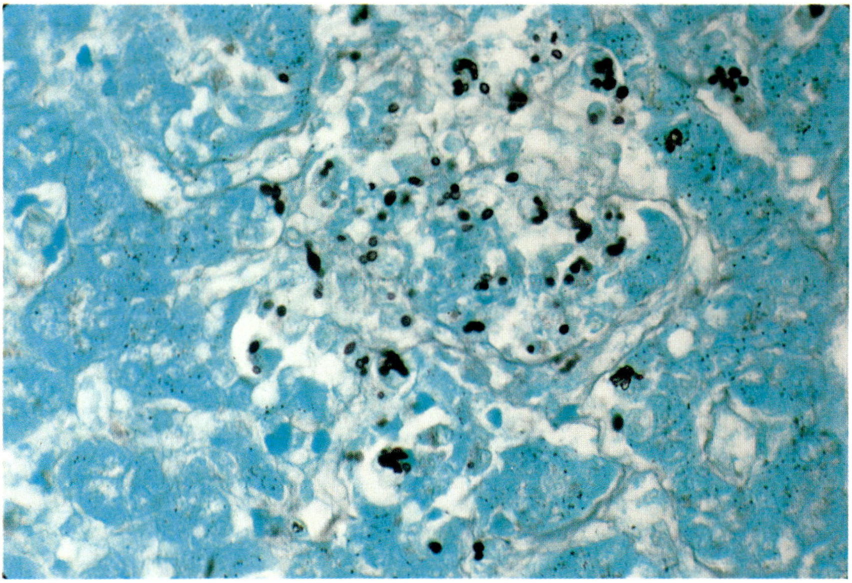

Figure 6 Liver biopsy specimen from an AIDS patient with histoplasma within a granuloma (Gomori's methenamine silver stain, × 250)

Typically hepatic mycoses produce granulomas without much inflammatory response. The organisms may be seen within microabscesses, granulomata or within the sinusoids of the liver[5,7,9,59]. Large collections of yeast-like organisms may be identified even in areas without granulomas or an inflammatory response[12]. Yeast can usually be identified on H&E stain but special stains including D-PAS, and methenamine silver (Figure 6) are recommended[7]. Treatment consists of prolonged therapy with amphotericin B[61].

Protozoal infections

Despite the frequency of protozoal infections, especially *Pneumocystis carinii*, *Toxoplasma* and *Isospora belli* in AIDS patients, hepatobiliary manifestations are rare. Cryptosporidium is probably the most common protozoon to produce hepatobiliary manifestations. This is discussed under biliary tract disease.

Careful study with the electron microscope led to the identification of Microsporidia (*Encephalitozoon cuniculi*) as the cause of fatal hepatocellular necrosis and jaundice in one HIV-infected individual[70]. Leishmaniasis (kala azar) is another example of an unusual infection involving the liver in HIV-infected individuals[71].

Biliary tract disease

Some opportunistic infections including CMV and cryptosporidium, play a role in extrahepatic bile duct disease. Controversy exists as to whether these organisms act as direct pathogens or actually represent superinfection upon devitalized tissue[72]. Acalculous cholecystitis, papillary stenosis and sclerosing cholangitis have all been described in persons with AIDS[72–80]. In addition, a recent report of primary bile duct lymphoma has been added as another cause of biliary disease in this population[81].

Acalculous cholecystitis

Acalculous cholecystitis may present with fever, right upper quadrant pain and fatigue. Diarrhoea often precedes the onset of these symptoms. On physical examination, Murphy's sign may be elicited[80]. CMV and/or cryptosporidium have been identified as aetiological agents[78–80].Ultrasound or CT scan demonstrate an absence of gallstones, sometimes with a distended and/or thickened gallbladder. Histologically, chronic inflammation with cytomegalic inclusion bodies may be seen lining the mucosal wall of the gallbladder. Symptoms usually resolve after cholecystectomy[72].

Papillary stenosis and sclerosing cholangitis

Papillary stenosis and a syndrome resembling primary sclerosing cholangitis have received much attention[73–77]. It has been estimated that between 3%

and 11% of AIDS patients with CMV retinitis or gastrointestinal disease will ultimately develop papillary stenosis and/or sclerosing cholangitis[76].

The finding of both CMV and cryptosporidia within bile and gallbladder ductal mucosa has led to a proposed pathogenesis. It has been postulated that these organisms cause oedema, spasm and fibrosis resulting in an incomplete biliary obstruction[74]. Some investigators suggest that CMV is primarily responsible for the cholestasis and cryptosporidia merely represents a secondary invader[73]. Polymicrobial bacterial infection, as well as *Candida albicans*, have also been reported to cause cholangitis in these patients[73,82].

Symptoms similar to those of chronic cholecystitis, including fever, right upper quadrant pain, nausea, vomiting and occasionally jaundice, have been described. A marked elevation of alkaline phosphatase activity and mild hyperbilirubinaemia are the most common laboratory findings. Intrahepatic sclerosing cholangitis with normal alkaline phosphatase activity, however, has been described[75].

Ultrasound examination may not be abnormal. Diagnosis is made by endoscopic retrograde cholangiopancreatography (ERCP). A typical 'beaded appearance', with focal stricturing, as noted with primary sclerosing cholangitis, is seen. Endoscopic sphincterotomy may provide symptomatic relief in some cases[73,74].

Neoplasms

An increased and atypical presentation of certain tumours is considered another hallmark of AIDS. The 1985 revision of the surveillance case definition of AIDS included Kaposi's sarcoma and non-Hodgkin's lymphoma. Other tumours, although not currently recognized as pathognomonic of AIDS, have also been suggested as having an association with AIDS[83]. These include Hodgkin's disease, leukaemias and squamous cell carcinoma of the anal/genital and oral tissues. Of these, Kaposi's sarcoma, non-Hodgkin's lymphoma and Hodgkin's disease may involve the hepatobiliary tract.

Additionally, because of the increased incidence of a hepatitis B carrier state, the risk of hepatocellular carcinoma may be increased in this population[84].

Kaposi's sarcoma (KS)

No longer a rare indolent skin lesion, a highly aggressive variant of KS has been recognized to occur in young white HIV-infected homosexual men. KS has been reported in approximately 9% of all individuals with AIDS[85]. Of the homosexual population with AIDS, KS has been reported in up to 30%[85]. KS is the most common intrahepatic neoplasm noted at autopsy[5,7,50].

Interestingly, the overall frequency of KS has been declining[85]. This seems to coincide with a change in the sexual habits of the homosexual population and a decline in venereal disease[16]. Thus the sexual transmission of KS or a sexually transmitted cofactor such as CMV has been suggested to play a role[86,87]. Furthermore, *in-situ* hybridization has identified CMV-DNA in

KS, again supporting the role of CMV in this tumour[7].

This multicentric neoplasm is usually diagnosed in either the lung or bowel prior to diagnosis of hepatic involvement[5,7]. The asymptomatic nature of intrahepatic KS makes its diagnosis more common at necropsy[7,9,10,49,50]. A mild elevation of alkaline phosphatase activity may be noted. KS has a non-specific appearance on CT scan, ultrasound and liver spleen scan.

Grossly, KS lesions are purple–brown soft nodules, frequently involving subcapsular regions of the liver[7]. Liver biopsy examination reveals multifocal haemorrhagic nodules of varying size, seen predominantly within expanded portal tracts. Spindle-shaped cells and atypical angulated vascular channels are seen with extravasated red blood cells and vascular lakes (Figure 7)[7,50,85]. Treatment of KS consists of either single-agent chemotherapy or radiotherapy, although treatment of primary intrahepatic KS is unusual and generally not necessary[85,88].

Non-Hodgkin's lymphoma (NHL)

Non-Hodgkin's lymphoma, in the setting of AIDS, has several distinctive characteristics[89]. First, lymphomas of high-grade malignancy and B-cell origin had previously been uncommon in young men. The second distinguishing feature is the high frequency of extranodal and diffuse disease, rather than the usual focal involvement; 64% of patients in one study had advanced disease on presentation[89]. Hepatic involvement has been noted to occur in 25% of patients prior to treatment[90]. Lastly, an especially aggressive course

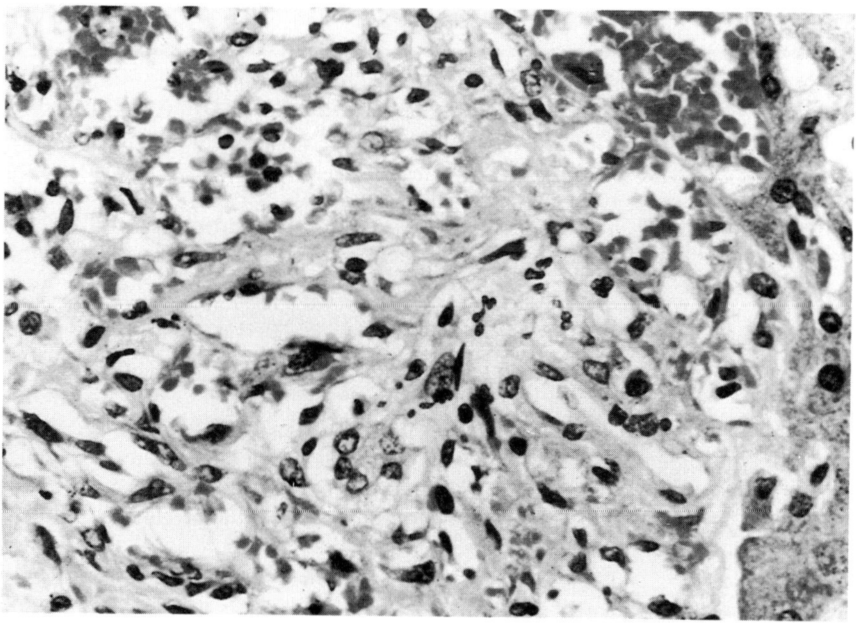

Figure 7 Spindle tumour cells admixed with red blood cell containing vascular channels in Kaposi's sarcoma (H&E, ×250)

of the disease has been noted. Primary lymphoma of the liver and biliary tract, although uncommon, has also been reported[50,81,90].

Considerable evidence exists that EBV has a role in the development of NHL. EBV genomic fragments have been identified in the majority of lymphomas examined in HIV-infected individuals. The proposed pathogenesis suggests that HIV-induced immunosuppression leads to unopposed proliferation of EBV transformed B-cell clones. This may be followed by c-Myc gene translocation resulting in malignant transformation[89].

Non-specific symptoms including fever, weight loss and malaise are common. When bulky disease exists right upper quadrant pain with elevations in alkaline phosphatase activity may be found[5,85]. The development of jaundice is dependent on the location of involved nodes or the presence of biliary duct lymphoma[85]. An elevated EBV-viral capsid antigen may be found in up to 100% of AIDS-related lymphomas and is thus useful for screening[17]. Ultrasound and CT scan may identify lesions greater than 1 cm in diameter. Percutaneous or skinny needle biopsy is necessary for definitive diagnosis.

Histopathological subclassifications reveal that the majority of NHLs are either (1) small, non-cleaved cell, (2) large cell immunoblastic–plasmacytoid or (3) large non-cleaved cell. Treatment consists of aggressive multi-drug chemotherapy[89]. Complete remission may be obtained for short durations although shortened survival is noted when compared to non-AIDS associated NHL[5,50,89]. By contrast with the usual non-fatal outcomes of Kaposi's sarcoma, NHL itself may be fatal in these individuals[85].

Hodgkin's disease (HD)

Though not currently included in the CDC criteria for the diagnosis of AIDS, some investigators have advocated inclusion of an atypical form of HD occurring in HIV-seropositive individuals[89,91–93]. HIV-infected individuals with HD have a more aggressive histological pattern and a greater likelihood of extranodal and metastatic disease[89]. Primary involvement of the liver with HD has not been reported. Standard therapy with multi-drug chemotherapy and radiation is recommended, although prognostically these individuals do worse[89].

Drug-induced changes

Drug hepatotoxicity has been estimated to account for varying degrees of hepatic injury in individuals with AIDS. At least 8% of the biopsies performed on individuals with AIDS have changes consistent with drug-induced injury[6]. Not surprisingly, drugs account for a significant percentage of observed liver disease in these patients, as one study found that at least 90% of hospitalized AIDS patients were taking one or more potentially hepatotoxic drugs[12]. Table 1 lists some of the many potentially hepatotoxic drugs commonly used in AIDS patients. Two of the most commonly used drugs in AIDS patients are zidovudine (AZT) and trimethoprim-sulphamethoxazole.

Table 1 Potentially hepatotoxic drugs commonly used in AIDS patients

Trimethoprin-sulphamethoxazole
Ketoconazole
Isoniazid
Rifampin
Zidovudine (AZT)
Pentamidine isethionate
Diphenylhydantoin
Prochlorperazine

AZT inhibits *in vitro* replication of HIV. Hepatotoxicity has not been noted to be a frequent or serious adverse drug effect in large trials[94]. Indeed, in one large multicentre trial of AZT, liver enzyme abnormalities were more frequent in the group receiving placebo[94]. Several reports of AZT-induced liver disease have appeared in the literature, although documentation of drug toxicity rather than AIDS-related disease has been difficult[95,96]. Acute cholestatic hepatitis due to AZT was documented in some cases by improvement after discontinuation of the drug and worsening after rechallenge[96].

Trimethoprim-sulphamethoxazole, frequently used in the treatment of AIDS-related infections, causes abnormalities in liver function more commonly in AIDS patients than in the general population[94–99]. Granulomas containing eosinophils have been described in studies of liver biopsies from AIDS patients and trimethoprim-sulphamethoxazole has frequently been implicated[6].

Recommendations

Hepatobiliary involvement occurs in the majority of AIDS-infected individuals. Specific pathogens or neoplasms may account for up to 50% of these abnormalities. Despite this, the role of liver biopsy in these patients remains controversial. Recommendations regarding liver biopsy have varied within the hepatology community. A general trend away from the aggressive diagnosis of diseases with liver biopsy examination to the present judicious use of liver biopsy in AIDS patients have been observed. The infrequent finding of disease confined to the liver makes diagnosis by less invasive methods preferable. A discriminating approach is also supported by the often low yield of diseases responding to specific treatment modalities. Lastly, the rare finding of single diseases causing abnormalities in the liver makes assessement of therapy difficult.

The other modality of diagnosis of hepatobiliary disorders is endoscopic retrograde cholangiopancreatography (ERCP). When symptomatic biliary tract disease is found, therapeutic ERCP may provide clinical improvement with possible prolongation of survival.

Outlined in Figure 8 is an algorithm for our approach to individuals with AIDS. Undefined signs, symptoms or abnormal biochemical parameters indicating liver disease often lead to further investigation. As mentioned above, liver biopsy is no longer used as a primary modality of diagnosis When other less invasive modalities including bone marrow aspiration/biopsy, skin

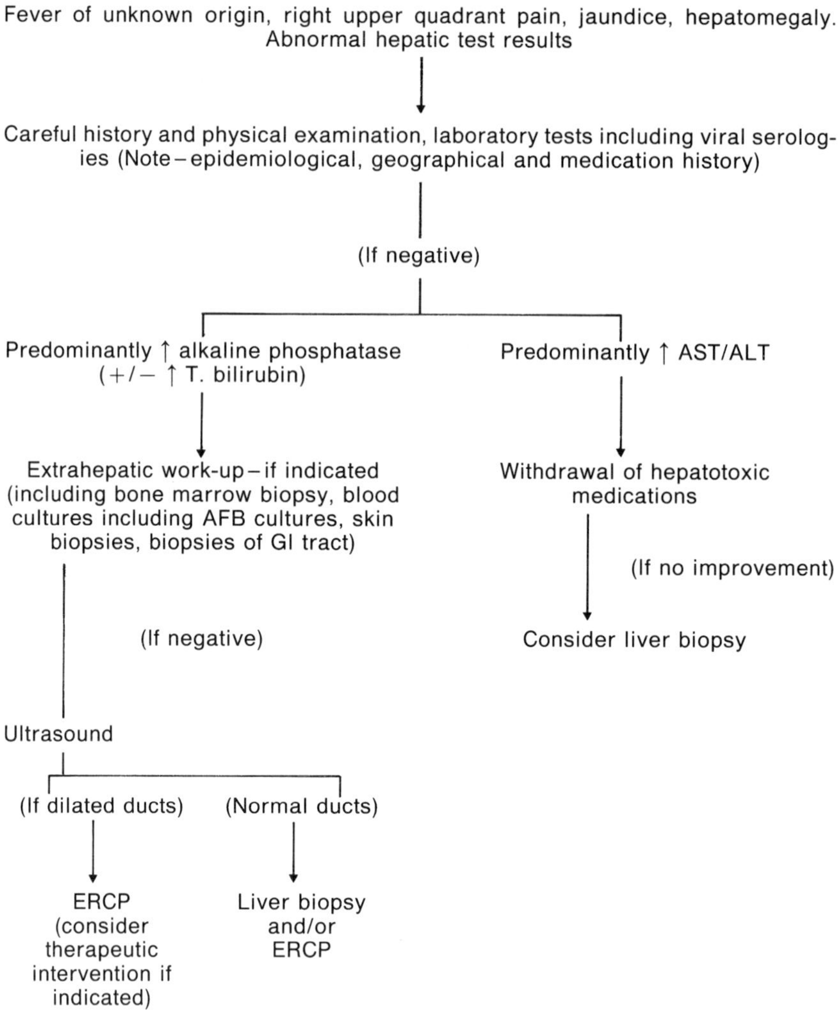

Figure 8 Algorithm for evaluation of hepatobiliary problems in HIV-infected individuals

biopsy and biopsies of the gastrointestinal tract are available, they are recommended. ERCP, however, may identify biliary tract complications, that are frequently symptomatic. With the potential for either curvative or palliative therapy a more aggressive use of ERCP is outlined. As more is learned about specific diagnosis, and more importantly about treatment of these disorders, this approach will certainly change again.

SUMMARY

Liver disease alone rarely leads to significant morbidity and mortality in HIV-infected individuls. Few fatalities in AIDS patients have been attributed to liver disease *per se*. Disseminated disease appears to be the rule for liver-related infections and neoplasms. Rarely primary disease involving the hepatobiliary tract has been reported. However, as the AIDS epidemic continues to grow, AIDS-related hepatobiliary disease will continue to plague gastroenterologists and hepatologists.

Acknowledgements

The authors thank Fenton Schaffner, MD for his continued assistance and help in preparing this manuscript, and Ms Mary Barrett for rapid and accurate preparation of the final typescript. Preparation of the review was supported in part by NIH grant DK-26438, and a generous gift from the Monique Weil-Caulier Bequest.

References

1. Rothenberg, R., Woelfel, M., Stoneburner, R., Milberg, J., Parker, R. and Truman, B. (1987). Survival with the Acquired Immunodeficiency Syndrome. *N. Engl. J. Med.*, **317**(21), 1297–1302
2. Quinn, T. C., Lacarias, F. R. K. and St John, R. K. (1989). Aids in the Americas: an emerging public health crisis. *N. Engl. J. Med.*, **320**, 1005–7
3. Statistics from the World Health Organization and the Centers for Disease Control (1989). *AIDS*, **3**, 113–17
4. Godwin, T. A. and Felix, J. C. (1987). Histopathology of the liver (abstr.) *Lab. Invest.*, **56**, 27A
5. Schneiderman, D. J., Arenson, D. M., Cello, J. P., Margaretten, W. and Weber, T. E. (1987). Hepatic disease in patients with the acquired immunodeficiency syndrome (AIDS). *Hepatology*, **7**(5), 925–30
6. Lebovics, E., Thung, S. N., Schaffner, F. and Radensky, P. (1985). The liver in the acquired immunodeficiency syndrome: a clinical and histologic study. *Hepatology*, **5**(2), 293–8
7. Glasgow, B. J., Anders, K., Layfield, L. J., Steinsapir, K. D., Gitnick, G. L. and Lewin, K. J. (1985). Clinical and pathologic findings of the liver in the acquired immunodeficiency syndrome (AIDS). *Am. J. Clin. Pathol.*, **83**(5), 582–8
8. Leevy, C. B., Nurse-Bey, H., Leevy, C. M. and Yu, J. (1988). Hepatic abnormalities in AIDS (abstr.). *Gastroenterology*, **94**, A561
9. Welch, K., Finkbeiner, W., Alpers, C. E., Blumenfeld, W., Davis, R. L., Smuckler, E. A. and Beckstead, J. H. (1984). Autopsy findings in the acquired immunodeficiency syndrome. *J. Am. Med. Assoc.*, **252**(9), 1152–9
10. Nakanuma, Y., Liew, C. T., Peters, R. L. and Govindarajan, S. (1986). Pathologic features of the liver in acquired immunodeficiency syndrome (AIDS). *Liver*, **6**, 158–66
11. Gordon, S. C., Reddy, K. R., Gould, E. E., McFadden, R., O'Brien, C., DeMedina, M., Jeffers, L. J. and Schiff, E. (1986). The spectrum of liver disease in the acquired immunodeficiency syndrome. *J. Hepatol.*, **2**, 475–84
12. Dworkin, B. M., Stahl, R. E., Giardina, M. A., Wormser, G. P., Weiss, L., Jankowski, R. and Rosenthal, W. S. (1987). The liver in acquired immunodeficiency syndrome: emphasis on patients with intravenous drug abuse. *Am. J. Gastroenterol.*, **82**(3), 231–6
13. Kahn, S. A., Saltzman, B. R., Klein, R. S., Mahadevia, P. S., Friedland, G. H. and Brandt, L. J. (1986). Hepatic disorders in the acquired immune deficiency syndrome: a clinical and pathological study. *Am. J. Gastroenterol.*, **81**(12), 1145–8
14. Scoazec, J. Y., March, C., Girard, P. M., Houtmann, J., Durand-Schneider, A. M., Saimot, A. G., Benhamou, J. P. and Feldmann, G. (1988). Peliosis hepatis and sinusoidal dilatation during infection by human immunodeficiency virus (HIV). *Am. J. Pathol.*, **131**(1), 38–47

15. Czapar, C. A., Weldon-Linne, M., Moore, D. M. and Rhone, D. P. (1986). Peliosis hepatis in the acquired immunodeficiency syndrome. *Arch. Pathol. Lab. Med.*, **110**, 611–13
16. Schneiderman, D. J. (1988). Hepatobiliary abnormalities in AIDS. In *Gastroenterology Clinics of North America*, Vol. **17**(3), 615–29. (Philadelphia: Saunders)
17. Palmer, M., Braly, L. F., and Schaffner, F. (1987). The liver in acquired immunodeficiency disease. *Semin. Liver Dis.* **7**(3), 192–202
18. Giesecke, J., Scalia-Tomba, G. and Furucrona, A. (1988). HIV infectivity – the hepatitis B lesion. *Scand. J. Infect. Dis.*, **20**, 385–7
19. Gerberding, J. L., Hopewell, P. C., Kaminsky, L. S. and Sande, M. A. (1986). Transmission of hepatitis B without transmission of AIDS by accidental needlestick (letter). *N. Engl. J. Med.*, **312**, 56
20. Uribe, M., Passarell, L., Arista, J., Schulz, E., Paez, O., Reyes, E. and Angeles, A. (1987). The liver in AIDS patients. Usefulness of liver needle biopsy. *Rev. Invest. Clin.*, **39**, 35–40
21. Laure, F., Zagury, D., Saimot, A. G., Gallo, R. C., Hahn, B. H. and Brechot, C. (1985). Hepatitis B virus DNA sequences in lymphoid cells from patients with AIDS and AIDS-related complex. *Science*, **229**, 561–3
22. Noonan, C. A., Yoffe, B., Mansell, P. W. A., Melnick, J. L. and Hollinger, F. B. (1986). Extrachromosomal sequences of hepatitis B virus DNA in peripheral blood mononuclear cells of acquired immune deficiency syndrome patients. *Proc. Natl. Acad. Sci. USA*, **83**, 5698–702
23. Levy, J. A. (1989). Human immunodeficiency viruses and the pathogenesis of AIDS (1989). *J. Am. Med. Assoc.*, **261**, 2997–3006
24. Hirschman, S. Z. and Zucker, M. L. (1988). Recombinant DNA related to hepatitis B and human immunodeficiency viruses in mononuclear cells of patients with AIDS. *J. Med. Virol.*, **26**, 145–52
25. Krogsgaard, K., Lindhardt, B. O., Nielsen, J. O., Andersson, P., Kryger, P., Aldershville, J., Gerstoft, J. and Pedersen, C. (1987). The influence of HTLV-III infection on the natural history of hepatitis B virus infection in male homosexual HBsAg carriers. *Hepatology*, **7**(1), 37–41
26. Rustgi, V. K., Hoofnagle, J. H., Gerin, J. L., Gelmann, E. P., Reichert, C. M., Cooper, J. N. and Macher, A. M. (1984). Hepatitis B virus infection in the acquired immunodeficiency syndrome. *Ann. Intern. Med.*, **101**(6), 795–7
27. Perrillo, R. P., Regenstein, F. G. and Roodman, S. T. (1986). Chronic hepatitis B in asymptomatic homosexual men with antibody to the human immunodeficiency virus. *Ann. Intern. Med.*, **105**(3), 382–3
28. Pastore, G., Santantonio, T., Monno, L., Milella, M., Luchena, N. and Angarano, G. (1988). Effects of HIV superinfection on HBV replication in a chronic HBsAg carrier with liver disease. *J. Hepatol.*, **7**, 164–8
29. McDonald, J. A., Harris, S., Waters, J. A. and Thomas, H. C. (1987). Effect of human immunodeficiency virus (HIV) infection on chronic hepatitis B hepatitic viral antigen display. *J. Hepatol.*, **4**, 337–42
30. Underhill, G. S., Jeffries, D. J., Forster, G. E. and Harris, J. R. W. (1986). Correlation between fulminant form of viral hepatitis and retrovirus infection associated with AIDS (letter). *Br. Med. J.*, **292**, 1080–1
31. Biggar, R. J., Goedert, J. J. and Hoofnagle, J. (1987). Accelerated loss of antibody to hepatitis B surface antigen among immunodeficient homosexual men infected with HIV (letter). *N. Engl. J. Med.*, **316**(10), 630–1
32. Collier, A. C., Corey, L., Murphy, V. L. and Handsfield, H. H. (1988). Antibody to human immunodeficiency (HIV) and supoptimal response to hepatitis B vaccination. *Ann. Intern. Med.*, **109**, 101–5
33. Lazizi, Y., Grangeot-Korosl, L., Delfraissy, J. F., Boue, F., Dubreuil, P., Badur, S. and Pillot, J. (1988). Reappearance of hepatitis B virus in immune patients infected with the human immunodeficiency virus Type I (letter). *J. Infect. Dis.*, **158**(3), 666–7
34. Carne, C. A., Weller, I. V. D., Waite, J., Briggs, M., Pearce, F., Adler, M. W. and Tedder, R. S. (1987). Impaired responsiveness of homosexual men with HIV antibodies to plasma derived hepatitis B vaccine. *Br. Med. J.*, **294**, 866–8
35. Harward, M. P., Kaiser, D. L. and Fedson, D. S. (1988). Acceptance of hepatitis B vaccine by medical and surgical residents. *J. Gen. Intern. Med.*, **3**, 150–5

36. Stevens, C. E., Taylor, P. E., Rubinstein, P. *et al.* (1985). Safety of hepatitis B vaccine. *N. Engl. J. Med.*, **312**, 375–6
37. Barre-Sinoussi, F., Nugeyre, M. T., Girard, M., Tron, F. and Chermann, J. C. (1985). Laboratory and serological studies argue against possible transmission of AIDS by hepatitis B vaccine (letter). *Lancet*, **2**, 274
38. Papaevangelou, G., Roumeliotou-Karayannis, A., Kallinikos, G. and Politou, K. (1985). Lack of antibodies to LAV/HTLV-III in hepatitis B vaccine recipients. *Eur. J. Epidemiol.*, **1**, 323–5
39. Novick, D. M., Farci, P., Croxson, T. S., Taylor, M. B., Schneebaum, C. W., Lai, M. E., Bach, N., Senie, R. T., Gelb, A. M. and Kreek, M. J. (1988). Hepatitis D virus and human immunodeficiency virus antibodies in parenteral drug abusers who are hepatitis B surface antigen positive. *J. Infect. Dis.*, **158**, 795–803
40. DeCock, K. M., Niland, J. C., Lu, H. P., Rahimian, A., Edwards, V., Shriver, K., Govindarajan, S. and Redeker, A. G. (1988). Experience with human immunodeficiency virus infection in patients with hepatitis B virus and hepatitis delta virus infections in Los Angeles, 1977–1985. *Am. J. Epidemiol.*, **127**, 1250–60
41. Solomon, R. E., Kaslow, R. A., Phair, J. P., Lyter, D., Visscher, B., Lyman, D., Vanraden, M. T. and Gerin, J. (1988). Human immunodeficiency virus and hepatitis delta virus in homosexual men. *Ann. Intern. Med.*, **108**, 51–4
42. Weisfuse, I. B., Hadler, S. C., Fields, H. A. *et al.* (1989). Delta hepatitis in homosexual men in the United States. *Hepatology*, **9**, 872–4
43. Grippon, P., Ribiere, O., Cadranel, J. F., Pelletier, S., Pillot, B., Emerit, J. and Opolon, P. (1987). Long-term delta antigenemia without appearance of delta antibody in two immunodeficient patients (letter). *Lancet*, **2**, 1031
44. Shattock, A. G., Finlay, H. and Hillary, I. B. (1987). Possible reactivation of hepatitis D with chronic delta antigenemia by human immunodeficiency virus. *Br. Med. J.*, **294**, 1656
45. Martin, P., DiBisceglie, A. M., Kassianides, C., Lisker-Melman, M. and Hoofnagle, J. H. (1989). Non-A Non-B hepatitis leads to rapidly progressive liver disease in patients with human immunodeficiency virus infection (abstract). *Gastroenterology*, **96**(5), A200
46. Libanore, M., Bicocchi, R., Sighinolfi, L. and Ghinelli, F. (1988). Fulminant NANB hepatitis in a patient with AIDS: a possible demonstration of direct hepatic injury by the viruses involved? (letter). *Infection*, **16**, 255
47. Quinnan, G. V. Jr, Masur, H., Rook, A. H. *et al.* (1984). Herpes virus infection in the acquired immunodeficiency syndrome. *J. Am. Med. Assoc.*, **252**, 72–7
48. Macher, A. M., Reichert, C. M., Strauss, S. E. *et al.* (1983). Death in the AIDS patient: role of cytomegalovirus (letter). *N. Engl. J. Med.* **309**, 1454
49. Guarda, L. A., Luna, M. A., Smith, J. L. *et al.* (1984). Acquired immune deficiency syndrome: postmortem findings. *Am. J. Clin. Pathol.*, **81**, 549–57
50. Reichert, C. M., O'Leary, T. J., Levens, D. L. *et al.* (1983). Autopsy pathology in the acquired immune deficiency syndrome. *Am. J. Pathol.*, **12**, 357–82
51. Guzda, L. A., Luna, M. A., Smith, J. L. *et al.* (1984). Acquired immunodeficiency syndrome: postmortem findings. *Am. J. Clin. Pathol.*, **81**, 549–57
52. Laskin, O. L., Cederberg, D. M., Mills, J., Eron, L. J., Mildvan, D. and Spector, S. A. (1987). Ganciclovir for the treatment and suppression of serious infections caused by cytomegalovirus. *Am. J. Med.*, **83**, 201–7
53. Beissner, R. S., Rappaport, E. S. and Diaz, J. A. (1987). Fatal case of Epstein-Barr virus-induced lymphoproliferative disorder associated with a human immunodeficiency virus infection. *Arch. Pathol. Lab. Med.*, **111**, 250–3
54. Duffy, L. F., Daum, F., Kahn, E. *et al.* (1986). Hepatitis in children with acquired immune deficiency syndrome. *Gastroenterology*, **90**, 173–81
55. Thung, S. N., Gerber, M. A., Benkov, K. J., Guttenberg, M. and Gordon, R. E. (1988). Chronic active hepatitis in a child with human immunodeficiency virus infection. *Arch. Pathol. Lab. Med.*, **112**, 914–16
56. Kamani, N., Lightman, H., Leiderman, I. and Krilov, L. R. (1988). Pediatric acquired immunodeficiency syndrome-related complex: clinical and immunologic features. *Pediatr. Infect. Dis. J.*, **7**, 383–8
57. Zimmerli, W., Bianchi, L., Gudat, F., Spichtin, H., Erb, P., von Planta, M. and Heitz, P. U. (1988). Disseminated herpes simplex Type 2 and systemic candida infection in a patient

with previous asymptomatic human immunodeficiency virus infection (letter). *J. Infect. Dis.*, **157**, 597–8

58. Mosca, J. D., Bednarik, D. P., Raj, N. B. K., Rosen, C. A., Sodroski, J. G., Haseltine, W. A. and Pitha, P. M. (1987). Herpes simplex virus type-1 can reactivate transcription of latent human immunodeficiency virus. *Nature*, **325**, 67–70
59. Orenstein, M. S., Tavitan, A., Yonk, B., Dincsoy, J. P., Zerega, J., Iyer, S. K. and Straus, E. W. (1985). Granulomatous involvement of the liver in patients with AIDS. *Gut*, **26**, 1220–5
60. Lebovics, E., Dworkin, B. M., Heier, S. K. and Rosenthal, W. S. (1988). The hepatobiliary manifestations of human immunodeficiency virus infection. *Am. J. Gastroenterol.*, **83**, 1–7
61. Glatt, A. E., Chirqwin, K., and Landesman, S. H. (1988). Treatment of infections associated with human immunodeficiency virus. *N. Engl. J. Med.*, **318**, 1439–48
62. Selwyn, P. A., Hartel, D., Lewis, V. A. *et al.* (1989). A prospective study of the risk of tuberculosis among intravenous drug users with human immunodeficiency virus infection. *N. Engl. J. Med.*, **320**, 545–50
63. Moreno, S., Pacho, E., Lopez-Herce, J. A., Rodriguez-Creixems, M., Martin-Scapa, C. and Bouza, E. (1988). Mycobacterium tuberculosis visceral abscesses in the acquired immunodeficiency syndrome (AIDS) [letter]. *Am. Intern. Med.*, **109**, 437
64. Weinberg, J. J., Cohen, P. and Malhotra, R. (1988). Primary tuberculous liver abscess associated with the human immunodeficiency virus. *Tubercle*, **69**, 145–7
65. Chin, K. P., Lowe, M. A., Tong, M. J. and Koehler, A. L. (1987). Vibrio vulnificus infection after raw oyster ingestion in a patient with liver disease and acquired immune deficiency syndrome-related complex. *Gastroenterology*, **92**, 796–9
66. Reddy, K. R., Chan, J. C., Smiley, D., Jeffers, L. J. and Schiffer, E. R. (1988). Spontaneous Group B salmonella enteritidis peritonitis in cirrhotic ascites and acquired immune deficiency syndrome. *Am. J. Gastroenterol.*, **83**(8), 882–4
67. Bonner, J. R., Dismukes, W. E., Alexander, W. J. *et al.* (1984). Disseminated histoplasmosis in patients with the acquired immune deficiency syndrome. *Arch. Intern. Med.*, **144**, 2178–81
68. Mandell, W., Goldberg, D. M., and Neu, H. C. (1986). Histoplasmosis in patients with the acquired immune deficiency syndrome. *Am. J. Med.*, **81**, 974–8
69. Wheat, L. J., Slama, T. G. and Zeckel, M. L. (1985). Histoplasmosis in the acquired immune deficiency syndrome. *Am. J. Med.*, **78**, 203–10
70. Terada, S., Reddy, K. R., Jeffers, L. J., Cali, A. and Schiff, E. (1987). Microsporidan hepatitis in the acquired immunodeficiency syndrome. *Ann. Intern. Med.*, **107**, 61–2
71. Falk, S., Helm, E. B., Hubner, K. and Stutte, H. J. (1988). Disseminated visceral leishmaniasis (kala azar) in acquired immunodeficiency syndrome (AIDS). *Pathol. Res. Pract.*, **183**, 252–5
72. Aaron, J. S., Wynter, C. D., Kirton, O. C. and Simko, V. (1988). Cytomegalovirus associated with acalculous cholecystitis in a patient with acquired immune deficiency syndrome. *Am. J. Gastroenterol.*, **83**, 879–81
73. Margulis, S. J., Honig, C. L., Soave, R., Govoni, A. F., Mouradian, J. A. and Jacobsen, I. M. (1986). Biliary tract obstruction in the acquired immunodeficiency syndrome. *Ann. Intern. Med.*, **105**, 207–10
74. Schneiderman, D. J., Cello, J. P. and Laing, F. C. (1987). Papillary stenosis and sclerosing cholangitis in the acquired immunodeficiency syndrome. *Ann. Intern. Med.*, **106**, 546–9
75. Stillman, A. E., Schmid, R. and Howe, J. B. (1987). Acquired immunodeficiency syndrome and biliary tract disease (letter). *Ann. Intern. Med.*, **106**, 634
76. Jacobson, M. A., Cells, J. P. and Sande, M. A. (1988). Cholestasis and disseminated cytomegalovirus disease in patients with the acquired immunodeficiency syndrome. *Am. J. Med.*, **84**, 218–24
77. Roulot, D., Valla, D., Brun-Vezinet, F. *et al.* (1987). Cholangitis in the acquired immunodeficiency syndrome: report of two cases and review of the literature. *Gut*, **28**, 1653–60
78. Pitlik, S., Fainstein, V., Rios, A. *et al.* (1983). Cryptosporidial cholecystitis (letter). *N. Engl. J. Med.*, **308**, 967
79. Kahn, D. G., Garfinkle, J. M., Klonoff, D. C., Pembrook, L. J. and Marrow, D. J. (1987). Cryptosporidial and cytomegaloviral hepatitis and cholecystitis. *Arch. Pathol. Lab. Med.*, **3**, 879–81

80. Blumberg, R. S., Kelsey, P., Perrone, T., Dickersin, R., Laguaglia, M. and Ferruci, J. (1984). Cytomegalovirus- and cryptosporidium-associated acalculous gangrenous cholecystitis. *Am. J. Med.*, **76**, 1118–19
81. Kaplan, L. D., Kahn, J., Jacobson, M., Bottles, K. and Cello, J. (1989). Primary bile duct lymphoma in the acquired immunodeficiency syndrome (AIDS). *Ann. Intern. Med.*, **110**, 161–2
82. Cockerill, F. R., Hurley, D. V., Malagelada, J. R. *et al.* (1986). Polymicrobial cholangitis and Kaposi's sarcoma in blood product transfusion-related acquired immunodeficiency syndrome. *Am. J. Med.* **80**, 1237–41
83. Centers for Disease Control (1987). Revision of the CDC surveillance case definition for acquired immunodeficiency syndrome. *Morbidity and Mortality Weekly Report*, **36** (Suppl. 15)
84. Sonnabend, J., Witkins, S. S. and Purtilo, D. R. (1983). Acquired immunodeficiency syndrome, opportunistic infections and malignancies in male homosexuals. A hypothesis of etiologic factors in pathogenesis. *J. Am. Med. Assoc.*, **249**, 2370–4
85. Friedman, S. L. (1988). Gastrointestinal and hepatobiliary neoplasms in AIDS. In: *Gastroenterology Clinics of North America*, vol. 17, pp. 465–86. (Philadelphia: Saunders)
86. Giraldo, G., Beth, E., Coeur, P. *et al.* (1972). Kaposi's sarcoma: a new model in the search for viruses associated with human malignancies. *J. Natl. Cancer Inst.*, **49**, 1495
87. Drew, W. L. (1986). Is CMV a cofactor in the pathogenesis of AIDS Kaposi's sarcoma? *Mount Sinai J. Med.* **53**, 622–5
88. Safai, B., Johnson, K. G., Myshowski, P. L. *et al.* (1985). The natural history of Kaposi's sarcoma in the acquired immunodeficiency syndrome. *Ann. Intern. Med.*, **103**, 744–50
89. Knowles, D. M., Chamulak, G. A., Subar, M. *et al.* (1988). Lymphoid neoplasia associated with the acquired immunodeficiency syndrome (AIDS). *Ann. Intern. Med.*, **108**, 744–53
90. Caccamo, D., Peruez, N. K. and Marchevsky, A. (1986). Primary lymphoma of the liver in the acquired immunodeficiency syndrome. *Arch. Pathol. Lab. Med.*, **110**, 553–5
91. Bear, D. M., Anderson, E. T. and Wilkinson, L. S. (1986). Acquired immune deficiency syndrome in homosexual men with Hodgkin's disease. *Am. J. Med.*, **80**, 738–40
92. Robert, N. J. and Schneidermann, H. (1984). Hodgkin's disease and the acquired immunodeficiency syndrome (letter). *Ann. Intern. Med.*, **101**, 142–3
93. Scheib, R. G. and Siegel, R. S. (1985). Atypical Hodgkin's disease and the acquired immunodeficiency syndrome (letter). *Ann. Intern. Med.*, **102**, 554
94. Richman, D. D., Fischl, M. A., Grieco, M. H., Gottlieb, M. S., Volberding, P. A., Laskin, O. L., Leedom, J. M., Groopman, J. E., Mildvan, D., Hirsch, M. S., Jackson, G. G., Durack, D. T., Nusinoff-Lehrman, S. and the AZT Collaborative Working Group (1987). The toxicity of azidothymidine (AZT) in the treatment of patients with AIDS and AIDS-related complex. *N. Engl. J. Med.*, **317**, 192–7
95. Melamed, A. J., Muller, R. J., Gold, J. W., Campbell, S. W., Kleinberg, M. L. and Armstrong, D. (1987). Possible zidovudine-induced hepatotoxicity (letter). *J. Am. Med. Assoc.*, **258**, 2063
96. Dubin, G. and Braffman, M. N. (1989). Zidovudine-induced hepatotoxicity. *Ann. Intern. Med.*, **110**, 85–6
97. Gordin, F. M., Simon, G. L., Wofsky, C. B. *et al.* (1984). Adverse reactions to trimethoprim-sulfamethoxazole in patients with the acquired immunodeficiency syndrome. *Ann. Intern. Med.*, **100**, 495–9
98. Wharton, J. M., Coleman, D. L., Wofsky, C. B. *et al.* (1986). Trimethoprim-sulfamethoxazole or pentamidine for pneumocystis carinii pneumonia in the acquired immunodeficiency syndrome: a prospective randomized trial. *Ann. Intern. Med.*, **105**, 37–44
99. Butkus Small, C., Harris, C. A., Friedland, G. H. and Klein, R. S. (1985). The treatment of pneumocystis carinii pneumonia in the acquired immunodeficiency syndrome. *Arch. Intern. Med.*, **145**, 837–40

27
Viral infections of the liver: safety of blood and blood products

H. J. ALTER

The past half-decade has seen major changes in blood transfusion practice. Measures, predominantly instituted as a response to transfusion-transmitted AIDS, have indirectly had a marked impact on transfusion-associated hepatitis (TAH). In this paper I will review these direct and indirect approaches to disease prevention, and do this primarily in the context of non-A, non-B hepatitis (NANBH), the most common serious complication of blood transfusion and the most common form of viral hepatitis in developed nations.

The current risk of TAH in the United States and in most other areas of the world is unknown, because prospective studies have not been performed since 1985 when profound changes in the blood supply began to occur. These changes in the donor base have had such a positive impact on reducing transfusion risk that prior measurements of TAH incidence are obsolete. There is a distinct need to initiate new prospective studies of TAH incidence, and such an initiative is being sponsored by the National Heart Lung and Blood Institute.

In the classical prospective studies of TAH incidence in recipients of volunteer donor blood (all conducted prior to 1980), TAH incidence ranged from 7% to 17% and generally from 7% to 12%[1]. These were predominantly studies in open-heart surgery patients and involved recipients of multiple blood units. Because there is not a linear relationship between hepatitis incidence and the number of units transfused it has been difficult to estimate a per-unit risk. However, early studies by Seeff *et al.* in the VA system looked at single-unit transfusions and projected a per-unit risk of 1.6% for volunteer donors and 5.4% for paid donors[2]. It is of interest that these projections are not far from estimates made utilizing the newly developed test for detection of hepatitis C virus (HCV) carriers; this assay suggests an HCV (NANBH virus) carrier rate of 0.5–1% in volunteer donors and a rate five times that in paid plasma donors. The assay for antibody to HCV (anti-HCV) will be described in detail below. Although the incidence of TAH varied in these early studies, there was great uniformity in the proportion of total hepatitis cases that were classified as NANBH, exceeding 90% in each of the studies. With the introduction of specific tests to identify carriers of the hepatitis B virus (HBV) in 1970, and with subsequent increases in sensitivity of the HBV screening assays, HBV has played a diminishing role in the causation of TAH[3], and HCV has been the predominant determinant of hepatitis incidence. In our NIH series, 98% of TAH cases are classified as NANBH, and in a Japanese study 100% of cases were NANBH.

In prospective studies conducted since 1980[4], the incidence of TAH has varied markedly according to geographical area. Rates of 2–3% have been observed in Australia and the Netherlands, while rates as high as 44% have been observed in Japan. An incidence of 20% was reported in Sweden and 14–17% in Italy and Spain. The most recent prospective study was reported by Feinman in Canada, where the incidence was 9%, virtually all classified as NANBH[5]. To emphasize the changing pattern of TAH, preliminary data from Canada indicate that the prior rate of 9% has fallen to approximately 2% in the 'post-AIDS' era. The specific reasons for this decline will be discussed subsequently.

Concern for NANBH derives from prospective studies of TAH which uniformly indicated that 40–60% of NANBH cases demonstrated alanine aminotransferase (ALT) elevations for more than 6 months and generally for more than 1 year after the acute episode[1]. The elevations of ALT were often intermittent; indeed a fluctuating pattern of transaminase elevations is characteristic of NANBH infection. These fluctuations have never been adequately explained, but are more likely related to bursts of viral replication than to variations in host immune response. Now that the virus has been identified, *in-vitro* indices of viral replication may be developed, and allow for correlative studies relating viral growth to hepatocellular inflammation. In addition to biochemical evidence of chronic hepatitis, most prospective studies include histological confirmation of chronic disease activity. Liver biopsies in transfusion-associated cases show that the majority of such patients have the lesions of either chronic active hepatitis (CAH) or cirrhosis, often with an overlap between the two[6]. The CAH is generally mild on initial biopsy and may not evolve on subsequent biopsy. However, almost every series with serial biopsies has revealed the histological progression from CAH to cirrhosis in a significant number of cases. In the NIH series[6], among 13 patients with CAH who were rebiopsied, generally within 3 years of initial biopsy, 46% showed a stable lesion, 15% showed histological improvement and 39% demonstrated progressively severe CAH and/or cirrhosis; four of 13 patients developed cirrhosis while under observation. In aggregate, 22% of the NIH patients had cirrhosis on the initial or subsequent biopsy. The number of chronic NANBH cases with histological confirmation of cirrhosis is remarkably constant from series to series, almost always about 20%.

Data on chronic NANBH are further confirmed in studies of haemophiliac patients who, because of therapy with commercial clotting factor concentrates, have been afflicted with virtually all transfusion-transmitted viral infections, particularly HBV, HCV, and HIV. It had been previously demonstrated in a composite of 10 studies performed in haemophiliac patients that 64% had chronic elevations of serum ALT[6]. Based on the absence of hepatitis B surface antigen, and on the histological pattern of the hepatitis, it had been presumed that most of these cases represented NANBH. That this presumption was correct is now supported by the specific HCV assay which uniformly indicates that 60–80% of haemophiliacs are anti-HCV positive. In the most comprehensive evaluation of liver disease among haemophiliacs, 155 biopsies were collated from multiple centres and read under code by a panel of expert hepatopathologists[7]. The majority of patients had only mild or moderate lesions, but 15% had cirrhosis and an additional 7% had severe CAH which would probably evolve into cirrhosis, again reaching the approximate 20% incidence observed in standard transfusion cases.

A large proportion of NANBH occurs outside the transfusion setting. This form of sporadic or community-acquired NANBH has been extensively investigated by Miriam Alter *et al.* at CDC[8]. Among 119 community-acquired cases, 48% had a history of parenteral exposure through blood transfusion, intravenous drug use or their occupation, but 50% had no known source of infection. The CDC study further indicated that the frequency of chronic hepatitis was the same in community-acquired cases as it had been in the prospective studies of TAH, namely 50%, and that the incidence of chronic hepatitis was the same in those with known parenteral exposure as in those without a known source of exposure[9]. This suggested that both parenterally acquired and sporadic NANBH were due to the same agent, an agent with an inordinate propensity to cause chronic liver disease. That such is the case is now being confirmed by the specific assay which reveals that up to 80% of community-acquired NANBH cases are anti-HCV positive.

One of the most dramatic outcomes of investigations with the anti-HCV assay is the probability that the agent of NANBH (HCV) is causally associated with the development of hepatocellular carcinoma (HCC). Such an association had been previously suggested by individual case reports, and then by retrospective evaluations in Japan which showed an epidemiological link between HCC and a prior history of blood transfusion[6]. A case study in Japan also histologically documented the progression from acute post-transfusion hepatitis through the sequential development of chronic active hepatitis, bridging necrosis, cirrhosis and finally HCC, the entire evolution requiring 18 years[10]. Many more studies will be required to establish causality, but now that a marker is available it should be possible to accrue data which will establish a link between HCV and HCC just as was done for HBV. Preliminary data suggest that in Japan, where HCC prevalence is very high, HCV is a more important aetiological determinant than is HBV.

The evolution of the specific HCV assay has been an extremely exciting event, and follows more than a decade of frustration in developing a serological approach to the study of this virus. The techniqe utilized to discover the NANBH virus was sophisticated, labour-intensive and unique[11]. It represents the first time that molecular biology has detected an infectious agent, not previously replicated *in vitro* or recognized by electron microscopy. Basically, a cDNA library was generated from whole nucleic acid derived from large volumes of chimpanzee plasma demonstrated to have a very high infectivity titre for the agent of NANBH. The cDNA was then inserted into an expression vector, gt11, and cloned, initially in *E. coli* and later, in yeast. Clones were screened with sera from patients with chronic NANBH or patients convalescing from NANBH. Using radioautography, a reactive clone was identified and subsequently subcloned. The protein derived from this clone was then used as the antigen in a radioimmunoassay, and subsequently an enzyme immunoassay to detect antibody to HCV[12]. The specificity of this assay was first evaluated in chimpanzees infected with HBV, hepatitis A virus (HAV) and NANBV (HCV). Not only was the test specific for HCV, but clear-cut anti-HCV seroconversion was demonstrated in chimpanzees that had been inoculated with sera from patients with NANBH. The specificity of the assay was next evaluated in the coded NIH NANBH panel which had previously demonstrated the non-specificity of 20 putative NANBH tests. The Chiron assay showed 100% reproducibility in coded duplicate samples and detected six of six patients with chronic hepatitis whose NANBH infection had been confirmed by chimpanzee inoculation. It failed to detect antibody in two patients with acute NANBH, but subsequent samples from these patients were anti-HCV positive. The assay was negative in well-pedigreed normal and disease controls. Hence this was the first assay to reproducibly 'break' this coded panel.

In the next phase of evaluation we examined the specificity and potential efficacy of the anti-HCV assay by utilizing sera from patients with 'classic' transfusion-associated NANBH, and their respective donors[13]. Because NANBH has been diagnosed by exclusionary criteria, and because such cases are often diagnostically nebulous, we felt it was essential to evaluate the anti-HCV assay in cases that were clinically unequivocal and histologically confirmed. We selected our 15 best-defined cases, all of whom had chronic hepatitis, 14 of whom had biopsy documentation of chronic hepatitis consistent with a viral aetiology, and four of whom had been proven to cause NANBH infection in the chimpanzee model. These patients had all been multiply transfused at the time of cardiac surgery. Anti-HCV seroconversion was demonstrated in each (100%) of these 15 cases[13]. Hence the anti-HCV assay served to confirm the clinical and histological diagnosis and, in turn, these cases verified the relationship between HCV and transfusion-associated NANBH. At the time of the Ortho clinical trial, additional chronic NANBH cases were evaluated to a total of 26; 24 of 26 (92%) showed anti-HCV seroconversion. We also evaluated five cases that appeared to have acute NANBH which spontaneously resolved; three of these five (60%) were anti-HCV positive. In aggregate, 27 of 31 cases (87%) had serological evidence of HCV infection. It appeared that chronic cases were more likely to be positive than acute cases, and that seropositivity correlated with the certainty of the clinical diagnosis. There are several possible explanations for why all NANBH cases are not anti-HCV positive.

1. As alluded to above, there is considerable room for diagnostic error utilizing the exclusionary criteria which now serve as the basis for NANBH diagnosis. The likelihood of diagnostic error increases in cases where the duration of ALT elevation is short, and where the magnitude of ALT elevation is slight. It is these transient, mild hepatitis cases which

are most likely to be anti-HCV negative.

2. The case may be due to a NANBH agent other than HCV. This is the most intriguing possibility, and there has been considerable indirect evidence to suggest that there may be more than one NANBH agent. However, the high frequency of anti-HCV seroconversion in well-defined cases of NANBH suggests that if a second agent exists, it will account for only a small proportion of the total NANBH spectrum. Whether a second agent exists can now be directly explored by selecting appropriate cases and employing the molecular biological techniques that were so successful in discovering HCV.
3. Some NANBH cases may spuriously appear to be anti-HCV negative because they have been inadequately sampled. Seroconversion following HCV infection may be very delayed and cases must be tested for 6–12 months before they can be classified as anti-HCV negative with reasonable serological certainty. In the early evaluations of the anti-HCV assay such late samples were often unavailable. Conversely, if the sample is obtained too late in transient cases, a previous positive result may no longer be manifest.
4. The sensitivity of the first generation anti-HCV assay is unknown, and it is probable that some cases test anti-HCV negative even though caused by the hepatitis C virus. This possibility can now be explored by immunofluorescence testing of liver tissue, by *in situ* hybridization and by polymerase chain reaction.

In prospectively followed and repeatedly sampled patients in the NIH series[13], the mean interval to anti-HCV seroconversion was almost 24 weeks from the time of transfusion; this interval was reduced to 21 weeks if one very long-duration case was excluded from analysis. Antibody, once developed, persisted in 14 of the 15 chronic cases and persistence has been documented for over 12 years. In contrast, anti-HCV disappeared in each of the three acute cases in whom it had developed; however, in these acute cases antibody remained detectable for a long interval after biochemical and clinical resolution of the disease (9 years in one case). It is probable that the presence of anti-HCV generally correlates with active viral replication and infectivity, but in some cases it appears to represent a convalescent state in which the blood would no longer be infectious. At present the replicative and convalescent stages cannot be easily distinguished, except perhaps by PCR, and it is safest from the transfusion standpoint to consider all anti-HCV positive donors potentially infectious.

An analysis of linked donor and recipient sera in the NIH study[13] revealed an anti-HCV positive donor in 14 of 16 HCV-related NANBH cases (87%). Other studies have not found this high a proportion of anti-HCV positive donors. There are many possible explanations for this discrepancy, including the certainty of the diagnosis and the time period in which the study was conducted. These discrepancies will be clarified as more cases are studied, as more rigid diagnostic criteria are applied and as more sensitive technology is developed. At present I think it is reasonable to say that the anti-HCV assay will detect at least 50% of donors capable of transmitting NANBH, and that it might detect as many as 85%.

A comparison of the direct and surrogate assays in the NIH study indicated that the surrogate assays (ALT, anti-HBc) would detect approximately 50% of the anti-HCV positive donors that had been implicated in hepatitis transmission. While less than 15% of surrogate marker positive donors are anti-HCV positive, this proportion increases to greater than 40% if one tests individuals with both surrogate markers or individuals that have only one marker, but have been shown to be implicated in a case of NANBH. In those countries which initiated surrogate testing there will be a need to reconsider whether such testing should be retained in light of the availability of a specific HCV assay. It is probable that the ALT test will be retained because of the long interval between the onset of infection and the development of detectable antibody, and because of the possibility that there might be a second hepatitis agent that would be detected by this index of hepatocellular inflammation. The anti-HBC assay is likely to be retained because it not only serves as a back-up for the detection of HCV carriers, but might detect HBV carriers who are HBsAg negative and also serve as an excellent surrogate marker for high-risk sexual and addictive behaviour which fosters the transmission of HIV.

Assays performed as part of the Ortho clinical trial revealed a fairly uniform prevalence of anti-HCV in Canada, Europe and the United States (0.34%, 0.57%, 0.60%, respectively) and a higher prevalence in Japan (1.5%) and Africa (6.0%). In Western nations donor loss will not be excessive , and the risk–benefit ratio of adopting this test appears to be very favourable. Licensure is anticipated in early 1990.

Although it has not yet been documented in prospective studies, it is the general impression, based on reported cases and preliminary prospective data, that the incidence of TAH has dramatically declined in recent years. This decline has been coincident with multiple measures designed to prevent transfusion-associated AIDS. These measures include:

1. the more judicious use of blood and blood products and a heightened awareness by patients and physicians of the deleterious and sometimes mortal risks of blood transfusion;
2. the increasing use of autologous blood by pre-deposit and intraoperative salvage;
3. the interdiction of donors at high risk for HIV transmission by information to encourage self-deferral, an intensified donor interview with direct questions regarding risk behaviour, increased donor accountability in the consent process and confidential post-donation unit exclusion;
4. the increased use of single donor platelets obtained by apheresis;
5. the routine viral inactivation of plasma products including clotting factor concentrates and
6. the introduction of surrogate assays.

Prospective studies of TAH in the United States and Canada in 1980–85 revealed a hepatitis incidence of 8–9%. Using 8% as the pre-1985 and pre-AIDS testing baseline, I believe that all the above-cited AIDS preventive measures have effected an approximate 40% decline in TAH incidence, reducing that incidence to under 5%. I estimate that surrogate markers have effected an additional 20% decline, bringing the current incidence below 4%. It is my prediction, based on the HCV data presented above, that the specific anti-HCV assay will reduce the existing hepatitis incidence by at least 50% or to an overall rate less than 2%. This is a remarkable decline considering that TAH rates in the United States prior to 1970 were as high as 33% and that they remained in the range of 10% throughout the 1970s and early 1980s. It is important to note, however, that although tests for HBV, NANBV and HIV have been and will be very important in hepatitis prevention, the most important elements are not test-related, but rather related to donor selection. It is my contention that the major elements responsible for hepatitis reduction were: first, the exclusion of paid donors and the development of an all-volunteer donor system; second, the intensified process of donor exclusion based on high-risk behaviour; and third, changes in blood usage engendered by the threat of AIDS, particularly the increasing use of autologous blood. This is not to minimize the importance of testing and the increasing importance of viral inactivation procedures, but it is to place such testing in perspective within the total realm of blood transfusion practice. It is also to emphasize that these donor-related measures have a generic potential to affect all disease transmission including viruses yet to be discovered rather than having the restricted specificity of the serological approach.

Overall, despite an increasing number of agents known to be transmitted by blood, the blood supply is paradoxically safer than it has ever been, and likely to become still safer as we enter the last decade of this century. While a zero-risk blood supply may never be achievable, I believe we soon will reach an asymptote which closely approximates zero.

References

1. Dienstag, J. L. (1983). Non-A, non-B hepatitis. I. Recognition, epidemiology, and clinical features. *Gastroenterology*, **85**, 439–62
2. Seeff, L. B., Zimmerman, H. J., Wright, E. C. *et al.* (1977). A randomized, double-blind controlled trial of the efficacy of immune serum globulin for the prevention of post-transfusion hepatitis: A Veterans Administration cooperative study. *Gastroenterology*, **72**, 111–21
3. Seeff, L. B. (1988). Transfusion-association hepatitis B: past and present. *Transf. Med. Rev.*, **2**, 204–14
4. Fagan, E. A. and Williams, R. (1984). Non-A, non-B hepatitis. *Sem. Liver Dis.*, **4**, 314–35
5. Feinman, S. V., Berris, N. and Bojarski, S. (1988). Posttransfusion hepatitis in Toronto, Canada. *Gastroenterology*, **95**, 464–9
6. Alter, H. J. (1989). Chronic consequences of non-A, non-B hepatitis. In Seeff, L. B. and Lewis, J. H. (eds), *Current Perspectives in Hepatology*, pp. 83–97. (New York: Plenum)
7. Aledort, L. M., Levine, P. H., Hilgartner, M. *et al.* (1985). A study of liver biopsies and liver disease among hemophiliacs. *Blood*, **66**, 367–72
8. Alter, M. J., Coleman, P. J., Alexander, J. *et al.* (1989). Importance of heterosexual activity in the transmission of hepatitis B and non-A non-B hepatitis. *J. Am. Med. Assoc.*, **262**, 1201–5
9. Alter, H. J. and Prince, A. M. (1988). Transfusion-associated non-A, non-B hepatitis: an assessment of the causative agent and its clinical impact. *Trans. Med. Rev.*, **2**, 288–93
10. Kiyosawa, K., Akahane, Y., Nagata, A. *et al.* (1984). Hepatocellular carcinoma after non-

A, non-B posttransfusion hepatitis. *Am. J. Gastroenterol.*, **79**, 777–81

11. Choo, O. L., Kuo, G., Weiner, A. J., Overby, L. R., Bradley, D. W. and Houghton, M. (1989). Isolation of a cDNA clone derived from a blood-borne non-A, non-B viral hepatitis genome. *Science*, **244**, 359–61
12. Kuo, G., Choo, Q. L., Alter, H. J. *et al.* (1989). An assay for circulating antibodies to a major etiologic virus of human non-A, non-B hepatitis. *Science*, **244**, 362–4
13. Alter, H. J., Purcell, R. H., Shih, J. W., Melpolder, J. C., Houghton, M., Choo, Q.-L. and Kuo, G. (1989). Detection of antibody to hepatitis C virus in prospectively followed transfusion recipients with acute and chronic non-A, non-B hepatitis. *N. Engl. J. Med.* (In press)

28
An outbreak of viral hepatitis A in Shanghai

M. HU, L. KANG and G. YAO

INTRODUCTION

Around 19 January 1988 the number of cases of viral hepatitis in Shanghai increased dramatically, doubling daily during the next few days. The outbreak peaked on 1 February and by 18 March 292 301 cases had been reported, with an incidence of 4082.6 per 100 000 individuals from 1 January to 18 March, twelve times the usual incidence during that time of year in Shanghai.

This severe outbreak of viral hepatitis A (HA) was unusual, even in the international history of such outbreaks. Epidemiological and virological studies linked this outbreak to consumption of hairy clams. This paper reports some of the important characteristics of this HA epidemic.

CHARACTERISTICS OF THE OUTBREAK

Epidemiology

Area

A proportion of 94.9% of all cases occurred in the 12 Shanghai urban districts (Table 1). Cases of viral hepatitis A were identified in 11% of city families (73 184/663 368), and two or more cases occurred simultaneously in 8.03% of the affected families with statistically significant family aggregation ($p < 0.01$).

Time of outbreak

In all urban districts an increase in the number of cases began on 14 January and reached a peak on 6 February. Period of highest incidence was about 20 days. The outbreak was characterized by a sawtooth curve, with three peaks occurring around 20 and 25 January and 1 February. A similar pattern was seen in all urban districts (Figure 1).

Table 1 Incidence of acute viral hepatitis in Shanghai (1 January–19 March, 1988)

Urban district	*No. of cases**	*Incidence* (10^5)
Nanshi	43 591	5686.26
Luwan	23 832	5020.13
Hwangpu	28 308	4097.34
Shuwei	27 908	4108.50
Zaipei	27 803	4138.99
Hongkon	33 179	4006.84
Changning	19 886	3882.90
Yangpu	38 150	3769.30
Jingan	18 304	3743.38
Puoduo	24 066	3460.20
Minghong	2788	2211.56
Wuxong	4486	2100.37
Total	292 301	4082.60

* Data were collected and confirmed from the notification report cards of notifiable infectious disease from various district hygiene and anti-epidemic centres

Age and sex

The outbreak largely affected young adults, with the highest incidence during the endemic period in the age group 20–29 years ($7996.52/10^5$), followed by 30–39 years ($7603.89/10^5$), and these two groups accounted for 83.5% of all cases. Fewer cases appeared in the ≥ 50 year age group (only 0.26–0.58% of the total) and these observations correlate well with the prevalence data of antibodies to hepatitis A virus (anti-HAV) in different age groups of this area just before the outbreak (Table 2). Factory workers were affected most (68.17%), followed by white-collar staff (8.5%) (Table 3). The male and female ratio of cases was 1.26:1.

Diarrhoea prior to the outbreak

An outbreak of diarrhoea, with 20 000 cases at the end of December 1987 and the beginning of January 1988, was related to the consumption of hairy clams. In most cases bacterial dysentery was diagnosed clinically, but this outbreak alerted the authorities to the possibility of clam contamination, and the municipal government banned sales of seafood on 4 January 1988.

Nature of the outbreak

In Shanghai, outbreaks of hepatitis A usually appear in February, reach a peak in March and decrease in April. This outbreak began 1 month earlier, and the number of cases at the peak was 53 times greater than the usual peak.

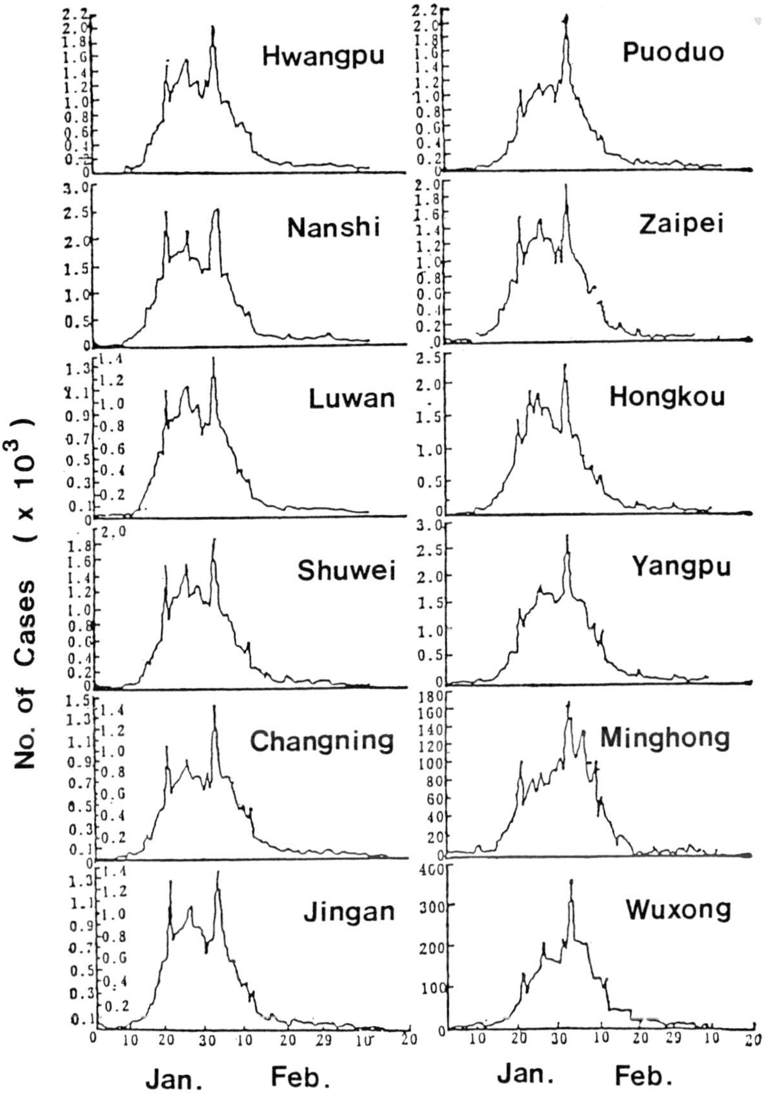

Figure 1 Endemic curve of acute viral hepatitis in Shanghai (1 January–18 March 1988, Shanghai)

This outbreak of viral hepatitis A was not water-borne

A total of 4354 water samples collected from 12 urban waterworks (including water samples from pipe systems and dwellings) from January to December 1987 met the national sanitary standards as determined by turbidity, residue of chlorine, and counts of *E. coli.* The distribution of cases was not related to areas supplied by particular waterworks, and incidences in students and soldiers living in universities or camps located in urban areas were similar

Table 2 Relationship between incidence of viral hepatitis A and consumption of hairy clams in different age groups

Age (years)	*Population*	*Negative rate for anti-HAV (%)*	*Consumption rate of hairy clams (%)**	*Incidence of HA (/10^5)†*
<15	1 048 048	71.28	10.56	2241.50
15~	356 246	72.41	13.80	3479.62
20~	1 684 033	40.83	22.30	7996.52
30~	1 406 662	26.02	20.00	7603.89
40~	668 897	15.62	13.20	991.91
≥50	995 790	5.23	13.10	233.68

$r_s = 0.9143$; $p < 0.025$
*Consumption rate of hairy clams in the last 10 days of December 1987, Shanghai
†Incidence during the period of January–February 1988, Shanghai

to those in the same period in other years ($480/10^5$ on average) but significantly lower than those in the general population in January to April 1988, even though water came from the same sources. In contrast, residents of a suburb 35 km from the city, with their own water supply, had an incidence of $3800/10^5$ during the same period, significantly higher than that in nearby suburbs but similar to that of city districts.

Food-borne spread

From the large-scale distribution of hepatitis cases, any food likely to be a source of contamination would have to have been available in large quantities within a relatively short period, eaten raw or semi-raw, and sold at a time equivalent to the average incubation period before the outbreak. The most likely source was contaminated hairy clams.

Epidemiological studies indicated a close relationship between consumption of hairy clams and the endemic

A paired study showed that 88% of patients with acute viral hepatitis A had eaten hairy clams, a two-fold greater incidence than in the control group. The difference was largely significant, with odds ratio of 9.47 (Table 4).

A sampling survey showed that 31.7% of a sample population had eaten hairy clams, so by extrapolation 2 260 000 people in Shanghai could have consumed the molluscs. The occurrence of hepatitis A in people who had eaten hairy clams was 11.92%, significantly higher than in those who had not eaten hairy clams (0.52%), indicating a 22.9 times higher risk (Table 5).

The incidence of hepatitis A paralleled the amount of hairy clams consumed, with a difference significant by X trend test ($p < 0.01$) (Table 6). Risk increased significantly when hairy clams were eaten raw or cooked lightly by washing with boiling water.

Hairy clams were delivered to markets at a time corresponding to the outbreak, and the peak of hairy clam consumption preceded the outbreak by a time equivalent to the incubation period of viral hepatitis A (Figure 2).

Table 3 Case distribution of acute viral hepatitis in different occupational groups (January–March 1988, Shanghai)

	Occupation											
	Factory worker	*White-collar staff*	*Food handler*	*Nursery children*	*Medical worker*	*Pre-school children*	*Pupil in primary school*	*Middle-school student*	*University student*	*Other*	*Unknown*	*Total*
No. of cases	170 961	21 340	6196	369	2607	6872	12 311	10 609	1389	14 470	3657	250 781
Percentage	68.17	8.51	2.46	0.15	1.04	2.74	4.91	4.23	0.55	5.77	1.46	100

Table 4 Paired study of acute viral hepatitis in Shanghai urban areas (1988)

	Patients' clam-consumption		*Controls' clam-consumption**			
District	*No.*	*Percentage*	*No.*	*Percentage*	χ^2	*Odds ratio*
Shuwei	112	93.3	60	50.0	55.48	13.93
Hongkou	52	91.2	25	43.9	29.16	13.24
Wuxong	77	90.6	24	43.6	72.46	12.47
Puoduo	227	89.4	111	43.7	117.18	10.87
Zaipei	80	87.0	51	55.4	13.46	5.39
Yangpu	81	77.9	58	55.8	11.46	2.65
Nanshi	103	96.3	41	38.3	81.62	41.93
Luwan	90	73.8	46	37.7	32.16	4.65
Jingan	50	92.6	20	37.0	26.28	21.31
Minghong	102	94.4	31	28.7	98.64	41.80
Railway	91	86.7	38	36.2	58.45	12.00
Total	1065	88.2	505	41.8	573.43	9.47†

* Matched controls were selected for an age difference of no less than 5 years, the same sex, similar occupation, and residence in the neighbourhood
† Mantel–Haenszel summary odds ratio

Table 5 Relationship between morbidity of viral hepatitis A and clam consumption by sampling survey (January–March 1988)

	Clam-consumption		*Non-clam consumption*		
District	*No. of individuals*	*Morbidity of HA (%)*	*No. of individuals*	*Morbidity of HA (%)*	*Relative risk*
Hwangpu	2374	16.22	6514	0.66	24.58
Nanshi	4260	7.58	6813	0.19	39.89
Luwan	4899	19.10	9928	0.89	21.46
Shuwei	735	17.96	855	0.35	51.31
Jingan	180	20.00	836	2.39	8.37
Puoduo	343	10.20	865	0.46	22.17
Zaipei	2066	12.10	3750	0.83	14.58
Hongkuo	4159	8.32	11 383	0.19	43.79
Yangpu	1422	9.84	1860	0.75	13.12
Minghong	614	3.91	1664	0.00	7.52
Wuxong	1155	4.76	2472	0.20	23.80
Changning	2190	11.32	5728	0.51	22.20
Total	24 397	11.92	52 668	0.52	22.92

Table 6 Paired study of amount of clams eaten

		No. of clams eaten					
	Nos.	1–	10–	20–	30+	χ^2	p value
Patients	638	79	136	194	229	19.18	<0.01
Controls	277	61	64	83	69		

Detection of hepatitis A virus (HAV) and HAV RNA in hairy clams

Hepatitis A virus (HAV) and HAV RNA were detected in pooled hairy clam samples from various markets in Shanghai urban areas at the beginning of January 1988, and from Qidong Beach, Jiang-Su Province where hairy clams

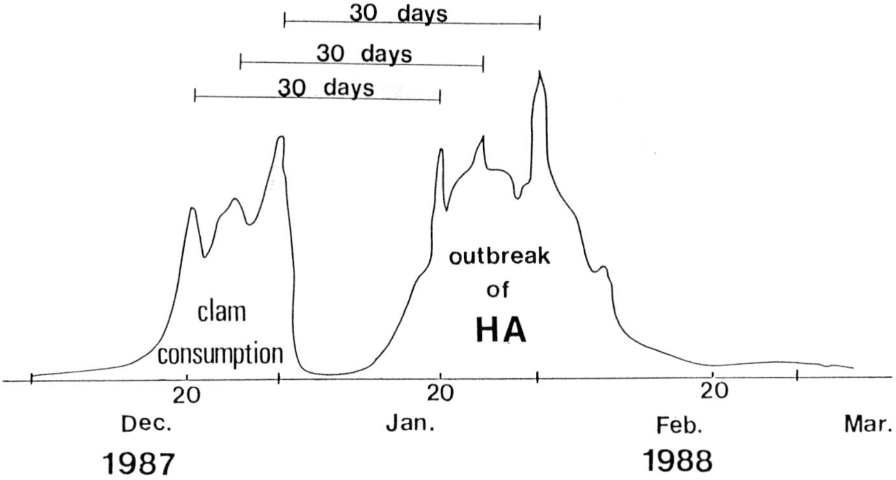

Figure 2 Time of consumption of hairy clams and outbreak of HA

were raised, and Ningbo city area (also in Jiang-Su Province) where the hairy clams were imported from Qidong in March 1988, corresponding to the late period of the outbreak. Tissue culture methods and hybridization assays were used for detection (Table 7, Figure 3).

Pooled alimentary gland and/or branchia extracts from 250–1000 hairy clams were homogenized and concentrated by ultracentrifugation. HAV was isolated in PLC/PRF/5 cells at 32 °C and HAAg was determined periodically by ELISA. Isolated HAV was identified further by immunofluorescence blocking test, neutralization assay and immunoelectromicroscopy with paired chimpanzee sera[1,2].

HAV cDNA recombinant clone 3831, which represents part of VPI, whole of P2 and part of P3 HAV coded genome extending about 3000–6000

Table 7 Detection of HAV in hairy clams by cell culture

Samples	*Virus isolation*	
	HAAg (ELISA)	*Incubation period (days)*†
1. Mixed hairy clam samples (collected from Shanghai markets, Jan. 1988)		
Alimentary gland	+(6.3)*	40
Branchia	+(6.6)	40
2. Mixed hairy clam samples (collected from Qidong, March 1988)	+(7.8)	60
3. Mixed hairy clam samples (collected from Ningbo, March 1988)	+(8.1)	60

*The data in parentheses are the ratios of OD value from infected cellular extracts to non-infected extracts (P/N) by ELISA as previously described[9]

†Incubation period is the time unit HAAg was first detected by ELISA (P/N > 2.1) in the infected cellular extracts

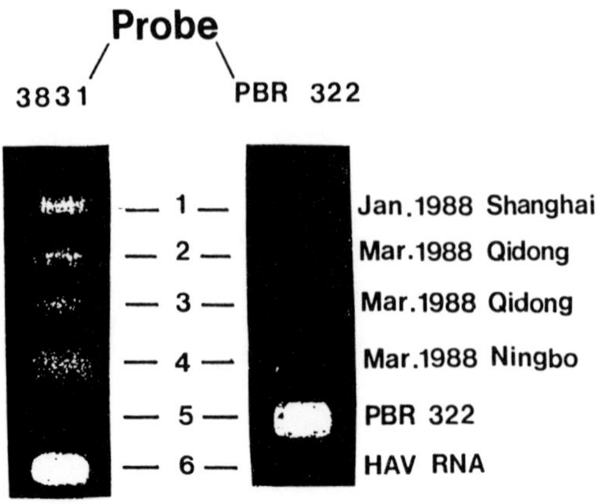

Figure 3 Hybridization of various hairy clam samples with HAV cDNA 3831 and PBR 322 DNA respectively. Hairy clam samples collected from the areas indicated were treated (see Table 3). Samples 2 and 3 were both collected from the hairy clam rearing area, Qidong but in different locations. PBR 322 DNA and purified HAV RNA were used as negative and positive controls (1 μg for each dot). Probes were 32P-labelled as 10^8 cpm/μg DNA. Autoradiograph exposure time was 4 days

nucleotide base pairs (kindly provided by Dr K. von der Helm, Max von Pettenkofer-Institute, Munich) and PBR 322 DNA were used as probes. RNA was extracted from the pooled, concentrated hairy clam pellets from different sources by proteinase-A treatment, phenolization, alcohol precipitation, and dotted on nylon paper (Gene Screen plus membrane, Dupont). ^{32}P-labelled HAV cDNA 3831 reacted with all the pooled hairy clam samples as well as with the purified HAV RNA positive control and the control ^{32}P-labelled PBR 322 probe did not react with the hairy clam preparations but only with its own DNA control. The hairy clams were heavily contaminated with HAV, with an average of 2–8 TCID 50 HAV in each hairy clam. A case–control study confirmed that in 638 cases about 12% of the patients had eaten only one shellfish. Detection of HAV and HAV RNA from samples collected directly in the clam-rearing area indicates that the source of contamination was probably the heavily polluted waters off the coast of Jiang-Su Province, bordering Shanghai.

Source of hairy clams and possible contaminating factors

Source of hairy clams

During September 1987, for the first time large quantities of hairy clams were discovered in Lusi port in Qidong county, Jiang-Su Province. By the end of 1987, 4000 tons of these hairy clams had been harvested, delivered to Shanghai, Nanton (a major city in Jiang-Su Province) and other locations, and sold mostly by private traders. From 9 December 1987, hairy clams produced in Qidong reached Shanghai, with the largest deliveries of about 2600 tons in the first days of January 1988. As mentioned above, the municipal government prohibited further sales of hairy clams in the markets on 4 January 1988.

Possible contaminating factors

1. Viral hepatitis A was widespread in Qidong with an incidence of $1611.7/10^5$ in 1987. By 10 March 1988, Qidong county had the highest number of cases of viral hepatitis A in Jiang-Su Province.
2. Faeces were not disposed of properly in Qidong. Toilet facilities were in poor condition, and it is possible that faeces drained directly, or after inadequate processing, into the sea. In addition, during the fishing season several hundred boats with thousands of fishermen working at sea could be a source of fecal contamination.

Clinical features

Clinical manifestation

The typical clinical manifestation of viral hepatitis A in the epidemic was an abrupt onset of disease after an incubation period of 2–6 weeks with an average of about 1 month. Ninety-one per cent of patients became icteric, and 93% had alanine aminotransferase (ALT) levels higher than 400–1000 u/dl. Anti-HAV IgM was present in 95.5% of cases, and faecal HAAg was detected in 62.8% of patients within 1 week after onset of illness. Overt jaundice with remarkable elevations of serum bilirubin (SB) (>1 mg/dl or 170 μmol/l) was present in a significant proportion of patients. Clinical pictures showed 2.05% of all cases were consistent with the diagnosis of cholestatic hepatitis.

Complications

Arthralgia, rash, gastrointestinal bleeding tendency and cardiac arrythmia were seen in some patients. Some uncommon complications were red cell aplasia, thrombocytopenic purpura, optic neuritis, polyneuritis, transversal myelitis, and haemolytic anaemia. Most complications responded to treatment and no permanent sequelae remained.

Hepatitis in pregnancy

Approximately 1.95% of patients with viral hepatitis A were pregnant. Infection in pregnancy neither aggravated the pathological process nor affected the fetus. The frequency of perinatal death associated with hepatitis was similar to that without hepatitis (2.3:1.9%) but pregnant women with hepatitis had more frequent complications with turbid amniotic fluid (I–III) (49–75%). No deaths occurred in these patients.

Double infection of viral hepatitis A and B

Of patients with hepatitis A 8.8% were positive for hepatitis B surface antigen (HBsAg) but the clinical and pathological pictures were similar to patients with only hepatitis A, except that values such as SB and ALT returned to normal after a slight delay. However, a previous history of chronic active hepatitis B or cirrhosis often led to more severe symptoms, resulting in ascites and hepatic failure. Laboratory studies showed that infection with HAV was associated with temporary suppression of replication for hepatitis B virus (HBV), resulting in lowered titres or even disappearance of HBsAg and HBV DNA, and shift of hepatitis B e-antigen (HBeAg)-positive to HBeAg-negative, and antibody to hepatitis B e antigen (anti-HBe) and/or antibody to hepatitis B surface antigen (anti-HBs) negative to positive. During recovery, HBV DNA and HBeAg became positive again.

Duration of disease

Follow-up of 1212 cases of hepatitis A in 18 factories and a central hospital showed that clinical recovery with normal liver function occurred in 63.4%, 20.4%, 8.6%, 4.8% and 1.5% of patients in 2, 3, 4, 5 and 6 months respectively. Only 1.3% of cases had not recovered at 6 months. In a few patients there was relapse of illness following a period during which the jaundice had improved notably or had disappeared. All cases recovered within 1 year.

During the outbreak, even though the number of hospital beds was increased ten-fold and all available space in schools, factories, clubs, etc., was used, 60% of patients had to be treated at home. There was no evidence of secondary transmission, nor were prognoses different for patients treated in hospital, in isolation or at home with either simple or complex therapies.

Death rate

Death occurred in 47 cases with a death rate of $16.07/10^5$ (22 male; 25 female: ages 8–60 years, with a mean age of 30.4 ± 10.9 years); 59.6% of deaths occurred in the group aged 20–35 years.

1. *Fulminant viral hepatitis A*: 25 patients with negative laboratory findings for HBV progressed to fulminant hepatic failure with a death rate of $8.55/10^5$. Liver tissue obtained in 12 cases after death showed subacute hepatic necrosis in 10 and acute necrosis in 2. Three cases had pure red cell aplasia confirmed by bone marrow puncture in combination with subacute necrosis.
2. *HAV infection of 15 patients with prior HBV infection:* all were positive for HBsAg; 11 of 15 patients were also positive for HBeAg. In this group the clinical features were similar to those of hepatitis A. Five deaths in patients with combined infection were autopsied: three had submassive hepatic necrosis in addition to cirrhosis, one had chronic active hepatitis with submassive necrosis, and one had massive hepatic necrosis.
3. *Deaths in viral hepatitis A cases from causes other than hepatic failures*: in seven cases of viral hepatitis A, coexistent disease or drug-related complications were considered to be causes of death. Two cases died of heart disease (congenital heart disease, chronic heart failure and

arrhythmia). Malignant histiocytosis, septic shock, infection of biliary tract with renal failure, or drug-related bullose dermatitis were causes of death in the other five cases. One case died of unknown cause (autopsy showed typical acute hepatitis).

From these results the prognosis of viral hepatitis A was good with a low death rate and no chronic sequelae. However, in the 292 301 HA cases 8.8% had been infected previously with HBV and were HBsAg-positive, and 15 deaths fell into this HAV and HBV coinfected group. In comparison to the 25 deaths in the remaining 91.2% of HA patients, the death rate in the group of HAV and HBV co-infections was 6.2 times higher than in patients only infected with HAV, indicating the importance during HA outbreaks of protecting patients possibly with chronic hepatitis B in areas with high prevalence of hepatitis B.

CONCLUSION AND DISCUSSION

This hepatitis A outbreak was the most severe known to have been caused by eating shellfish[3–8]. Epidemiological and virological studies related this epidemic to the consumption of contaminated hairy clams harvested in Chidong county, Jiang-Su Province, a neighbouring area of Shanghai. Contamination probably resulted from insufficient processing of raw faeces and waste water in the local endemic area. Previous studies showed that shellfish can ingest and concentrate HAV to more than 15–1000 times[9,10]. In this epidemic, hairy clams collected in Shanghai urban markets were heavily contaminated with around 2–8 TCID 50 of HAV in each hairy clam, a level almost certain to cause hepatitis A infection in man. A case–control study confirmed that among 638 cases about 12% of the patients had eaten only one clam (Kang *et al.*, data not shown); epidemiological studies estimated that around 2 260 000 people in Shanghai consumed the molluscs, and most people ate the hairy clams either semi-raw or raw. The prevalence data of antibodies to HAV in different age groups measured before the outbreak indicated that a severe epidemic of viral hepatitis A could occur in the area, especially in the younger age groups, but the possibility of virulent mutation of HAV cannot be excluded at present. HAV isolations from this endemic are being studied further.

This outbreak brought high economic losses, and emphasized the urgent need for improving environmental hygiene. It is important to establish hygienic standards and controls for shellfish production and to support this control with legislation. In addition, developing a sensitive, rapid surveillance assay, e.g. a polymerase chain reaction, for detecting even small amounts of viral contamination in seafood could be very helpful; the habit of eating clams raw or slightly cooked should be discouraged. Last, but very important, the development of a hepatitis A vaccine for mass immunization in China should be accelerated.

Acknowledgements

The authors acknowledge the efficient cooperation of the staffs of the Shanghai Hygiene and Antiepidemic Center and the various Shanghai Urban Hygiene and Antiepidemic Centers and municipal hospitals. They also thank Professor F. Deinhardt (Max von Pettenkofer-Institute, Munich) for the useful criticism and suggestions.

References

1. Hu, M., Lu, X., Sun, B., Shen, R., Fu, J., Meng, C., Chen, M., Wang, C. and Dong, X. (1984). Isolation of 3 strains of HAV directly from human feces by human diploid fibroblasts. *Chinese J. Infect. Dis.*, **2**, 109–13
2. Hu, M., Scheid, R. and Deinhardt, F. (1982). Isolation of hepatitis A virus in cell culture from human stool specimen collected in China. *J. Shanghai Med.*, **5**, 171–4
3. Roos, B. (1956). Hepatitis conveyed by oysters. *Svensk Lakartidn*, **53**, 989–1003
4. Communicable Disease Centre, Public Health Service, Department of Health, Education and Welfare (1961). *Morbidity and Mortality Weekly Reports*, 10 (no. 17)
5. Mason, J. O. and McLean, W. R. (1962). Infectious hepatitis traced to the consumption of raw oysters: an epidemiologic study. *Am. J. Hyg.*, **75**, 90–111
6. Goldfield, M. (1976). Epidemiological indicators for transmission of viruses by water. In Berg, G., Bodily, H. L., Lennette, E. H., Melnick, J. L. and Metcalf, T. G. (eds), *Viruses in Water*, pp. 70–85. (New York: American Public Health Association)
7. Kang, L., Shao, J., Nu, G., Huang, Y., Qu, J., Fu, T., Wu, J., Qian, W., Shu, J., Hu, S., Wang, C., Xu, D., Zhou, T., Yan, L., Qia, Y., Wei, Y., Yuan, G., Xiong, Q. and Hu, S. (1983). Epidemiological study of an epidemic of viral hepatitis A. *Chinese J. Infect., Dis.*, **1**, 168–72
8. Maretic, Z., Bürek, V., Alambasic, K. and Golobic, B. (1986). An epidemic of hepatitis A conveyed by mussels in Pula. *Sixth International Congress of Infectious Diseases*, abstracts, no. 186. (München: Futuramed Verlag)
9. Enriquez, R., Frösner, G. G., Hochstein-Mintzel, V., Riedemann, S. and Reinhardt, G. (1986). Concentration of hepatitis A virus in mussels from surrounding water. *Sixth International Congress of Infectious Diseases*, Abstracts. no. 185. (München: Futuramed Verlag)
10. Hu, M., Li, T., Hu, X., Deinhardt, F., Jiang, Y. and Yin, B. (1986). Isolation of HAV from experimentally infected shellfish. *Sixth International Congress of Infectious Diseases*, Abstracts, no. 688. (München: Futuramed Verlag)

29
Specific prophylaxis against hepatitis A

S. IWARSON

GAMMA GLOBULIN PROPHYLAXIS

Today administration of gamma globulin (immune serum globulin) is the only commercially available means of preventing hepatitis A. Gamma globulin may provide protection against hepatitis A if given during the incubation period up to approximately 2 weeks before the onset of symptoms, but of course, the earlier it is given the greater the chance for protection. Immunity persists for approximately 8 weeks following a standard dose of 0.02 ml/kg.

Gamma globulin prophylaxis may work either by preventing the hepatitis A virus infection or by weakening the symptoms of hepatitis A. If given before virus exposure gamma globulin is at least 90% effective in preventing jaundice. Prolonged protection following gamma globulin prophylaxis is attributed to so-called 'passive–active immunization' which means a subclinical or asymptomatic infection leading to later permanent immunity.

The administration of recommended doses of gamma globulin usually does not result in serum antibody levels detectable by available assays. This means that usual serodiagnostic criteria may be applied also to persons receiving gamma globulin prophylaxis. Neutralizing anti-HAV antibodies may be found in low titre in the sera of recipients of gamma globulin by the use of sensitive neutralization assays. Such assays should be useful for standardizing passive immunoprophylaxis against hepatitis A and for evaluating the potential efficacy of new hepatitis A vaccines.

In 1976 Krugman *et al.*[1] found that inoculation with a mixture of infectious HAV-containing serum and gamma globulin did not cause hepatitis in seronegative recipients. In contrast, recipients of the same virus-containing serum not mixed with gamma globulin contracted hepatitis A, demonstrating the presence of neutralizing antibodies in gamma globulin.

Population studies on anti-HAV antibodies suggest that the prevalence of this antibody is gradually declining in the US and in Western Europe, yet anti-HAV titres in products from these countries have not decreased substantially over the past 20 years. This probably reflects, at least in the USA, the increased use of plasma from paid donors, who tend to have a higher prevalence and titre of anti-HAV.

In Western Europe and the USA two major groups benefit from gamma globulin prophylaxis against hepatitis A. These are foreign travellers and close contacts of hepatitis A patients. For travellers from low endemicity countries the risk of exposure to HAV varies with the prevalence of hepatitis A in the areas visited, and the length of stay.

A single dose of gamma globulin equal to 0.02 ml/kg body weight is recommended as *pre-exposure prophylaxis* prior to travel anticipated to last no longer than approximately 2–3 months. For prolonged travel 0.06 ml/kg body weight is recommended to be given prior to initiating travel and regularly every 4–6 months thereafter.

In all situations in which *postexposure prophylaxis* is indicated, the same single intramuscular dose of 0.02 ml/kg body weight is recommended. Such prophylaxis is recommended for close personal contact (household and/or sexual) with a person with hepatitis A, for staff and attendees of day-care centres where HAV is being transmitted, and for staff and residents in certain other institutions where HAV transmission is occurring. Gamma globulin is also indicated for postexposure prophylaxis in common source exposures to food or water contaminated with HAV when recognized within 2 weeks of the exposure.

HEPATITIS A VACCINES

Even if gamma globulin is safe and effective it provides only temporary protection against hepatitis A, and today the interest is focused on the development of vaccines against the disease. Three major approaches to the development of an HAV vaccine have been considered. These include live attenuated vaccines, inactivated or killed vaccines, and recombinant or synthetic peptide vaccines. The observation that the virulence of HAV decreases following repeated passages of the virus in cell culture led to the development of attenuated HAV vaccine candidates already the 1970s by Provost and others at the MSD Research Laboratories[2]. The most attenuated of these vaccine strains did not appear to be infectious in humans. Less attenuated variants of the same strain, however, caused a rise in aminotransferases of human volunteers, suggesting that there is a delicate balance between attenuation and infectivity when dealing with attenuated vaccine candidates.

Some years later a group at the NIH in Bethesda[3] reported on the preparation of two prototype live virus vaccines which were given i.v. to chimpanzees and marmosets. One of these vaccine strains appeared to be less virulent than the other, especially in marmosets, but challenge studies in the animals were considered inconclusive.

The Bethesda workers concluded that an oral live HAV vaccine would be preferable in humans, since it would imitate the natural route of infection and would be easy and inexpensive to administer.

More recently a study from the People's Republic of China, by Dr Mao and his colleagues in Zheijang, was reported[4]. They had studied an attenuated live hepatitis A vaccine which had been grown in human diploid cells. The strain, called H-2, was given subcutaneously to 12 human volunteers, who all developed neutralizing antibodies in low titre. No-one had any ALT elevation. This study is probably the most encouraging one at present using an attenuated vaccine.

One drawback to the use of attenuated HAV vaccines is the potential for reversion of the vaccine strain to full virulence, with possible transmission of the revertant virus to contacts. Furthermore, there is no marker for differentiating wild-type virus from attenuated strains of HAV. The biological basis of attenuation is not yet fully understood.

These difficulties and potential risks with attenuated vaccines against hepatitis A have encouraged researchers to focus their interest on inactivated or killed vaccines. In 1978 Provost and Hilleman, at Merck, showed that formalin-inactivated HAV prepared from the liver of infected marmosets was a useful vaccine when tested in marmosets. In the mid 1980s Provost and his group[5] presented a highly purified, formalin-inactivated vaccine prepared from cell culture grown HAV, demonstrating that inactivated as well as attenuated HAV vaccines can be produced in cell culture.

Recently, a group at the Walter Reed Army Institute of Research in Washington[6] has produced a formalin-inactivated HAV vaccine from infected cell cultures that evoked a protective antibody response when administered to owl monkeys. Professor Flehmig and his colleagues in Tübingen have presented an interesting approach, namely a combined vaccine preparation against hepatitis A and B. This has been achieved by mixing a commercially available hepatitis B vaccine produced in yeasts with their own cell culture-produced hepatitis A virus vaccine[7].

Flehmig *et al.* vaccinated 15 seronegative volunteers with three doses of the combined hepatitis A and B vaccine at intervals of 1 month. After the first dose all volunteers had developed neutralizing antibodies against hepatitis A, and antibody titres against hepatitis A remained stable during a 6-month follow-up period with this killed hepatitis A vaccine made from HAV propagated in human diploid cells.

Apparently inactivated vaccine candidates may be immunogenic and safe. One problem associated with inactivated vaccines is that they may be relatively expensive because of the relatively poor yields of virus obtained with current cell culture techniques. In recent years, however, a better understanding of viral replication and better techniques has improved the yields of virus currently achieved in cell cultures. Furthermore, based on our past experience with gamma globulin, it is likely that a very small amount of serum neutralizing antibody is necessary for protection against hepatitis A.

A potential disadvantage of using an inactivated HAV vaccine administered parenterally is that secretory immunity may not be induced. Secretory immunity plays an important role in protection against many viral infections of the gastrointestinal tract. For instance, with inactivated poliovirus vaccine production of secretory IgA is not stimulated and enteric infection with poliovirus may occur. A live, attenuated oral polio vaccine, on the other hand, stimulates secretory IgA and prevents intestinal infection. Whether a similar effect will occur with an oral HAV vaccine is uncertain, since the question as to whether replication of HAV occurs in the gut still has to be answered.

In spite of these potential drawbacks major vaccine producers such as Merck, Sharp & Dohme, and Smith-Kline French, today develop inactivated vaccines as a first priority. Both manufacturers at present have such vaccines in clinical trials. This probably means that we will have a first generation of inactivated hepatitis A vaccines on the commercial market within a short period.

Alternative approaches to HAV vaccine development involve the application of new concepts in molecular biology and recombinant DNA technology. A complementary DNA copy of an antigenic segment of viral RNA may, for instance, be inserted into a bacterial plasmid vector in a position downstream from a bacterial gene promoter. The resultant peptide encoded by the cloned DNA is produced by the bacterium and can be purified and used for vaccine production. However, stable expression of cloned genes cannot easily be obtained in bacteria, necessitating the recloning of the DNA vector systems.

DNA coding for antigenic determinants of HAV could also be spliced into cDNA copies of existing attenuated polio or vaccinia virus to generate polyvalent strains suitable for vaccine use.

Another modern approach is to synthesize oligopeptides representing critical neutralization sites of the virus. These new techniques will probably be useful for the second generation of hepatitis A vaccines which may possibly reach the market in the next 5–10 years.

To summarize, inactivated hepatitis A vaccines are on their way to the market. In view of this fact it should be pointed out that hepatitis A will probably be the least severe disease we will be vaccinating against. This means that a very high degree of safety is required for these vaccines. Also, there is an excellent effect of passive immunization with gamma globulin against hepatitis A, which further stresses the safety aspect.

Some questions concerning the behaviour of HAV still remain to be answered, but further improvements in current methods of vaccine production, and a better understanding of the mechanisms of HAV replication and infection, will probably provide the basis for further progress in the development of new hepatitis A vaccines.

References

1. Krugman, S., Ward, R., Giles, J. P. *et al.* (1960). Infectious hepatitis: Studies on the effect of gamma globulin and on the incidence of inapparent infection. *J. Am. Med. Assoc.*, **174**, 823–30
2. Provost, P. J., Bishop, R. P., Gerety, R. J., Hilleman, M. R. *et al.* (1986). New findings in live attenuated hepatitis A vaccine development. *J. Med. Virol.*, **20**, 165–75
3. Karron, R. A., Daemer, R., Ticehurst, J., D'Hondt, E. *et al.* (1988). Studies of prototype live hepatitis A virus vaccines in primate models. *J. Infect. Dis.*, **157**, 338–45

4. Mao, J. S., Dong, D. X., Zang, H. Y., Chen, N. L., *et al.* (1989). Primary study of attenuated live hepatitis A vaccine (HS strain) in humans. *J. Infect. Dis.*, **159**, 621–4
5. Provost, P. J., Hughes, J. V., Miller, W. J., Giesa, P. A. *et al.* (1986). An inactivated hepatitis A viral vaccine of cell culture origin. *J. Med. Virol.*, **19**, 23–31
6. Binn, L. N., Bancroft, W. H., Eckels, K. H., Marchwicki, R. H. *et al.* (1988). Inactivated hepatitis A virus vaccine produced in human diploid MRC-5 cells. In Zuckerman, A. J. (ed.) *Viral hepatitis and Liver Diseases*, pp. 91–3. (New York: Alan R. Liss)
7. Flehmig, B., Heinricy, U. and Pfisterer, M. (1989). Paper presented at the Basel Liver Week, October 12–17, 1989 (Abstract)

Index